The Parent's
AUTISM
SOURCEBOOK

The Parent's
AUTISM
SOURCEBOOK

A Comprehensive Guide to
Screenings, Treatments, Services,
and Organizations

KIM MACK ROSENBERG

Skyhorse Publishing

Skyhorse Publishing books may be purchased in bulk at special discounts for sales promotion, corporate gifts, fund-raising, or educational purposes. Special editions can also be created to specifications. For details, contact the Special Sales Department, Skyhorse Publishing, 307 West 36th Street, 11th Floor, New York, NY 10018 or info@skyhorsepublishing.com.

Skyhorse® and Skyhorse Publishing® are registered trademarks of Skyhorse Publishing, Inc.®, a Delaware corporation.

Visit our website at www.skyhorsepublishing.com.

Cover design by Brian Peterson

10 9 8 7 6 5 4 3 2 1

Library of Congress Cataloging-in-Publication Data is available on file.

Print ISBN: 978-1-63220-263-5
Ebook ISBN: 978-1-63220-938-2

Printed in the United States of America

CONTENTS

OVERVIEW

Introduction

If you are concerned that your child may have Autism Spectrum Disorder (ASD) or if your child is recently diagnosed with ASD, you likely are emotional, overwhelmed, frightened, and unsure of the future for your child and family. This sourcebook is designed to provide parents information about the diagnosis process as well as some of the treatment options available to help your child with ASD reach his or her greatest potential. If you are concerned about your child's development, it is important to act right away. Talk to your pediatrician as soon as you suspect an issue. You know your child best; if something seems wrong, do not accept a wait-and-see approach from your doctor or anyone else—no matter how well intentioned. Seek help in getting your child evaluated right away.

There are many choices for parents to make, and usually not unlimited financial resources, so understanding options is critical in the decision-making process. While the scope of this book is broad, there are so many options available and new treatments developing all the time that it is impossible to catalog all of them. At the end of this book is a resource directory compiled by the editors at Skyhorse containing many national and state resources for families. Every effort has been made by Skyhorse to provide accurate information at the time of publication. For more in-depth descriptions of many treatments discussed here as well as additional treatment options, an excellent resource for parents is *Cutting Edge Therapies for Autism*, another Skyhorse publication. Inclusion in this book is not an endorsement of any particular treatment or practitioner (nor is exclusion meant to imply a negative opinion). This book is for informational purposes only and does not constitute medical, legal, or other professional advice. Parents should determine, along with the trusted professionals with whom they work, the most appropriate course of treatment for their child.

Understanding your child's diagnosis and determining the most appropriate of educational interventions, therapies, and medical or other interventions to meet your child's unique needs can be daunting, especially to the parents of a child newly diagnosed. In part this is because, as the name implies, there is not one "ASD." It is a spectrum with a wide range of skills and functional levels. The learning, thinking, problem-solving, and daily life skills abilities of people with ASD can range from gifted to severely challenged, and any individual can also have skills that range widely–for example a child with ASD may be very verbal but have significant repetitive behaviors. Each individual with ASD has a unique constellation of strengths and challenges. The diversity in ASD, both within the ASD population and within each individual, creates challenges for parents and practitioners in determining the most appropriate course or courses of treatment for an individual with ASD.

About Autism Spectrum Disorder

Traditionally, autism spectrum disorder was described as a developmental disability. More recently, many who diagnose and treat individuals with ASD are recognizing it as a bio-neurological condition. Many individuals with ASD have medical conditions such as mito-chondrial disease or dysfunction, immune system disorders, gastrointestinal disease/digestive disorders, autoimmune issues, allergies and sensitivities (including allergies and/or sensitivi-ties to many foods), asthma, epilepsy/seizure disorders, persistent viral infections, sensory inte-gration dysfunction, feeding issues, sleeping issues, hypothyroidism, adrenal function issues, and other conditions. Consequently, along with traditional therapeutic and educational inter-ventions, more treatments are being offered medically (including integrative treatments) and nutritionally to help improve the health and well-being of individuals with ASD. Practitioners and parents report that when these other conditions are treated, symptoms associated with autism often improve, and in some cases resolve.

Regardless of how one categorizes it, ASD can cause significant social, communication, behavioral, and learning challenges for the affected individual.

Early Signs & Symptoms

Parents are often the first to notice something unusual about a child's behavior or develop-ment. It may be that the child is not meeting developmental milestones or it may be that when a parent compares a child's development to that of other children, the child's development or behavior is unusual or concerning. If you are worried about your child's development, raise your concerns with your pediatrician or other healthcare practitioner right away. Do not take a wait-and-see approach and don't allow your concerns to be discounted or dismissed. Trust your "mommy gut" or "daddy gut" if you feel that something is wrong. You should work with your healthcare practitioner, but always remember that you spend the most time with your child and will notice things that, in short check-ups, may not be apparent to someone else. The sooner your child can be evaluated to determine if intervention is appropriate, the better. The earlier your child begins to receive services and treatments, the better. The human brain has remark-able plasticity (the ability to heal and change) but plasticity may be greatest at younger ages. That said, there is no window that closes on brain plasticity, so if your child is not diagnosed until a later age, they still have great potential.

At what age do children with ASD show signs of atypical development? There is no one answer. For some infants, development seems atypical from birth or early infancy—as they go through their first year they are not responsive to normal social cues (for example, they have incon-sistent eye contact), they don't exhibit typical pre-language skills, or they are intensively focused on certain objects. Other children appear to develop normally (often for the first 18–36 months) and then lose skills or plateau in the development of skills and begin exhibiting symptoms of ASD. This is called regressive autism. For some children the regression is slow, for others it is dramatic. For some children, regression appears linked to environmental factors, including vaccinations.

While each child with ASD will present with different symptoms, symptoms generally fall into the following categories: social impairments, verbal and non-verbal communication challenges, and behavior challenges, including repetitive or stereotyped behavior.

Social Impairment

For most children with ASD, everyday social interactions are challenging and communications difficulties exacerbate these social challenges. For example, some children with ASD may:

- Make little eye contact, have inconsistent eye contact, or glance sideways rather than straight on;
- Not respond to their name or other basic social overtures (such as "hello" or "how are you");
- Not engage in typical reciprocal behaviors such as sharing a toy or pointing something out to someone else;
- Have difficulty transitioning to new activities or environments or have difficulty in accepting or adapting to a change in an expected schedule, and;
- Have highly restrictive interests.

According to the National Institute of Mental Health:

> Recent research suggests that children with ASD do not respond to emotional cues in human social interactions because they may not pay attention to the social cues that others typically notice. For example, one study found that children with ASD focus on the mouth of the person speaking to them instead of on the eyes, which is where children with typical development tend to focus. A related study showed that children with ASD appear to be drawn to repetitive movements linked to a sound, such as hand-clapping during a game of pat-a-cake. More research is needed to confirm these findings, but such studies suggest that children with ASD may misread or not notice subtle social cues—a smile, a wink, or a grimace—that could help them understand social relationships and interactions. For these children, a question such as, "Can you wait a minute?" always means the same thing, whether the speaker is joking, asking a real question, or issuing a firm request. Without the ability to interpret another person's tone of voice as well as gestures, facial expressions, and other nonverbal communications, children with ASD may not properly respond.

However, there also are reports from parents and others that when children or adults with ASD, particularly those with significant verbal challenges, are able to communicate (through the use of assistive technology, for example), they demonstrate that they were far more observant than studies might suggest. Therefore, important advice to parents of children with

ASD is to assume that your child understands what is being said around her and to never say anything about the child in her presence that you would not want her to hear (and don't allow doctors, teachers, therapists, or others to speak about your child in her presence as if she is not there).

"Theory of mind" also may present social and communicative challenges to individuals with ASD, regardless of verbal skills. Many children with ASD have difficulty understanding that other people have their own points of view, opinions, and feelings that may differ from those of individuals with ASD. As a simple example, a child with ASD may assume that his favorite scene in a movie is also your favorite scene and have difficulty accepting that this may not be the case. This makes it difficult for children with ASD to understand other people's behavior when it differs from what the child expects based on her own point of view.

Communication Impairments

In addition to social challenges, children with ASD often face significant communication challenges. Language skills for children with ASD range from highly verbal to non-verbal, but even highly verbal individuals often have difficulty communicating.

Previously it was thought that if a child was not speaking by approximately kindergarten age, he likely would not acquire independent verbal language skills. However, consistent with growing knowledge of brain plasticity, more recent research suggests that many non-verbal children may acquire some language skills in later childhood or even in adolescence.

Non-verbal individuals who do not have an effective means of communication may become increasingly frustrated, act out to try to get their needs met and to communicate, and may become anxious or depressed. Thus it is important to try to find a way for individuals with ASD to communicate if possible. Interestingly, the use of augmentative and alternative communicative devices, in particular iPads, also seems to help some individuals eventually speak independently. Some theorize that these devices decrease frustration and anxiety, creating an environment more conducive to speech development. However, even if a child does not develop independent verbal skills, these devices give them the opportunity to communicate and interact in ways they previously could not. Using these devices, many people with ASD have shown not only keen intellect but also thoughts, feelings and observations that the outward symptoms of ASD might mask.

Even where a child with ASD has verbal language, she may have delays or non-typical speech patterns such as:

- Delayed language acquisition;
- Delayed use of simple phrases or the inability to combine words into simple phrases;
- Loss of language skills or a plateau in the acquisition of language skills;
- Pronoun reversal issues in older children (note that even typically developing toddlers may have pronoun reversal issues);
- Echolalia or "scripting"—repeating words or phrases that they have heard. For example, some children with ASD have incredible abilities to memorize and repeat large portions of movies or television shows. Also parents should be alert for a child using echolalic language

to communicate independently (i.e., a child appears to be speaking appropriately but actually is using scripted language). Often a parent may be the only one to realize the echolalic speech in those instances, which could mask a speech delay or the severity of the delay. Other children may use echolalic language to express something where they don't have the actual language to do so (e.g., describing something that happened in a video, such as "the train went into the roundhouse" to express that he is tired and wants to go to sleep). Thus, echolalic language may serve as an important means of communication or a bridge to more independent speech for some children and, if your child is echolalic, it is important to discuss how to address echolalia with your speech professional;

- Use of unusual words or phrases that do not seem echolalic but seem out of place.

Even individuals with ASD who have relatively strong verbal skills often have difficulties with social aspects of language, such as back-and-forth conversation, discussing topics that are non-favored topics, or accepting attempts by others to steer conversation away from the individual's often narrow interests. These individuals also have difficulty recognizing that their favorite topic may not be of interest to the person with whom they are speaking. Further, some people with ASD present with very flat affect in facial features and voice. Others may communicate in a sing-song voice. The prosody of speech may not only be atypical but also may not match the person's actual feelings, presenting further communication challenges.

Behaviors

Individuals with ASD may face many behavior challenges including repetitive behaviors, narrow interests, difficulties adapting to change or unpredictability in their environment, and aggression.

Many children with ASD engage in repetitive or stereotyped behaviors. These behaviors can be physical or verbal and range from very noticeable or disruptive to quite subtle. These behaviors are often referred to as self-stimulatory behaviors, or stimming. The following is a non-inclusive list of examples of stimming:

- Hand flapping, finger flicking, moving fingers in front of the eyes;
- Repeating words or making unusual noises (e.g., screeching, grunting, humming);
- Rocking;
- Head banging, scratching, or other self-injurious behaviors;
- Jumping;
- Toe-walking;
- Lining up toys (instead of playing with them appropriately) or other objects (e.g., shoes, household objects);
- Rolling toys back and forth in the absence of play;
- Spinning objects or intense focus on objects that spin or move;
- Staring at lights or ceiling fans;

- Turning lights on and off repeatedly; and
- Repeatedly pressing buttons on electronic toys, in the absence of meaningful play.

If a child's stimming activity is disrupted (for example, a ceiling fan turned off or their organization of objects is changed) they may become upset. A child may engage in stimming for various reasons, including to calm himself if his sensory system is overloaded; to excite his system if his system is understimulated; or even to express pain or discomfort (for example, some children with severe gastrointestinal pain may bend themselves over furniture to try to relieve the pain or a child may bang his head in an attempt to relieve severe pain). For any self-stimulatory behavior (or other behaviors, including aggression), it is important to get to the root cause of the behavior rather than to simply try to "unteach" or stop the behavior, particularly in those instances where a behavior is written off as an autism symptom when the child is actually trying to communicate a medical need.

Many individuals with ASD also have highly focused or narrow interests or persistent preoccupations. While anything can become a focused interest for someone with ASD, some common examples of topics upon which individuals with ASD may focus include trains and train schedules/transit maps, vacuum cleaners, lights/light switches, numbers, and ceiling fans. People with ASD may obtain incredible amounts of knowledge about the subject with which they are preoccupied and may have difficulty accepting that others may not be as interested. Academically, many (though not all, of course) children with ASD gravitate toward numbers/mathematics or science-related topics.

Individuals with ASD may be challenged by changes in expected routines, transitions from one activity to another, or moving from one environment/location to another. Changes to these routines can be very upsetting and some children may be distraught during these difficult periods. Examples of this inflexibility include needing to take the same route between two places, eating the same foods, and doing activities in a certain order. For this reason, many schools use picture calendars to show a daily routine and review with children each day to prepare for any changes to the routine. Families can also incorporate these picture schedules into the home routine. Individuals with autism also may be distressed by unpredictable movements. For example, movements or noises by unknown dogs are frequently concerning to people with ASD because they may be unexpected and cannot be anticipated. This difficulty could be behavioral but may also have a visual processing or auditory component.

Some individuals with ASD also have aggressive behaviors. These behaviors may be directed toward themselves and involve self-injurious behaviors such as head banging, hitting, scratching, or pulling out hair/eyebrows/eyelashes. Behavior may also be directed toward others. When a person with ASD exhibits aggression it is critical to not only work toward controlling the behavior but also to try to determine its root cause. Aggression may be the result of physical pain, frustration, anxiety or other underlying reasons and it is important to try to address the cause not just the symptom (the behavior) in order to resolve aggression and address the needs of the individual with ASD.

What is the Risk?

How common is ASD? While results of ASD prevalence studies vary, they show that more and more children are being diagnosed with ASD. Boys are at about a four to five times higher risk for ASD than are girls.

Currently, the most commonly relied upon statistic of autism prevalence in the United States is 1 in 68 (1 in 42 boys and 1 in 189 girls), announced in early 2014 by the United States Centers for Disease Control and Prevention (CDC). This prevalence rate was calculated based on a 2010 survey by the CDC of health and school records of 8-year-old children in eleven U.S. communities. The 1 in 68 prevalence rate is a 30 percent increase over the 1 in 88 rate announced by the CDC in 2012 and an enormous increase over the prevalence rates (as low as 1 in 10,000) in the 1980s.

Some experts do not acknowledge a true increase in autism, arguing that changes to autism diagnostic criteria, diagnostic substitution, and awareness, among other things, have led to more children being diagnosed with ASD. While these factors likely play some role, many other experts believe that they cannot fully account for the huge increase in the autism prevalence rate over the past few decades and that a significant part of the increase cannot be explained by these factors. Anecdotally, many teachers (and other professionals) report that, until recent years, they did not see in their classrooms (or elsewhere) children with the constellation of symptoms found in ASD. It seems incredible that parents, doctors, and teachers all would have missed massive numbers of children with the severe communication, social, and behavioral challenges frequently seen with ASD.

Causes

As the prevalence of ASD continues to rise, causation remains uncertain. Current research suggests that both genetics and environmental exposures contribute to the development of ASD. Epigenetics examines how environmental factors may affect genes, including causing new (not inherited) mutations to genes. This area of research may provide important information concerning both the development of ASD and treatment.

Prior conventional wisdom held that autism was primarily an inherited genetic condition. While there is still much research to be done on the role of environmental factors in the development of autism, it is becoming more apparent that autism is not solely an inherited genetic condition. Studies in the past several years support the hypothesis that the environment plays a significant role in ASD causation or suggest that environmental factors are important and that heritability (the "proportion of observed variation in a particular trait . . . that can be attributed to inherited genetic factors in contrast to environmental ones" [www.merriam-webster.com]) is not the sole determinant in ASD causation. Here are just a few examples of recent research. In 2011, a large twins study—the California Autism Twin Study (CATS)—calculated a heritability rate of 37 percent for autism and 38 percent for ASD—rates much lower than prior (and much smaller) twins studies. Importantly, even this rate may be an overestimate because the researchers did not account for the interaction between genes and the environment. More recently, researchers from the University of Chicago examined medical records from more than 100 million people living in the United States and found a strong correlation (at the county level) between autism and intellectual disability rates and incidences of genital malformations in newborn males (which suggest an in-utero exposure altering normal development), suggesting a more significant role for environmental factors in the development of ASD. A study by Canadian researchers just published in January 2015 showed far less genetic similarity than expected by the researchers between siblings who each have ASD. The study involved whole-genome sequencing of siblings and parents and found that in less than a third of cases did siblings share gene variations thought to be relevant to ASD. While this study was not looking at environmental factors, and while the study was relatively small, the results suggest that factors other than heritability are significant in autism causation.

Genetic Factors

While genetic factors play a role in the development of autism, it does not appear that, as a general rule, autism can be defined as a solely inherited genetic disorder. The rapid increase in the rate of autism over the past two decades also suggests otherwise. Moreover, despite extensive research, scientists have had limited success in identifying genes or genetic mutations (a change to a gene's DNA sequence) linked to autism. Currently, only approximately 10 percent of autism cases appear to be related to genetic or chromosomal disorders, including Fragile X Syndrome, Down Syndrome and Tuberous Sclerosis. For the vast majority of individuals with autism, there is no clear cut genetic cause. Even where genetic mutations can be identified, impact by environmental factors cannot necessarily be ruled out because genetic mutations are not only inherited but may arise independently, and may be related to environmental factors.

It is important to remember that having an increased genetic risk or predisposition does not mean that an individual necessarily will develop autism.

Environmental Factors

"Environmental factors" broadly means anything outside our bodies, including, for a developing fetus, the womb. These factors include, for example: food; medications; air; pollutants and toxins; fertility issues, pregnancy complications, and birth trauma; family history of autoimmune disease; allergies; and stress. Some people are more susceptible to the effects of environmental factors than others. Developing fetuses, infants, and young children are particularly vulnerable to environmental insults because they are undergoing rapid physical and developmental growth and changes.

A number of environmental factors have been or are being studied in connection with autism including pesticides; vaccines; certain pharmaceuticals; freeway proximity; mercury, aluminum, and other heavy metal exposure (including maternal exposure); and lack of or limited use of prenatal vitamins or nutritional deficiencies in pregnancy. It is also important to keep in mind that there are literally thousands of chemicals in our environment, many of which have not been well-studied for harmful effects in general. Moreover, the effects of chemicals in combination often are not well-studied.

How may these environmental factors be related to ASD? While many more studies of environmental factors need to be done, the total load theory is one possible way to explain the role of environmental factors in ASD causation or contribution. The total load theory posits that each person has a tipping point (and it varies from individual to individual) at which their body can no longer handle the stressors placed on it. For some, the manifestation of having reached the tipping point is ASD.

Because not much is known yet about who is most susceptible to harm from which particular environmental factors or combinations of factors, some experts recommend minimizing exposures to the extent possible—living a more "green" lifestyle, for example, and choosing, when possible, clean, organic food, cleaning products without harmful chemicals, chemical-free beds and other furniture, low-or no-VOC paints, and non-fluorescent lighting. We cannot control everything in our environment, but addressing issues we can control can have a big impact. Moreover, for some individuals who are sensitive to environmental factors, reducing these environmental stressors may help in reducing the symptoms of ASD. Remember, we are all susceptible to negative impact from environmental factors. If you suspect that your child has ASD or has recently been diagnosed, you are probably under tremendous stress. Reducing negative environmental factors within your control also may help you stay healthy to help your child.

SCREENING & DIAGNOSIS

While children can reliably be diagnosed with ASD by approximately age two (and even younger in some cases) many children still are not diagnosed until they are more than four years old. In some instances, diagnosis is delayed because children are not being screened properly, or because parents are encouraged to take a "wait and see" approach, or because some parents are concerned with labeling their child with ASD or another label. However, the sooner your child is evaluated and can begin receiving services, the better. Early intervention may help improve a child's outcome and may prevent further worsening of some autism symptoms.

If you are concerned about your child's development, push for further evaluation. At the same time, if your child is under three, your pediatrician should refer you to your state's early intervention program. You also may be able to self-refer to early intervention. You do not need an autism diagnosis to begin receiving early intervention services. Generally, eligibility for early intervention services is based on the significance of a delay in an assessed area or areas rather than a diagnostic label.

ASD evaluations are often done by a team of professionals that may include a doctor (a developmental pediatrician, a neuropsychologist, a child psychiatrist or psychologist, or a neurologist) and professionals in a wide range of fields, including speech therapy, occupational therapy, physical therapy, audiology, and vision.

A clinician diagnosing your child relies on the diagnostic criteria in the most recent edition of the *Diagnostic and Statistical Manual of Mental Disorders* (the *DSM-5*). Our focus here is on warning signs to parents, but you should be familiar with the formal criteria as well. Parents also should be aware that—unlike prior versions of the *DSM*, which had separate diagnosis criteria for autism, Pervasive Developmental Delay - Not Otherwise Specified (PDD-NOS), and Asperger Syndrome, among others—in the *DSM-5* there is a single umbrella diagnosis for ASD. You can learn more about the *DSM-5* criteria at autism .about.com/od/diagnosingautism/a/What-Are-The-New-Criteria-For-Diagnosing-Autism-Spectrum-Disorders.htm.

It is important to note that, while the *DSM-5* provides the diagnostic criteria for ASD, there is no one "test" for ASD. Different assessment tools may be used depending on where you live or who conducts the assessment(s). This section is meant to provide information concerning some commonly used assessments and does not represent all possible screening and diagnostic tools.

A developmental history taken from parents and caregivers also should be a part of the screening and diagnosis process for ASD. This type of history may be taken during an interview or you may be asked to provide it in writing. If you are asked to provide it in writing, you may be asked for a follow-up interview to obtain more detailed information. The following areas are generally covered:

- Family medical history (both immediate and extended family), including developmental disabilities, learning differences, emotional/behavioral issues, and medical conditions (particularly autoimmune disorders).
- Child's birth and maternal pregnancy history, as well as any fertility issues and/or treatments)
- Child's medical history, including:
  - Diagnosed medical conditions
  - Hospitalization and surgical procedures
  - Sensory differences
  - Current and past medications and supplements
  - Any other medical concerns
- Developmental milestones, including:
  - Language/Communication
  - Social/Emotional
  - Physical
  - Cognitive
  - Any regressions or loss of acquiring or emerging skills or other developmental red flags
- Results of previous evaluations, if any
- History of interventions, if any

Developmental Surveillance and Screening

Screening for ASD is usually a multi-step process beginning with developmental surveillance done by your child's pediatrician during well-child visits. During any well-child visit, your child's doctor should determine if your child is meeting developmental milestones across several categories—social and emotional; language; cognitive; and physical—as well as look for signs of atypical development. The doctor should examine your child, engage with the child, and ask you questions regarding the child's development. If your child's doctor does not appear to routinely check your child's developmental milestones, ask that it be done. In addition to regular developmental surveillance at well-child visits, the American Academy of Pediatrics (AAP) currently recommends developmental screenings at 9 months, 18 months, and 24 or 30 months. The AAP also recommends screening specifically for ASD during regular well-child visits at 18 and 24 months. If a child shows signs associated with ASD, if another family member (particularly a sibling) has ASD, or if the child otherwise might be at risk, additional screening might be warranted.

As a parent, you should also familiarize yourself with developmental milestones. You know your child best and in a short well-child visit your doctor may not get the full picture. There are comprehensive lists of developmental milestones and red flags at http://www.cdc.gov/ncbddd/actearly/pdf/checklists/all_checklists.pdf. While there is a range of "typical" development, these lists are helpful in identifying what children generally are expected to have achieved at

2 months, 4 months, 6 months, 9 months, 12 months, 18 months, 2 years, 3 years, 4 years, and 5 years. In addition, these lists highlight behavior or developmental concerns for parents at each age. You should always let your doctor know if you have concerns about your child's development. For example, you should alert your pediatrician if:

- By 4 months, your child is not smiling at people;
- By 6 months, your child is not affectionate with caregivers/familiar people, laughing, or responding to sounds;
- By 9 months, your child doesn't recognize familiar people, doesn't babble, doesn't engage in back-and-forth play, or doesn't respond to his or her name;
- By 12 months, your child is not pointing, is not using simple gestures like head shaking or waving, or does not have simple single words (such as "mama" or "dada");
- By 18 months, your child is not showing things to others by pointing, doesn't have at least six words, is failing to gain new words, and does not seem to notice or care if a parent/caregiver leaves/returns;
- By 24 months, your child does not use meaningful, independent (not echolalic) two-word phrases or cannot follow simple instructions;
- Any time your child loses skills she previously had acquired.

Screening Tools

Screening tools do exactly what the name implies—they screen for possible issues and risk factors and help determine if further diagnostic evaluation is needed. Screening tools are not diagnostic and should not be used to diagnose ASD. If someone makes a diagnosis based only on the results of a screening tool, ask that your child be referred for a comprehensive evaluation. There are many different screening tools available. Some tools are disorder-specific (in this case, ASD), others screen for delays in a particular area of development (such as screens for social challenges), and others are more general developmental screening tools. Screening tools may be administered in a variety of settings including pediatricians' offices, homes, schools, and therapists' clinics or offices. Generally, though not universally, screening tools are relatively short questionnaires completed by parents and scored and explained by a professional (doctor, therapist, etc.).

The following list is not exhaustive, and other tests may be available and may be appropriate depending on particular developmental concerns. Organizations such as the American Academy of Pediatrics and First Signs (http://firstsigns.org/screening/tools/rec.htm) also have information on their websites about available screening tools.

The Modified Checklist for Autism in Toddlers, Revised with Follow-Up (M-CHAT-R/F)™

The M-CHAT-R/F™ targets 16- to 30-month-olds and is designed to be administered during pediatric well-child visits but can also be administered by other professionals. It is a quick screening tool that also can be scored in just a few minutes. It does have a relatively high rate of false positives, meaning that not all children who screen positive will later be diagnosed with ASD. It is a two-stage test and depending on the results of the first stage (a 20-question parent-answered questionnaire) the child can be classified as low risk (no additional action recommended other than later rescreening for children under two at the initial screening); medium risk, which warrants administering the more specific follow-up screen to determine if the child should be referred for diagnostic evaluation and early intervention services; or high risk, which warrants immediate referral for diagnostic evaluation and early intervention services. While this tool is available online and parents can self-administer the screen, professional administration and scoring still is recommended to help the parents understand the results and to make appropriate recommendations.

Ages & Stages Questionnaires® (ASQ)

ASQ-3® (ASQ Third Edition) is a screening tool for children from 1 to 66 months of age and is designed to be used both in the home and in medical or clinical settings. The parent fills out an age-appropriate questionnaire (approximately 30 items), which can be scored in just a few minutes. The ASQ-3® screens for a variety of issues associated with ASD including communication, gross and fine motor skills, problem-solving abilities, and social/emotional issues.

In addition to ASQ-3®, parents can complete the Ages & Stages Questionnaires®: Social-Emotional, Second Edition (ASQ:SE-2™), which focuses on social/emotional issues.

Brief Infant Toddler Social Emotional Assessment (BITSEA™)

The BITSEA™ is a screening tool appropriate for children ages 12 to 36 months and is designed to evaluate social and emotional behavior. This parent-completed screening tool can be used in a home or office setting and is quick (approximately 42 items) to complete. The BITSEA™ can be followed up with a more comprehensive screen if the results raise concerns.

Communication and Symbolic Behavior Scales Developmental Profile™ (CSBS DP™) Infant-Toddler Checklist

The CSBS DP™ Infant-Toddler Checklist screens in seven areas that may indicate a language delay and is designed to assess children whose communicative abilities (not actual age) range from 6 to 24 months. The CSBS DP™ Infant-Toddler Checklist can be completed by parents or by a professional and is scored by a professional. The entire CSBS DP™ takes approximately an hour to complete.

Parents' Evaluation of Developmental Status (PEDS) and Parents' Evaluation of Developmental Milestones (PEDS:DM)

PEDS and PEDS:DM are screening tools designed for children from birth to approximately eight years old. PEDS screens for issues concerning language, motor skills, self-help, behavior, social/emotional issues, and academic skills, while PEDS:DM is designed to be more accurate than informal developmental milestone checklists. These screens can be administered together. Parents complete the short questionnaires, which are scored and explained by the professional providing the screening assessment.

Temperament and Atypical Behavior Scale (TABS)

TABS is a screening tool for children between 11 and 71 months of age. The 15-item questionnaire can be completed by parents in just a few minutes and scored quickly by a professional. TABS particularly looks at behavior and regulatory issues.

Child Development Inventory (CDI)

The CDI is targeted for preschoolers and toddlers. Unlike a number of the screening tools discussed above, the CDI is a longer, approximately 300-item questionnaire. The CDI is completed by parents and is designed to measure eight different areas relating to motor skills, language, social, self-help, and cognitive to provide parents information on a child's skills and possible challenges as well as to help assess school readiness.

Diagnosis

If a screening assessment raises concerns and/or other risk factors exist, a child should be referred for a comprehensive ASD evaluation. Often a team of professionals evaluates a child to determine if an ASD diagnosis is appropriate. That team may include a doctor (developmental pediatrician, neuropsychologist, child psychiatrist or psychologist, or neurologist) and likely also will include professionals in a wide range of fields, including speech therapy, occupational therapy, physical therapy, audiology, and vision, depending on the child.

These professionals will use a variety of methods in determining if your child meets the *DSM-5* diagnostic criteria for ASD. They will obtain information from you, likely including a comprehensive family history, as discussed above, and will interact with your child. Certain testing may be performed including:

- Hearing tests to determine if a child has a hearing impairment that requires further intervention and could impact communication, socialization, and even behavior;
- Vision evaluation;
- Speech evaluation;
- Occupational and/or physical therapy evaluations;
- An electroencephalogram (EEG) to assess for seizure activity or other unusual brain wave activity;
- Magnetic Resonance Imaging (MRI) and/or Computer Assisted Axial Tomography (CAT SCAN) to assess for neurological issues or structural changes in the brain;

- Genetic testing for conditions such as Fragile X; and
- Testing for possible metabolic or mitochondrial issues that may warrant more comprehensive evaluation.

The professionals diagnosing your child likely also will use one or more of various standardized and specialized tests. These assessments are designed to cover multiple domains to provide a comprehensive picture of an individual's challenges and strengths. The most commonly used diagnostic tools include:

The Autism Diagnostic Observation Schedule, Second Edition™ (ADOS™-2)

The ADOS™-2 is a standardized assessment that takes approximately an hour to administer. It consists of a series of structured or semi-structured interactions between the child and the professional administering the ADOS™-2, giving the evaluator a chance to observe social issues, behaviors, and communication issues potentially associated with ASD. The ADOS™-2 has multiple modules to allow for a choice appropriate to the child's developmental level and communication abilities. It was revised in 2012 and, among other things, can now be administered to children as young as 12 to 30 months. A highly trained clinician should administer this evaluation.

The Autism Diagnostic Interview,™ Revised (ADI™-R)

ADI™-R is a companion instrument to the ADOS™-2. ADI™-R focuses primarily on social issues, behaviors, and communication issues. The assessor administering the ADI™-R conducts a structured interview with the parents of the child being assessed. The interview includes a full developmental history, as well as current observations concerning development. Like the ADOS™-2, this assessment is standardized.

Childhood Autism Rating Scale™, Second Edition (CARS™-2)

CARS™-2 consists of a 15-item questionnaire completed by a professional evaluator (scores are standardized) and a parent/caregiver questionnaire. There are two different CARS™ questionnaires—a standard form and a high functioning form (used when evaluating children six and older who are more verbal). The parent/caregiver questionnaire is not scored.

Vineland Adaptive Behavior Scales, Second Edition (Vineland™-II)

This standardized tool measures how a child is performing in four domains: daily living skills, communication, socialization, and motor skills. Additionally there is an optional index to measure maladaptive behaviors. The assessment can be conducted through an interview form or a parent/caregiver-completed form. There also is an expanded interview form as well as a teacher rating form that can be administered.

Regardless of which assessment tools and tests are administered, you likely will receive written reports from the various professionals evaluating your child or a comprehensive report combining testing results and providing information about your child's diagnosis. You also can expect to meet with either the professional overseeing the evaluation or the team of evaluators to discuss the results and their recommendations for your child. This is an important chance for you to ask questions. No question should be off-limits—you are working to determine the most appropriate course of action to help your child and this is also an opportunity for you to gain more knowledge about the evaluation processes and how results are analyzed. This may be the first time your child is evaluated, but chances are that it will not be the last time. As your child ages, he will likely be evaluated for preschool-aged special education services and re-evaluated regularly to determine appropriate school-aged services. You might also have your child evaluated at later dates to help you determine whether his diagnosis still is accurate or to help you independently determine appropriate interventions.

Evaluations can be stressful for both children and parents. Children may be in an unfamiliar environment and, even if evaluated at home, will be working with an unfamiliar adult. For children who do not adapt well to change, the pressure can be tremendous and a child's behavior during evaluations can be challenging for parents as well. Moreover, as parents, we want to paint our children in the best light but it is important to be honest and not aspirational in your responses to parent questionnaires and interviews. Even though it is difficult and emotional to admit to someone the significant challenges your child may be facing, your honesty will help your child to receive the most accurate diagnosis and access to services he may need to help him reach his fullest potential.

Educational Assessments

As your child gets older and enters the school system, you will also need to learn to navigate a new set of rules. Based on federal law, including the Individuals with Disabilities Education Act (IDEA), children with disabilities are entitled to a free and appropriate public education. Your child's eligibility for services from your school district is not based merely on a diagnosis of ASD, rather it is based on your child's educational needs. Therefore, it is possible that a child would be categorized differently from ASD (for example, speech and language impaired) for educational purposes or, less commonly, could be determined to be ineligible for special education services despite having an autism diagnosis.

The IDEA was enacted to provide children access to evaluation for and receipt of appropriate educational services. Under IDEA, whether the parent or another person recommends that a child be evaluated, the parent must provide informed written consent. This means that if a school recommends evaluation for your child, the school must explain why, how the evaluation will be conducted, and alternatives considered, and it must provide the parents with information to learn more about their rights and their child's rights.

If a parent consents to evaluation and a school district refuses to evaluate or, after evaluation, refuses to provide services at all or at an appropriate level, the parents may avail themselves of their due process rights to attempt to resolve the dispute. Often this may begin with a voluntary resolution session or mediation but may ultimately result in the parents commencing litigation against a school district to attempt to resolve the parties' differences. The procedure may vary somewhat in different states. For example, in some places there is one level of administrative review before a lawsuit moves to civil court and in some places there are two levels of administrative review. There may be options in addition to public school placement in your school district if your district is unable to offer your child an appropriate program. Some districts will facilitate placement in another public school district that can provide an appropriate placement for your child, districts may agree to fund placement in a private school program, or, if you believe the district has not offered your child an appropriate placement, you may consider placing your child in a private program and litigating against your school district for reimbursement. An attorney who practices in this area of law can be very helpful in the process of negotiating with your district and, particularly, if you eventually need to litigate against the school district. Some parents also use advocates to help guide them through this process. Professionals familiar with your school district can help you navigate this process and provide practical and realistic advice about working with your district. Each district is different and it is important that parents understand their child's rights to ensure that their child is receiving an appropriate education.

THERAPIES & INTERVENTIONS

When a child is diagnosed with ASD, parents are, justifiably, overwhelmed. While they now have a name to put to the issues they have seen in their child and the challenges they have been experiencing as a family, the ASD label does not automatically provide a clear course of action. In fact, each child's needs are specific to that child's constellation of strengths and challenges. However, the sooner your child begins to receive services, the better. Keep in mind though that intervention at any age can help a child, so do not think that if you did not get early intervention that your child cannot make significant strides—children can and do make gains at any age.

For children whose delays are noted before they are three, early intervention is an important avenue to access treatment. Children under three who are at risk of developmental delays may be eligible for services such as speech therapy, physical therapy, occupational therapy, and special education. These services are provided through state early intervention programs. Through your state's system, you can ask for an evaluation to determine if your child qualifies for services. Your pediatrician should be able to provide relevant contact information. Whether these services are provided for a fee, on a sliding fee scale, or at no cost to the family varies from area to area. A formal ASD diagnosis is not needed to begin early intervention treatment where a particular symptom is noted, such as language delay. Eligibility for early intervention services is dependent on the significance of a child's delay or delays across multiple domains. Therefore, don't wait for a formal autism diagnosis to request an early intervention evaluation.

Depending on the child's age, you may be requesting services through early intervention, preschool, or school-aged services. Services may be provided in the home, in a therapist's office, at a school or center-based location, or some combination of these settings, depending on your child's age and needs and the availability of services in your area. In addition, parents may privately pay for therapy services (possibly seeking insurance reimbursement where available). Many parents also seek additional treatments for their children including medical/biomedical treatments, nutritional approaches, and other therapeutic modalities.

Types of Treatments

There are many different types of treatments available for individuals diagnosed with ASD, including:

- Educational, behavioral, and communications programs and therapies;
- Dietary approaches;
- Medical and biomedical approaches, including integrative medicine (we are using this term to broadly describe integrative, complementary, and so-called alternative approaches)

There are many interventions that parents and professionals have found help may help some children with ASD. As with treatments (whether traditional or more cutting edge) for many health conditions, not every individual with ASD will benefit from every treatment option. Some modalities or treatments have peer-reviewed research to support them but some may not. Many have anecdotal evidence of positive results. With so many options to choose from, families should research which approach or combination of approaches is appropriate for their child and their family. Consideration needs to be given to the cost of various approaches (especially where interventions are not provided through early intervention or school districts and where they may not be covered or reimbursed by insurance), the time commitment for various treatment modalities, and the impact of interventions—time, money, and emotional—not just on the child with ASD but on the whole family. You can consult books and websites about treatment options. Read with a critical eye, especially if something sounds too good to be true. Dig for unbiased sources where available. Ask "tough" questions of practitioners you are considering—legitimate practitioners should welcome the chance to share with an interested parent information about the treatment modality or modalities in which they practice. Some sample questions include:

- What is a typical treatment like?
- What is required of the child during treatment?
- What range of results does the practitioner see?
- Are there categories of individuals who seem to respond (or not respond) to the treatment and why?
- Are there people for whom the treatment would be inappropriate or contraindicated?
- What are the true costs of the treatment (for example, are there add-ons a parent will be encouraged to buy that increase the cost)?
- How long is treatment expected to last?
- How soon do patients/clients generally see results?
- Is there any carryover therapy to do at home? If so, is specialized equipment needed? What is the time commitment? Cost?
- Does the practitioner have any patients you can speak with about their experiences?
- Are there studies of this treatment? If not, what support is there for the effectiveness and safety of the treatment?

When you are exploring treatment options, other parents also can be a very good resource but you also need to consider that each child and family is unique and what works for one family may not work for yours. Nonetheless, valuable insight can be gained from other parents. Many times, parents are able to provide a tip, a resource, a new therapist or modality that you might otherwise not have heard about. When discussing a treatment, ask other parents for specific information. Try to determine how your child is similar or dissimilar from their child. Ask what changes they saw and why they attribute the changes to the intervention you are considering. Ask for the positives and negatives about the treatment from the parent perspective—this can provide a balance to information the practitioner provides. For example, if there is a home carryover component, the practitioner may share what he truly believes is the time commitment or compliance level required but a parent may have a different experience. Ask parents about the costs, in terms of time, money, and balancing family life.

Another note of caution: It is tempting to want to start to do many things all at once so that your child can make progress as quickly as possible. However, it is important to keep in mind that you want to be able to, as best you can, determine which treatments work and which do not. If several new treatments are started at once, you will be less able to attribute either good or poor results to one thing and determine what you should keep in your program and what should be changed. Work with your trusted professionals to determine for each intervention how to approach introducing that intervention and subsequent treatments.

Every effort has been made to accurately describe the treatment modalities discussed herein. However, if you are considering any of the modalities, please discuss them with professionals trained in those areas, who are able to provide the most accurate and timely information. Keep in mind that many individual practitioners also will adapt methods or protocols in their practices. The descriptions herein are provided for informational purposes only and not as medical, educational, or otherwise professional advice. In some instances, we have provided websites for general information but also encourage you to explore further.

Educational and Behavior Approaches

Applied Behavior Analysis (ABA)

Perhaps the most well-known treatment approach with respect to ASD is applied behavior analysis (ABA). There is not one "ABA," rather ABA provides basic principles designed to reward positive and reduce negative behaviors. ABA programs can be used to change negative or maladaptive behaviors and establish positive behaviors, teach new skills, and generalize skills or behaviors between different environments. ABA providers take data to track progress toward specific goals.

Some children receive comprehensive ABA programs. These programs can take place in a school or center-based setting, in the home, or in some combination thereof. Comprehensive ABA can take 20 or 30 (or more) hours a week and last for years. A comprehensive program will work toward improved functioning overall.

In addition, some children, either as part of a comprehensive ABA program or separately, receive focused ABA to address discrete issues, such as a difficult to resolve behavior. These programs may be shorter in both regular time commitment and duration needed.

Discrete Trial Training (DTT) is perhaps the best-known form of ABA. As its name implies, DTT uses a series of trials designed to teach each step of a learning objective. DTT takes place in a very controlled one-on-one student-to-therapist teaching environment. Trials are repeated to teach the objective. DTT uses positive reinforcement to reward a student for a correct answer or positive response/behavior. ABA therapists use instructions, prompting, and other methods to help students reach their established goals.

In addition to in-person ABA instruction, ABA programs are available through web-based programs. While live ABA instruction is preferable, it is not always available for the amount of time needed or may not be available in some geographic areas. These programs can be valuable resources, for example, to parents who live in under-served communities or parents who want to augment the school or home services a child already receives.

Parents should make sure of the qualifications of their ABA providers and those who supervise the therapists. Many insurance companies that may provide coverage for ABA may expect supervisors and/or therapists to have certain qualifications, such an advanced degree or board certification in ABA. You should determine what your insurance requirements are if this is an issue for you. Moreover a qualification like board certification helps to ensure (but of course cannot guarantee) that ABA is being appropriately implemented with your child.

More information about ABA can be found at www.abainternational.org.

Pivotal Response Treatment (PRT)®

PRT® is based on ABA principles but is a more natural method designed to, in particular, improve socialization and communication for children with ASD. PRT® "targets pivotal areas of a child's development, such as motivation, responsivity to multiple cues, self-management, and social initiations. These skills are pivotal because they are the foundational behaviors upon which learners with ASD can make widespread and generalized improvements in many other areas. By targeting these critical behaviors, PRT® results in widespread, collateral improvements in communication, social, and behavioral domains." (http://www.autismprthelp.com/about-prt.php). While ABA frequently relies on reinforcers such as candy or another treat to reward positive behavior, PRT promotes the use of natural reinforcers related to an activity. For example, if a child is working toward requesting a specific object, the reinforcer is that object, rather than something unrelated to the task.

Family plays an important role in PRT, providing insight into what motivates an individual learner and also in providing social situations that allow the child to generalize skills.

More information is available at www.autismprthelp.com.

Verbal Behavior Intervention (VBI) or Verbal Behavior Therapy (VBT)

VBI/VBT focuses on communication skills, such as the purposeful use of verbal and non-verbal language to communicate requests (known in VBI/VBT as "mands") and communication to share information (known in VBI/VBT as a "tact"). VBI/VBT applies the work of B. F. Skinner and principles of ABA in developing communication skills. As with ABA, reinforcers are an important part of VBI/VBT. Learners are given positive reinforcement not just for communicating but also for efforts toward communicating. Prompting is also an important part of VBT, scaffolding for the learner and reducing prompts over time, so that she can work incrementally to reach a language goal.

Developmental, Individual Differences, Relationship-Based Approach (DIR® and Floortime methods)

Floortime-based therapies (such as DIR/Floortime® and the Greenspan Floortime Approach™), based on the work of Dr. Stanley Greenspan and Dr. Serena Wieder, generally are designed to help children reach six key developmental milestones, focusing on the social-emotional and intellectual, to help children form relationships and encourage intellectual/cognitive growth. These milestones relate generally to self-regulation and interest in the world around the child rather than an inward focus; engagement with others; and increasingly more complex communication and social-emotional involvement, including more creative play, problem-solving skills, logical thought, and forming links between ideas for more complex learning. While the Floortime methods are not themselves speech therapy, occupational therapy, or educational methodologies, many professionals with specialized training in speech, OT, special education, and child psychology also receive training in Floortime methods and Floortime methods often are incorporated with these therapies.

Learn more about DIR® and Floortime methods at www.icdl.com and www.stanleygreenspan.com.

Early Start Denver Model (ESDM)

As its name suggests, ESDM is a method focused on early development in the infant and toddler years. It is based on ABA as well as developmental psychology and, like ABA, usually focuses on one-on-one teaching. It also emphasizes parent training and involvement to generalize learning. Therapists and parents use ESDM not only in a clinical setting but also as part of a child's daily life, with the goal of improving overall function. ESDM encompasses more natural, play-based activities.

Learn more about ESDM at www.ucdmc.ucdavis.edu/mindinstitute/research/esdm.

Relationship Development Intervention (RDI®)

RDI®, developed by psychologist Steven Gutstein, PhD, aims to improve a child's social/emotional well being, her life skills, cognitive function, and relationships, especially with parents and caregivers. RDI® capitalizes on brain plasticity and challenges the brain to grow and develop to help those with ASD (and other challenges) to be able to function in a more "typical" way. As such, it does not just seek to teach mechanisms to help those with ASD cope despite their challenges but to actually change the brain. Certified RDI® consultants can develop a child-specific plan, provide therapy and also teach parents and caregivers ways to apply RDI principles in daily living.

More information is available at www.rdiconnect.com.

Son-Rise Program®

The Son-Rise Program® was created by Barry Neil Kaufman and Samahria Lyte Kaufman initially to help their son, who was diagnosed with severe autism. The program developed from the premise that autism is a neurological disorder affecting a child's ability to relate, not merely a behavioral disorder. The program is heavily dependent on parent involvement. Therefore, parent training is a key component of the Son-Rise Program®. Ideally the program takes place in a space created in the home to minimize distractions and sensory overstimulation. Son-Rise® is play-oriented and focuses on socialization and building relationships. Under the Son-Rise Program®, you identify a child's motivators and then use those to encourage the child's participation. The program does not discourage a child's stimming but instead encourages the parent to join the child in stimming—meeting the child where he is as a way for him to begin to relate to the world. Many families recruit a team of volunteers or staff to help immerse the child in the Son-Rise Program®.

More information is available at www.autismtreatmentcenter.org.

Treatment and Education of Autistic and related Communication-handicapped Children (TEACCH®)

TEACCH® is a structured approach to education for those with ASD. It provides a framework for learning but is not a specific curriculum. The TEACCH® approach focuses on acceptance and support to help people with ASD achieve the most independence possible. Using visual and written information to teach skills, and providing support for socialization and communication, it is individualized and can be adapted to a person's age and developmental level.

More information is available at www.teacch.com

Rapid Prompting™ Method (Soma® RPM)

Soma® RPM was developed by Soma Mukhopadhyay, the mother of a severely affected young man, to allow learners with ASD to improve academic skills. In the process, students also are able to better communicate using the teaching tools of Soma® RPM, which can simply be paper and pencil. Soma® RPM encourages increasingly sophisticated responses as the learner's cognition and motor skills improve. Soma® RPM is based on the presumption that individuals with ASD are able to learn. Using Soma® RPM, students are given exposure to a wide variety of interesting and appropriate information and a way to learn and communicate what they have learned.

While Soma® RPM uses prompting, it is not facilitated communication. A teacher using Soma® RPM provides a variety of intensive prompts (non-touching) designed to get the student to respond and to compete with the student's self-stimulatory behaviors.

More information is available at www.halo-soma.org.

The Miller Method®

The Miller Method®, developed by Dr. Arnold Miller, PhD, and Eileen Eller-Miller, M.A., focuses on what it sees as a challenge to those with ASD in building systems and organizing behavior in increasingly complex ways, which is necessary for development. The Miller Method® determines the significance of atypical behaviors and turns those behaviors into functional ones. The Miller Method® uses activities designed to fill gaps in a child's development. It is an approach that also relies heavily on parent involvement for generalizing what is learned into the home and other environments.

More information is available at www.millermethod.org.

Communications

Even students with relatively strong verbal skills frequently require speech and communication interventions. Further, finding an effective means for individuals with limited verbal capacity to communicate is important to reduce stress, frustration, and possibly anxiety and depression. There are a number of communication methods that may help children with ASD.

Speech Therapy

Speech therapy is an integral part of services for children with ASD. Children with ASD often need help with both the production of speech and the pragmatic use of language. Even children who have relatively strong speech skills often struggle with social language. Speech therapy is intended to improve communication skills. For some, this may be verbal speech; for others, it may be speech through assisted or augmentative communication devices, or gestures. Speech therapy can be delivered in a wide variety of settings and may be 1:1, dyads (2 children with one therapist), or a small group, depending on a child's needs and goals.

Many speech therapists also work with children using oral motor exercises and tools. This is especially helpful for children who have low tone or motor planning difficulties that may inhibit speech production. Oral motor activities often use simple items or food found around the home (e.g., straws, bubbles, whistles) and there also are more specialized oral motor tools (e.g., chewies, vibrating tools, horns, texturized tools, brushes, special straws) that a therapist may recommend. Activities can include: blowing, sucking, and other lip-related activities, tongue-related activities (such as licking and other tongue movements, sound activities), and activities to strengthen the jaw (such as chewing).

Some speech therapists also are trained in a method known as PROMPT©. PROMPT© stands for "Prompts for Restructuring Oral Muscular Phonetic Targets." PROMPT© therapy involves touching cues to the jaw, tongue, and lips to help a child develop motor control and teach the movements necessary to articulate phonemes, words, phrases, and sentences. PROMPT© is used for a wide variety of communication-related challenges including ASD and apraxia/dyspraxia. Learn more about PROMPT© at www.promptinstitute.com.

The Picture Exchange Communication System (PECS™)

PECS™ uses picture symbols to systematically teach communication skills. Students are taught to initiate communication by giving a picture in exchange for an object—encouraging the child to make a connection between the two. As skills build, the use of pictures in exchange for objects is made more sophisticated and more demands are placed on the child. While initially PECS™ is often taught without use of verbal language, language is introduced to provide prompts to the child as demands increase, as well as to model language. PECS™ can be used to teach students increasingly complex and abstract communications skills, including emotions. PECS™ is often used both in homes and schools/centers to help children navigate their daily schedule.

Learn more about PECS™ at www.pecs-usa.com.

Augmentative/Assistive Communication Devices

There are a variety of devices, software programs, and apps that enable individuals with no or limited verbal communication to effectively communicate. These include devices solely devoted to language output as well as smart phones, computers, and tablets. In particular, iPads have become very popular communication devices and there are many apps and programs available for the iPad to provide communication support for individuals with ASD. Some apps and programs are as simple as a two-choice option where a child can choose yes or no, or can choose from milk or juice when asked what they want to drink. Other apps and programs are very sophisticated programs allowing conversational communication with a huge variety of words/symbols available. Moreover, there are many apps and software programs geared toward improving sentence structure, conversational language, vocabulary, and other aspects of speech that can support verbal children with language challenges. As noted above, some non-verbal children become verbal (to varying degrees) while using these devices. Use of these devices also can lessen frustration, anxiety, and even depression, that may be experienced by those who want to communicate but cannot.

Occupational Therapy

Occupational therapy can be use to help individuals with ASD develop important life skills and skills of daily living. In children this may include things like dressing, eating and use of utensils, cutting with scissors, writing, bathing/showering, and personal hygiene. Occupational therapists also work on helping individuals to improve socialization and therapy may be delivered with a peer for this purpose. Occupational therapy is provided in clinical offices, in schools, in homes and in sensory gyms, which contain equipment to help address sensory integration challenges faced by many individuals with ASD.

Sensory integration therapy is a critical aspect of occupational therapy for many individuals with ASD. Many children with ASD have difficulty processing and reacting to various sensory stimuli. Individuals can be hypersensitive to some things—such as a tag on a shirt, noise, and lights—or hyposensitive causing them to seek stimulus, like jumping or other movement. Among other things, sensory integration therapy uses the person's vestibular (balance and spatial orientation), tactile (touch/texture), and proprioceptive (where your body is in space and where your body parts are in relation to each other) systems to help regulate sensory processing.

Some tools used in sensory integration therapy may include swings, brushing, weighted vests, and stability balls, among many others.

Often children with ASD use a sensory diet to help them better function. A sensory diet is a plan of sensory activities custom designed to address a person's sensory needs in the situations in which they are challenged. A sensory diet can be used at home and in school, as well as in other environments. Sensory diets can address a wide range of issues including: proprioceptive, auditory, tactile, smell, taste, visual, and vestibular challenges. Classrooms may have sensory toolkits with various tools to address children's sensory needs to help them better attend and learn.

Physical Therapy

Some children with ASD also require physical therapy to address challenges relating to movement, including walking, stair climbing, coordination, and balance. Therapy can be delivered in a clinical setting, at school, or at home.

Other Therapeutic Interventions

Vision Therapy

Vision is more than just how well you see, it also includes how well your visual processing skills function. In fact, some of the symptoms of autism in a child may be related to difficulties with visual processing, including, but not limited to poor eye contact, side glancing rather than looking straight forward, hyperfocus, academic struggles, difficulties with transitions, difficulties with unpredictable movements, awareness of one's body in space, sensory sensitivity to light, and impulsivity. While different providers use different methods of testing, as a general rule, a patient's visual acuity will be tested along with a variety of tests to determine eye tracking, whether or how well the eyes work in tandem, and other issues. Some of the tests may be conducted using testing equipment, computers, or physical tests that allow the clinician to observe adaptive behaviors and other indicators in the child that suggest vision challenges. Some tests also may be conducted using lenses, such as prism lenses, that disrupt vision. Recommended therapy will vary both depending on the clinician and the testing results. Some therapies may be computer-based and other therapies may involve hands-on or physical activities. In some cases, therapies may involve a combination of the two. Therapy may take place at home or in a clinician's office or both. As a general rule, programs are closely monitored and regularly adjusted to meet the patient's changing needs.

Neurofeedback

Neurofeedback is a treatment modality that provides direct training to help improve efficiency of brain and central nervous system function and self-regulation. Neurofeedback can be used to treat many issues that involve brain disregulation, including ASD and ADHD. Individuals often are assessed prior to neurofeedback and at intervals during treatment using a specialized form of an EEG called a QEEG, a type of "brain mapping" that may assist in administering more targeted treatment. In neurofeedback, electrodes are attached to particular spots on the scalp and brain activity is analyzed and the neurofeedback program then provides feedback, often targeting specific frequencies, to the brain, which uses that feedback to improve efficiency and self-regulation. This training and repetition allows the brain to change, taking advantage of brain plasticity. There are several different types of neurofeedback used; some require the active participation of the patient—for example, manipulating an object on a computer screen—and others are more passive.

Service Dogs

Many families of children with autism are finding that trained autism service dogs are a true asset to their families. These dogs can help reduce the stress that people with ASD are under in interacting in a world that assaults their sensory systems and often places stressful social and communications demands on them. Some service dogs are able to sense when a child may have a seizure or, if a seizure begins, can alert those nearby. Dogs also can help with sleep issues. Service dogs can help prevent wandering, a serious and life threatening issue for children with ASD. Unlike people, who may, even unintentionally, make judgments about individuals with ASD, dogs do not judge. As a general rule, trained service dogs can enter public places and travel with the person they assist. In some instances, autism service dogs may be able to attend school with the child they assist, helping to reduce stress and encourage social relationships with peers.

Individuals with ASD may also benefit from interactions with a therapy or companion dog, either individually or in a group setting. These dogs can provide non-judgmental companionship, reduce anxiety, and help with socialization/communication and other issues but do not have the same extensive training and skill sets as service dogs and do not have the same public access rights as service dogs.

Art, Music, Dance and Drama Therapies

Art, music, dance, and drama can be powerful tools in helping individuals with ASD both in a clinical, therapeutic setting and as a creative outlet. It is not unusual for people with ASD to be artistically or musically talented or gifted. Many parents, for example, report that their child with ASD has perfect pitch.

Trained music, art, dance, and drama therapists can use their artistic modalities in a therapeutic setting to address some core challenges faced by individuals with autism, including social-emotional challenges, communication, sensory issues, gross and fine motor skills, organization and attention, and cognitive issues. Moreover, the therapy may also capitalize on and strengthen artistic skills that an individual may have. In this more formal, clinical setting, patients are assessed and individual treatment protocols developed to address individual challenges and goals.

Moreover, art, music, dance, and drama can be used in non-clinical settings to help individuals with ASD address some of their challenges as well as to capitalize on their strengths (for example, children who are verbal but echolalic may succeed at memorizing lines in a drama class and children with musical talent might feel more comfortable and have more fluency while singing). These inclusive programs can help children develop stronger communication skills, social-emotional connections, improve their self-esteem, and simply have fun in a safe and sensory-sensitive environment.

Hippotherapy and Therapeutic Horseback Riding

Hippotherapy and therapeutic horseback riding are two different treatment modalities both using horses to benefit children with ASD.

Hippotherapy is used by a variety of therapists (such as speech, occupational, and physical therapists), integrating movements of a horse in providing sensory and motor input while the therapist provides therapy to the patient within their practice area. Therapists who incorporate hippotherapy should have additional training beyond their core practice area.

Rather than operating as an adjunct to other therapeutic modalities, therapeutic horseback riding focuses on teaching equestrian skills. Horses are gentle, non-judgmental companions for children in therapeutic riding programs and this environment helps children to not only learn equestrian skills but also to work toward additional rider-specific goals such as balance, coordination, focus/attention, and socialization and communication.

Social Skills Interventions

There are numerous methodologies and tools available to address social challenges, one of the core issues faced by individuals with ASD.

Social Stories™ and similar programs use simple stories and illustrations to help individuals with ASD understand a myriad of social situations and can often be personalized to help make the lessons more concrete. Many parents and professionals use these stories to help teach individuals what to expect and how to behave appropriately in social situations, which is often not intuitive for individuals with ASD. It may also benefit children with ASD to act out scripts, facilitated by therapists, teachers, or parents, addressing particular social situations. The scripts can be used to show children different options in a social situation and what might happen depending on choices made.

There are a number of books and workshops for parents and professionals to learn ways to improve social skills for those with ASD. Two of the most well-known experts are Michelle Garcia Winner, MA, CCC-SLP, and Jed Baker, PhD.

Social Thinking® is a program developed by Michelle Garcia Winner to improve social thinking in individuals, including those with ASD, who face challenges in their social thinking abilities. Social Thinking® is often used in school settings to help students learn to process complex social information, but books and workshops make the program accessible to parents and all types of professionals as well, allowing it to be used in many situations.

Dr. Baker is the director of the Social Skills Training Project and gives presentations and workshops internationally focusing on social skills and challenging behaviors. He has authored several books, including *The Social Skills Picture Book* and *Social Skills Training for Children and Adolescents with Asperger Syndrome and Social Communication Problems*.

Programs and apps available for computers and mobile devices can help teach social and communication skills, including reading visual (facial expressions/body language) and verbal (such as tone of voice) cues in interpreting social situations. Videos also can be used to teach social skills and include videos that model social interactions. Moreover, in addition to the social scripts mentioned above, children can be videotaped while enacting a social situation and the video can be used as a teaching tool for the child.

Professionally moderated/guided social skills groups also may benefit children with ASD. These groups can be conducted in a school setting or privately and can be comprised of children with social challenges or be an integrated group including typically developing children and children with ASD. Many activities can be used in a group setting to facilitate social skills development—for example, board games, cooperative activities, role playing social scripts, and brainstorming on how to address a social challenge that arises in the group.

Auditory Therapies

Similar to our visual system—which is more than just visual acuity—our auditory system is more than just our ability to hear well. In addition to hearing well, a person must be able to process what she hears. Many children with ASD have difficulty with auditory processing, sound sensitivity and other sensory issues, attentional issues, speech and communication, and executive function. Auditory therapies may help by stimulating the brain in specific ways to help an individual better process sensory input.

There are a number of auditory therapy programs available, including but not limited to: Tomatis, Auditory Integration Training, Berard AIT, The Listening Program®, Solisten®, Therapeutic Listening®, Samonas™, Fast ForWord®, Earobics®, EnListen®, Rhythmic Entrainment Intervention (REI®), Interactive Metronome®, and EASe listening programs. Some auditory therapies are delivered in a clinical setting, others in a home setting, though even many of the home programs are overseen by a therapist trained in auditory therapy to ensure that the program is properly implemented. Often auditory therapy is based on music that has been manipulated (such as filtering the music or adjusting frequencies) but not all therapies are music based. Specialized headphones also may be used (such as bone-conducting headphones).

Brain Gym®

Brain Gym® is a program based on a series of 26 activities that work on coordinating the eyes, ears, hands, and body. These movements are intended to help coordinate the right and left brain hemispheres. Many exercises are done on each side of the body or across the midline. Brain Gym® can help with a variety of challenges faced by children with ASD including attentional issues, academics, coordination, organization, anxiety, and others. Some schools even incorporate Brain Gym® activities in the classroom. Brain Gym® was developed by Paul E. and Gail E. Dennison.

HANDLE®

HANDLE® is an acronym for Holistic Approach to Neurodevelopment and Learning Efficiency. In the HANDLE® model, behaviors are treated as communications and provide insight into which systems of the body, particularly challenged neurological systems, need to be treated. HANDLE® practitioners do thorough assessments to determine the root cause of challenges presented by an individual and, based on the results, develop a highly individualized program of HANDLE® exercises. HANDLE® believes in a system of Gentle Enhancement® to address challenges to systems, strengthen them, and avoid undue stress, thereby reducing the behaviors with which an individual presents. HANDLE® was developed by Judith Bluestone.

Craniosacral therapy (CST)

Craniosacral therapy may help relieve stress, improve the function of the nervous system, and improve immune system function, all of which are challenges for many individuals with ASD. The practitioner gently uses her hands to balance cerebrospinal fluid as well as membranes and tissues surrounding the spine and brain by releasing restrictions in the tissues. CST is not massage, it is done with a much lighter touch. Parents of children who receive this therapy often report that their children are more relaxed and socio-emotionally connected following therapy.

Chiropractic and Chiropractic Neurology

Most people hear the word chiropractor and think of manipulation or adjustment of the spine or other joints and soft tissue either by hand or using specialized instruments, and this treatment is an important part of what chiropractors do and may benefit some with ASD. Chiropractic corrections can be used to positively impact neurological function, relieve pain, and treat other conditions. But chiropractic care extends further. Chiropractors frequently also advise patients on nutrition, nutritional supplements, and general healthy lifestyle counseling.

Chiropractic neurology is a specialty within chiropractics requiring additional training and it focuses on the treatment of the brain and central nervous system. In addition to traditional chiropractic treatment methods such as manipulation/adjustment and nutritional consultation, chiropractic neurologists may use a combination of eye/vision exercises, physical activities (especially those aimed toward improving balance and coordination), activities for sensory regulation, cognitive activities, and others. There are many independent practitioners in this field who treat patients with ASD. Some well-known practitioners include Dr. Scott Theirl in Wisconsin, and Dr. Robert Melillo, who established the Brain Balance® Achievement Centers, which are located around the country.

Kinesiology/Applied Kinesiology

Applied Kinesiology uses manual muscle testing to evaluate patients. Essentially the practitioner is looking for feedback from the body to show where there are imbalances or other issues, looking at structural, chemical, and mental aspects of health. The practitioner may find issues related to one or more of these aspects. Treatments are patient-specific and can include joint manipulation, nutrition, lifestyle counseling, acupuncture or acupressure techniques based on the meridians, myofascial release (a hands-on technique involving stretching of the fascia), craniosacral therapy, and other treatments.

Reflex Integration

Some parents find various therapies that address integration of primitive reflexes helpful. There are a variety of automatic movements in infants that are necessary for the development of more controlled movement and postural reflexes. These primitive reflexes are some of the building blocks of a well-functioning central nervous system. As infants and young children grow and develop more control over movement, these primitive reflexes should integrate. For many children this happens naturally, but for some children these primitive reflexes fail to integrate and the failure of these reflexes to integrate may contribute to ASD and other related disorders. Primitive reflexes may fail to integrate for many reasons, including birth trauma, lack of movement during infancy, and stress or trauma to the body (including illness, environmental insults, or injury). There are a variety of methodologies practiced to help children integrate these primitive reflexes. These therapies may be delivered as a stand-alone therapy or may be introduced as part of other therapies, such as occupational therapy.

Additional Therapies

Additional therapeutic modalities that families have found helpful include:

- Acupuncture
- Acupressure
- Anat Baniel Method℠
- BodyTalk™
- EFT™ – Emotional Freedom Technique
- Light therapies (or phototherapies)
- Movement therapies

- Reiki
- Reflexology
- Various forms of energy medicine

Nutritional Approaches

Like anyone else, individuals with ASD should eat a healthy diet. Food can be an important means of providing a child with critical nutrients. This can be a real challenge for a family whose child is a "picky" eater, as many children with ASD are. There are many reasons for food difficulties. Some "pickiness" is sensory, some is resistance to change, which is often difficult for individuals with ASD. Some may stem from food allergies or sensitivities. Children may also experience gastrointestinal issues that are caused or exacerbated by the foods they are eating. These challenges make the introduction of new foods difficult.

Speech and occupational therapists may be able to help address certain feeding issues so be sure to mention any feeding issues to your therapy team. In more extreme cases, a child may require out-patient or in-patient feeding therapy.

Special diets are very popular for children with ASD and many children with ASD improve with dietary interventions. Working with a nutritionist familiar with a wide variety of diets and ASD is very helpful in making the right choices and ensuring that your child is getting the nutrients she needs. Allergy testing can be an important first step in determining foods that should be removed from or reduced in a person's diet. In addition to food allergies, many children with ASD also have food sensitivities, which can affect digestion, behavior, and cognition. It is not uncommon for a child with food allergies or sensitivities to have dark circles under their eyes. These are known as "allergic shiners." Some practitioners will run laboratory tests for food sensitivities, yeast overgrowth, and related imbalances. Others use different approaches such as NAET (an allergy elimination protocol), or eliminate likely offending foods and then, after a period of time, challenge with those foods one at a time to see if any cause a reaction.

Parents often report improvements in many of the symptoms of autism as well as improvements in gastrointestinal health when dietary changes are made. In addition to dietary changes, many doctors and nutritionists may recommend vitamins, minerals, and other supplements, such as probiotics, to support a child's nutritional status. Many children also improve when dietary enzymes are introduced. There are many different types of enzymes, targeting a narrow or broad range of foods. A nutritionist or doctor familiar with enzyme therapy can help you make the right choices and establish a sound protocol to address your child's particular needs.

While each child is unique, some foods that commonly cause problems for children with autism include gluten (a protein found in wheat and elsewhere), casein (a dairy protein), soy, corn, potato, foods containing phenols and salicylates, and foods containing artificial colors and flavors. There is no one "autism diet" that is right for every child but there are many choices. Again, working with a professional familiar with dietary interventions for children with ASD can help cut through much of the guesswork and help you to a establish the appropriate protocol for your child and adjust that protocol as needed over time. Some of the diets used with children on the autism spectrum include:

The Gluten-Free/Casein-Free Diet

The Gluten-Free/Casein-Free (GFCF) Diet (also frequently soy-free) is probably the most popular "autism" diet and is a usual starting point for families trying nutritional intervention. This diet removes wheat and other gluten-containing foods and casein (a protein in dairy). Many foods popular with children contain one or both of these proteins, including crackers, breads, cookies, pasta, milk, cheese, butter, yogurt, and ice cream. Many families also find it is necessary to remove soy from their child's diet to see more complete benefits of the GFCF diet. If you remove soy, it is important to recognize that many packaged food products that are "GFCF" contain soy. While there are many gluten-free and casein-free substitutes for favored foods now available, some families also find it possible to move toward a more whole-food diet such as the Paleo Diet or the Weston A. Price Diet (both discussed below) and avoid packaged foods, even if the packaged foods are diet compliant.

The Body Ecology Diet™ (BED™)

The Body Ecology Diet™ was created by Donna Gates and is a diet that helps to establish healthy gut flora. Many families find it particularly useful for children who have yeast overgrowth, finding that the diet's focus on principles such as low sugar foods, cultured foods, food combining, and balancing acid and alkaline foods helps to establish a healthier balance of gut flora. BED™ is implemented in stages, with foods being added in as gut health improves. The initial stage of the diet is the most restrictive.

The Feingold Diet

The Feingold Diet, developed by Dr. Ben F. Feingold, removes phenols and salicylates. For some children, these compounds—which occur both naturally in some plants, especially fruits, and artificially in artificial flavors, coloring, and preservatives—cause behavioral, learning, and health issues. The FAILSAFE Diet (Free of Additives, Low in Salicylates, Amines, and Flavor Enhancers), is another low salicylate diet and removes salicylates and additives, as well as amines (some of which occur in foods, others are a result of the breakdown of protein or fermentation) and glutamates.

The FODMAPs Diet

FODMAPs are Fermentable Oligo-Di-Monosaccharides and Polyols—certain short-chain carbohydrates/sugars. It is important to note that not all carbohydrates are FODMAPs. FODMAPs may cause gastrointestinal symptoms such as cramping, gas, diarrhea, and bloating—common symptoms in many children with ASD. The list of foods high in FODMAPs is quite long and different individuals may be more sensitive to some than others. The FODMAPs diet is also used to treat irritable bowel syndrome and similar gastrointestinal disorders.

Ketogenic Diet and Modified Atkins Diet

The Ketogenic and Modified Atkins diets are both used to improve seizure control, often in the case of intractable seizures, and should be implemented under medical/dietary supervision after determining that they are an appropriate intervention to ensure that proper caloric requirements, fat to carbohydrate/protein ratios, and nutritional needs are being met and to otherwise monitor the patient's health. The "classic" ketogenic diet generally calls for a 4:1 ratio (or sometimes a 3:1 ratio) of fats to carbohydrates and protein. Fat sources may include oils, creams, and butter. In addition to high fat intake, the diet eliminates sugary foods and high carbohydrate foods such as grains and potatoes. Food preparation and consumption is critical in successfully implementing a strict ketogenic diet—down to weighing out food. There are modifications to the classic version of the diet with 2:1 or 1:1 fat to carbohydrate/protein ratios and the modified Atkins diet is approximately a 1:1 ratio of fat to carbohydrates/protein. The modified ketogenic and Modified Atkins diets are more liberal than the classic ketogenic diet and are sometimes tried before a strict ketogenic diet or used as a step-down from a strict ketogenic diet.

The Low Oxalate Diet

The Low Oxalate Diet as used in children with ASD is based on the work of Susan Owens and reduces intake of high oxalate foods. A low oxalate diet typically limits or omits foods such as many beans, beets, nuts, spinach, raw carrots, fruits (such as certain berries and kiwi), buckwheat and millet, sweet potato, and chocolate/cocoa. Children with a leaky gut may absorb more oxalates than most people, which may result in oxidative damage, inflammation, glutathione depletion, and painful urination. Oxalates also may exacerbate an already leaky gut.

The Paleo Diet

The Paleo diet avoids a number of categories of foods including grains, dairy, legumes (such as peanuts and beans), soy, refined sugar, certain vegetables (potatoes, corn, and peas, for example), and processed foods. This diet encourages eating "whole foods." The Paleo diet currently is very popular generally (not just with respect to ASD) and there are many books and websites available both explaining the diet and providing recipes (including kid-friendly recipes). There is some variation from Paleo sources about what may or may not be included/excluded from the Paleo diet, particularly with respect to some starchier vegetables. There also are many versions of the Paleo diet tailored to address specific health concerns such as inflammation, autoimmune conditions, gastrointestinal issues, fat loss, neurologic health, and heart issues—to name just a few.

Specific Carbohydrate Diet™ (SCD™) and Gut and Psychology Syndrome™ (GAPS™) Diet

The SCD™ and the GAPS™ Diet both eliminate certain carbohydrates in order improve gastrointestinal healing and health. These diets probably have fewer carbohydrates than most people's standard diets but are not traditonal low carb diets. These diets are very popular for families with children with ASD. Elaine Gottschall (*Breaking The Vicious Cycle*) made SCD™ famous and Dr. Natasha Campbell McBride, expanding on SCD™ with, among other things, additional healthy foods and supplements, created GAPS™. These diets seek to eliminate foods that gut pathogens feed on, such as starches and complex sugars.

The Weston A. Price Foundation® Diet

The Weston A. Price Foundation® Diet, sometimes called the Nourishing Traditions diet (after the book *Nourishing Traditions*, written by Sally Fallon, who founded the Weston A. Price Foundation®), encourages a return to eating whole foods and avoiding additives, most soy, and refined sugar. Followers of this diet eat animal protein from high-quality sources (pasture-raised or grass-fed), good oils and saturated fats, fermented foods, bone broths, raw dairy, and soaked and sprouted grains/beans/seeds. Even if you do not follow the Weston A. Price Foundation® Diet specifically, many techniques (such as making bone broths, soaking/sprouting nuts and seeds) recommended under this diet are helpful to followers of other diets as well.

In addition to the diets above, many families also incorporate elements of raw diets and juicing of fruits and vegetables into their children's dietary regime for the health benefits of those protocols. There are many sources, both online and in books, for information about these diets. A good starting place online for learning about nutritional interventions for children with ASD is www.nourishinghope.com, the website of Julie Matthews, a certified nutrition consultant, who works with many families of children with autism and related conditions. Her descriptions of many of the diets available helped inform the descriptions above.

Integrative Approaches for the Treatment of Autism

Many parents of children diagnosed with ASD use integrative medical approaches in treating their children. Many different types of practitioners treat children on the autism spectrum including MDs, osteopaths, psychiatrists, naturopaths, homeopaths, practitioners of eastern medicines, nutritionists, and herbalists, among others. It follows that there are many treatment options addressing numerous conditions that appear to be more prevalent in children with autism. Some conditions treated may include:

- Adrenal dysfunction
- Allergies/sensitivities
- Anxiety, including social anxiety
- Autoimmune conditions

- Behavior issues, including repetitive behaviors and self-injurious behaviors
- Epilepsy/seizure disorders
- Gastrointestinal issues
- Hypothyroidism or other thyroid dysfunction
- Immune system dysfunction
- Low cholesterol
- Lyme disease and related conditions
- Mitochondrial disease or dysfunction
- Parasites
- Sleep issues
- Yeast overgrowth and other "gut bugs"/pathogens

Every practitioner uses different protocols and treatments. We have tried to include many of the commonly used integrative approaches to treating children with ASD. Keep in mind that these modalities may be used differently by different practitioners and, in addition to the uses listed below, may be used by practitioners for additional or different purposes. Some treatments may show beneficial results for some patients across multiple domains.

This compilation is intended for informational purposes only and is not medical advice. Whenever a practitioner recommends a treatment for your child, discuss with the practitioner why he or she is making the recommendations, details about what to expect from the treatment, what the targets are for the treatment recommended, cost of the treatment (many are not covered by insurance), anticipated length of treatment, and any side effects of which you should be aware. Many children with ASD receive multiple interventions and you should work with your provider(s) to ensure that treatments are added in an appropriate manner—both the order in which treatments are introduced as well as how and when to introduce treatments to allow you and your practitioner the best opportunity to assess which interventions are helping, are not showing any effects, or are causing an adverse reaction.

Integrative approaches used in treating individuals with ASD may include (note that some modalities, like herbs, used to treat a wide range of issues, are listed separately from more issue-specific treatments):

- Anti-seizure therapies: prescription drugs, hemp-derived CBD oils and similar products, dietary changes (including ketogenic and modified Atkins diets)
- Allergy treatments: sublingual immunotherapy, Nambudripad's Allergy Elimination Technique (NAET®), BioSET™, LDA (Low Dose Allergen) injections, nasal immunotherapy, supplements, and others
- Anti-Viral Treatments: prescription and natural treatments
- Anti-Parasitic Medications: prescription, over the counter, and natural treatments
- Anxiety, social anxiety, socialization challenges, and related issues: hemp-derived CBD oils and similar products, baclofen, oxytocin, Piracetam, citicholine, secretin, sulforaphane
- Detoxification protocols: There are many detoxification protocols including: homotoxicology, chelation therapy (available in many different forms and using different agents),

glutathione (including intravenous glutathione), methyl B-12 injections, NDF®, various supplements that promote detoxification

- Enzyme therapy
- Essential oils
- Gastrointestinal issues: anti-inflammatory medications, steroids, secretin, immunosuppressive medications, enzymes, probiotics
- Gut microbiome repair and restoration: Biofilm protocols, helminths, fecal transplants, probiotics
- Herbs
- Homeopathy: including classical homeopathy and sequential homeopathy, and CEASE therapy as well as over-the-counter homeopathic remedies
- Homotoxicology
- Hyperbaric Oxygen Therapy (HBOT), both hard chamber and soft chamber
- Immune system/immunomodulatory treatments: including intravenous immunoglobulin (IVIG), GcMAF, trichuris suis ova (TSO), hymenolepis diminuta cysticercoids (HDC) and other helminthes, Low Dose Naltrexone (LDN)
- Lyme disease treatments: prescription medications and natural treatments
- Melatonin for sleep issues
- Methyl B-12 injections: among the numerous reported benefits of MB12 are improvements in speech, communication, and socialization
- Mitochondrial treatments, including Coenzyme Q10, l-carnitine, B vitamins, antioxidants, and others.
- Omega-3 Fatty Acids, particularly fish oils
- PANDAs treatments: antibiotics, IVIG, and others
- Probiotics
- Thyroid-supporting or regulating medications and supplements
- Vitamin and mineral supplementation, nutraceuticals, and other supplements either for general support or targeting specific issues.
- Yeast and other gut pathogen treatments: prescription medications and natural treatments

Medications

There currently are no prescription drugs approved by the U.S. Food and Drug Administration (FDA) for treating the core challenges of ASD. The only approved drugs—risperidone (Risperdal®) and aripiprazole (Abilify®)—are approved for the treatment of irritability. Risperidone is an antipsychotic primarily used to treat schizophrenia and other disorders. In children with ASD, risperidone may reduce aggression (including self-injurious behaviors), tantrums, and rapid mood changes. However, serious potential side effects exist including significant weight gain, gynecomastia (development of large breasts in boys and young males), metabolic issues (including diabetes mellitus type 2), and tardive dyskinesia (involuntary, repetitive body movements). Moreover, there is not much data on use of risperidone treatment for autism in adolescents and young adults (as opposed to children). Aripiprazole is an atypical antipsychotic primarily used in the treatment of schizophrenia and bipolar disorder. Aripiprazole may reduce irritability, hyperactivity, and repetitive behaviors in children with ASD. Adverse effects from Aripiprazole seen in individuals with ASD taking aripiprazole include weight gain, drowsiness/sleepiness, tremors, and drooling. There is no long-term efficacy and safety data on use of these drugs for children with ASD.

Additionally, many treating doctors use a variety of other drugs off-label to treat children with autism. In particular, many of the drugs used to treat ADHD are prescribed for children with ASD.

Use of medications of any sort is a very personal decision for parents. Your child and your family need to consider the most appropriate choice for your unique situation. When considering use of anti-psychotic medications in particular, it is important to work with a doctor who will closely monitor your child (including changing doses or changing medications/weaning off a medication) and who is familiar with the serious potential side effects of these medications. If parents are concerned about potential side effects, they also may consider asking their doctor if there are alternative treatments to try before considering these medications.

New Therapies

There are many new therapies developing for the treatment of autism. Promising new treatments include:

Magnetic Resonance Therapy (MRT)

MRT is a neuro-modulation treatment developed by the Newport Brain Research Lab (The Brain Treatment Center). MRT is non-invasive and is a form of trans-cranial magnetic stimulation using a proprietary algorithm to modulate brain frequencies. Using QEEG and electro-cardiography (ECG), MRT is tailored to individual patients. This treatment shows promise not just for ASD but also for a variety of conditions including Alzheimer's Disease and Post-Traumatic Stress.

Stem Cells

Treatment of autism through the use of transplanted stem cells, particularly from cord blood (though some clinics use fetal stem cells), is relatively new and many families seeking this therapy travel outside the United States to obtain treatment. Clinical trials for this treatment are taking place in the United States and, among other things, they hope to flag which patients seem to respond best to the treatment. The theory behind this treatment is that the stem cells will help repair damaged cells and tissues, improve the function of normal cells and tissues, and create or repair connections. In particular, it is hypothesized that the cord blood stem cells will cross the blood-brain barrier and develop into specialized brain cells.

A Final Note on a Critical Safety Issue: Wandering

Parents of children with autism face an additional lifelong worry—the risk of their children wandering (also called elopement) and being injured, taken advantage of, or killed. Studies have shown that approximately half of individuals with ASD will engage in wandering behaviors. Wandering is something that everyone who lives with, cares for, or works with children or adults with autism needs to be aware of. Wandering-related factors, including drowning and prolonged exposure to outdoor conditions, remain among the top causes of death for those with autism.

The reasons that a person with ASD may wander are many but often a person with ASD will wander either to escape a situation or to try to get to something he or she desires. Many people with autism have deep, hyperfocused interests in particular things and may gravitate towards items of interest. That interest may be trains, a pool or other water source, a particular store, a particular person—the options are endless—and the person with autism may wander to try to reach that item of interest, potentially entering a dangerous situation. Other times, a person may want to escape a situation. Again, there can be many reasons for this but common reasons for escape include sensory overload and fear/anxiety, especially in new or unfamiliar situations.

Parents should be aware to the extent possible of potential wandering triggers for their child and make sure that others (teachers, therapists, caregivers, relatives, neighbors) know these triggers as well. Among the most valuable tools with respect to wandering are those put in place to prevent or minimize wandering in the first place. Parents also should explore various tracking device options that may be available in their communities—everything from iPhones, to GPS in shoes or clothing, to bracelets or other devices. Should your child wander, a tracking device may enable first responders to locate him quickly, increasing the chance that your child is safely returned home. There is excellent information available to parents, first responders, and others affected by autism from the National Autism Association and the AWAARE Collaboration at http://awaare.nationalautismassociation.org/.

DIRECTORY

Note: This directory is provided for reference and informational purposes only and is not intended to list all practitioners and providers who provide services to individuals with autism. The editors at Skyhorse have provided numerous resources and have endeavored to provide a starting place for families, but there are many additional services available and new providers begin offering treatment all the time. Every effort has been made to provide current, accurate information from publicly available sources for those individuals and entities listed, but please note that information can change and you should confirm all information, including, but not limited to, contact information, credentials, areas of practice, experience, and training, with the listed practitioner or provider.

We have not independently investigated education or credentials of those listed in this directory. Listing in this resource directory is not an endorsement or qualification as to competence, skill, or effectiveness of any practitioner or provider listed herein, and you should conduct a thorough investigation of any practitioner or provider before determining whether their services are appropriate for your family. Neither the author nor Skyhorse Publishing are responsible in any way for the background, education, licensure, scope of practice, or clinical experience of any practitioner or provider listed in this directory nor are they responsible for any unsatisfactory outcome as a result of contacting a practitioner, provider or resource listed herein.

There are many resources for additional practitioners and providers available online. For example, families can also consult:

> For medical and therapeutic modalities:
> http://www.epidemicanswers.org/providers
> http://www.medmaps.org/clinician-directory/

For additional school programs consult your state department of education website or AutismSpeaks for state-specific school listings (which may list additional early intervention, preschool, and school-aged programs in your community). You can begin that search here:
> https://www.autismspeaks.org/family-services/resource-guide.

Moreover, your state department of health, department of education, local entities charged with service coordination, and local autism organizations may be able to provide additional resources of all types available in your area.

NATIONAL

Academy of Special Needs Answers
Academy of Special Needs Planners
150 Chestnut Street
4th Floor, Box #15
Providence, RI 02903
Tel: (866)-296-5509
Website: http://www.specialneedsanswers.com

The Academy of Special Needs Planners consists of special needs planning professionals such as attorneys, financial planners and trust officers. It also provides a website and a monthly email newsletter available to consumers.

ACES ABA
Locations in CA, CO, HI, TX and WA
(800) 515 5016
Website: http://www.acesaba.com/

ACES provides services in the home, school, and community in several western states.

Act Today!
Autism Care & Treatment Today!
6330 Variel Ave., Ste. 102
Woodland Hills, CA 91367
Tel: (818)-340-4010
Toll Free: 877-9ACT-TODAY
Email: Info@act-today.org
Website: http://www.act-today.org

A national nonprofit 501(c)(3) organization, ACT Today raises awareness and provides treatment and support to families to help their children with autism achieve their full potential.

The Arc of the United States
1825 K Street NW, Suite 1200
Washington, DC 20006
Tel: (202)-534-3700
Toll Free: (800)-433-5255
Email: info@thearc.org
Facebook: facebook.com/thearcus
Twitter: twitter.com/thearcus
YouTube: youtube.com/user/thearcoftheus

The Arc promotes and protects the human rights of people with intellectual and developmental disabilities and actively supports their full inclusion and participation in the community throughout their lifetimes.

Arrowsmith Program
Various locations
www.arrowsmithschool.org

Premised on the concept of neuroplasticity, the program identifies weak cognitive capacities and provides specific cognitive exercises to intervene and strengthen those areas and improve learning. The website identifies programs across the United States incorporating the Arrowsmith Program.

Association of People Supporting Employment first (APSE)
416 Hungerford Dr., Suite 418
Rockville, MD 20850
Tel: (301) 279 0060
Email: membership@apse.org
Find your local chapter: Website: http://www.apse.org/about/chapter-directory/
Website: http://www.apse.org/

APSE advocates and educates concerning employment and self-sufficiency for people with disabilities.

Autism Risk & Safety Management
Dennis Debbaudt
2338 SE Holland St.
Port St. Lucie, FL 34952
Tel: (772) 398 9756
Fax: (772) 398 2428e) Fax: (772) 398 2428
Email: ddpi@flash.net
Website: www.autismriskmanagement.com

Training and resources for first responders, parents and others in the autism community.

AutisMate365
Website: autismate.com/AutisMate-Comprehensive-App-For-Autism/

AutisMate365 is a learning platform for individuals with ASD using a tablet device. This app allows a high degree of personalization to aid in learning.

AutismOne
Toll Free: (800) 908 5803
Website: http://www.autismone.org

Provides education and supports advocacy efforts for individuals affected by ASD and their families including an annual multi-day conference in the Chicago area featuring ASD experts in a wide range of fields from around the world.

Autism Service Dogs of America
5232 N Interstate Ave
Portland OR 97217
Email: info@autismservicedogsofamerica.org
Website: http://autismservicedogsofamerica.com/

Autism Society of America
4340 East-West Hwy, Suite 350
Bethesda, Maryland 20814
Tel: (301) 657 0881
Toll Free: (800).3AUTISM (Toll Free: (800).328.8476)
Email: info@autism-society.org
Website: http://www.autism-society.org

Autism Speaks
Email: familyservices@autismspeaks.org
Website: www.autismspeaks.org

Endeavors to raise public awareness about ASD and its effects on individuals, families, and society; provides resources and information on its website for individuals to learn about ASD, including information about treatment options and information to assist families in accessing resources in their communities; provides funding for various projects and research.

AvaTalker AAC
Website: avatalkeraac.com/

AvaTalker AAC is a two level customizable communication app for those with verbal challenges with an intuitive interface that makes it easy to build phrases and sentences.

Benefit Eligibility Screening Tool
Email form: Website: http://www.benefits.gov/ssa

The Benefit Eligibility Screening Tool (BEST) helps you find out if you could get benefits that Social Security administers. Based on your answers to questions, this tool will list benefits for which you might be eligible and tell you more information about how to qualify and apply.

Brain Balance Achievement Centers
Tel: (800) 877 5500
Find your location: www.brainbalancecenters.com/locations
Website: http://www.brainbalancecenters.com/

Brain Balance Achievement Centers offer the Brain Balance Program® in 54 nationwide locations. The Brain Balance Program® is an individualized and comprehensive approach to helping children with neurobehavioral and learning difficulties.

Butterfly Effects
500 Fairway Drive, Suite 102
Deerfield Beach FL, 33441
Toll Free: (800) 880 9270
Website: http://butterflyeffects.com/

Butterfly Effects provides therapy and tutoring services to individuals of all ages addressing challenges in the areas of academics, behavior, communication, daily living, social and life skills.

CARD: Center for Autism and Related Disorders
6 North Main Street Suite 110
Fairport, NY 14450
United States
Tel: (585) 377 6590
Contact Name: Denise Rhine
D.Rhine@centerforautism.com
Website: http://www.centerforautism.com

CARD's goal is to teach children functional skills, enabling them to live independent and productive lives to the fullest extent possible. CARD has over 17 international offices.

Challenger Division of Little League Baseball
Website: www.littleleague.org/learn/about/divisions/challenger.htm

Enables children with physical and mental challenges, ages 4–18, or up to age 22 if still enrolled in high school, participate in baseball. Challenger Division leagues are available in many areas.

Community Housing Network (CHN), Inc.
570 Kirts Blvd. Suite 231
Troy, MI 48084
Tel: (248) 269 1346
Contact Name: Linda Ronan Brown
Email: lbrown@chninc.net
Website: http://www.communityhousingnetwork.org

CHN is a nonprofit housing agency that assists people with disabilities with affordable housing and provides resources/referrals.

Cool Cuts 4 Kids (60 locations nationwide)
Hairdresser
Toll Free: (800).345.7811

Cool Cuts 4 Kids is attentive to special needs and sensory challenges and aims to provide a safe, trusting, and fun environment.

Council of Parent Attorneys and Advocates – COPAA
Legal Resource
PO Box 6767

Towson, MD 21285
Tel: (844)-426-7224
Website: http://www.copaa.org/

The Council of Parent Attorneys and Advocates, Inc. (COPAA) is an independent, nonprofit, 501(c)(3) tax-exempt organization of attorneys, advocates, parents and related professionals working to ensure civil rights and education rights of individuals with disabilities.

Department of Housing and Urban Development
Website: http://portal.hud.gov/hudportal/HUD?src=/localoffices

Dungarvin
2000 Randolph Rd. SE Suite 205
Albuquerque, NM 87106
Tel: (505) 998 1060
Website: http://www.dungarvin.com

Dungarvin provides a variety of individually tailored services and supports under the Medicaid Home and Community Based Waiver. Services provided include day services, supported employment, case management, supported foster care, children's services, respite care, host homes and supports for persons with disabilities.

Easter Seals Inc. (multiple locations in each state)
233 South Wacker Drive
Suite 2400
Chicago, IL 60606
Toll Free: (800)-221-6827
Find your local branch: Website: http://www.easterseals.com/connect-locally/

Easter Seals provides services, education, outreach, and advocacy for individuals with autism and other disabilities.

Elizabeth Birt Center for Autism Law & Advocacy
1930 Old Tustin Avenue, Suite A
Santa Ana, CA 92705
Email form: http://www.ebcala.org/contact
Website: http://www.ebcala.org

Educates lawyers, advocates and parents about the legal challenges relating to ASD, including special education, insurance, healthcare, family law, criminal law and tort law, as well as vaccine injury.

Epidemic Answers
PO Box 191
West Simsbury, CT 06092
Website: www.epidemicanswers.org

Provides educational resources for parents (and others) to help parents learn about causes and healing modalities to help children affected by ASD and other chronic illnesses. Tools include resources on their website, a free parent guide available online, online webinars and other learning opportunities, and a provider directory.

Fragile X Alliance
1615 Bonanza St. Suite 202
Walnut Creek, CA 94596
Toll Free: (800) 688 8765
Find your local branch: csn@fragilex.org
Email: natlfx@fragilex.org
Website: www.fragilex.org

Fragile X Alliance is a nonprofit organization of families that are affected with Fragile X Syndrome and associated disorders. Fragile X Alliance has a Houston chapter that can offer assistance to those that have gotten a diagnosis of Fragile X Syndrome.

Generation Rescue
13636 Ventura Blvd. #259
Sherman Oaks, CA 91423
Toll Free: (877)-98-AUTISM
Email Form: http://www.generationrescue.org/about/contact-us
Website: http://www.generationrescue.org

Generation Rescue provides information (through a variety of sources including their website, an annual multi-day conference featuring international experts in a many fields relating to ASD as well as smaller events and online learning opportunities, and a network of "Rescue Angels" mentor program) and immediate treatment assistance, including a grant program, to families affected by ASD, including.

GRASP419 Lafayette StreetNew York, NY 10003
Tel: (888) 474 7277
Email: info@grasp.org
Website: www.grasp.org

Organization providing a variety of services to the autism community, including advocacy & outreach, support groups, and programming.

The HANDLE Institute
Website: www.handle.org/

HANDLE is an acronym for Holistic Approach to Neurodevelopment and Learning Efficiency and is a non-drug, non-invasive and individualized modality to address learning and other challenges faced by those with ASD and other conditions.

Innovative Piano, Inc.
Locations in NY, NJ, TX, VA, MD, OH, GA, SC, PA, AL, ID, AZ, CO, MA, IL, NC, WA, CT, MI, FL
Toll Free: (800) 997 7093
Contact Name: Tammy

Email: contacts@innovativepiano.com
Website: http://www.innovativepiano.com

ABA-style piano lessons for special needs students.

KEEN (Kids Enjoy Exercise Now) USA
1301 K Street, NW
Suite 600, East Tower
Washington, DC 20005
Toll Free: (866)-903-KEEN (5336)
Email: info@keenusa.org
Website: http://www.keenusa.org/

KEEN is a national, nonprofit volunteer-led organization providing no-cost one-to-one recreational opportunities for children and young adults with developmental and physical disabilities.

Lindamood-Bell Learning Centers
Website: http://www.lindamoodbell.com

With approximately 50 locations around the United States, Lindamood-Bell programs focus on developing sensory-cognitive processes underlying reading and comprehension as well as other academic skills. Centers provide evaluation, consultation and instruction programs individualized to address each learner's needs.

May Institute
1409 Kingsley Avenue, Suite 1A
Orange Park, FL 32073
Tel: (904) 269 0773
Contact Name: William Flood
Email: wflood@mayintitute.org
Website: http://www.mayinstitute.org

The May Institute provides educational, rehabilitative, and behavioral healthcare services to individuals with autism spectrum disorder and other developmental disabilities, brain injury, mental illness, and behavioral health needs. The May Institute operates more than 160 service locations in more than a dozen states across the country.

Mentor Network
Sheridan Building 125 South 9th Street
Philadelphia, PA 19107
Tel: (215) 925 3461
Website: http://www.thementornetwork.com

The MENTOR Network is a national network of providers offering a variety of community-based services to adults and children with a variety of illnesses, disabilities, and challenges.

MetLife Center for Special Needs Planning
Toll Free: (800) 638 5433
Email form: https://www.metlife.com/individual/service/index.html

https://www.metlife.com/individual/planning/special-needs/index.html?WT.mc_id=vu1125#overview

Focuses on the concerns of families with children and other dependents with special needs through a nationwide network of MetLife Financial Services specialists.

Military Tool Kit for Special Needs
Toll Free: (800) 342 9647
Website: http://www.militaryhomefront.dod.mil

The DoD Special Needs Parent Toolkit has comprehensive information and tools that are geared towards helping military families with special needs children navigate the maze of medical and special education services, community support and benefits and entitlements.

The Miracle Project
Website: www.themiracleproject.org

Inclusive theater and expressive arts programs welcoming children, regardless of challenges, to perform and improve communication and social skills as well as their self-esteem. The Miracle Projects has a variety of options to participate.

National Association for Child Development (NACD)
Various locations
National Headquarters:
549 25th Street
Ogden, Utah 84401
Tel: (801) 621 8606
Fax: (801) 621 8389
Website: www.nacd.org

NACD's services—utilizing a wide variety of treatment modalities—are based on the neurodevelopmental assessment of each individual client. Treatment plans are implemented by family and caregivers with support and regular re-assessments by NACD.

National Autism Association (NAA)
Website: www.nationalautismassociation.org
NOTE: NAA has a number of local chapters (see nationalautismassociation.org/resources/naa-local-chapters.

Empowering and assisting families affected by autism through a variety of programs, funded research, resources available on their website, and an annual national conference featuring autism experts. The leading organization on issues concerning wandering prevention and response, including providing education and resources for parents, first responders and professionals working with children with autism. Also see awaare.nationalautismassociation.org/ for wandering-specific resources.

National Center on Institutions and Alternatives (NCIA)
7222 Ambassador Road
Windsor Mill, MD 21244
Tel: (410) 265 1490
Website: http://www.ncianet.org

NCIA provides individual care, concern, and treatment for intellectually and emotionally disabled youth and adults and those involved in the criminal justice system.

Navigating College
Website: http://navigatingcollege.org/

Navigating College provides information from adults with autism on the college experience.

NeuroSensory Centers of America
Website: www.neurosensorycenters.com/

Treatment providers use a battery of diagnostic tests called Sensory View™ to diagnose the source of patients' challenges and customize treatment modalities for each patient. Centers are located around the United States.

Operation Autism
2000 North 14th Street
Suite 240
Arlington, VA 22201
Toll Free: (866) 366 9710
Email form: http://www.operationautismonline.org/about-operation-autism/contact-us/

Operation Autism directly supports U.S. military families touched by autism and autism spectrum disorders.

Opportunity Services
2740 Oak Ridge Ct. Unit 301
Fort Myers, FL 33901
Tel: (239) 936 2773
Website: http://www.oppserv.org

Opportunity Services is a nonprofit organization serving adults with disabilities seeking job assistance or community immersion as well as employers.

Proloquo2Go and Proloquo4Text
Webiste: www.assistiveware.com

Proloquo2Go is a symbol-supported communications app and Proloquo4Text is a text-based app. Both give voice to individuals, including those with ASD, who have significant verbal communication challenges.

Pyramid Educational Consultants, Inc.
13 Garfield Way
Newark, DE 19713
Tel: (302) 368 2515
Toll Free: (888) 732 7462
Email: pyramidus@pecs.com

Provides information and products relating to PECS (Picture Exchange Communication System) and the Pyramid Approach to Education.

Rethink
Website: www.rethinkfirst.com

Web-based program of ABA-based curriculum including assessment tools, teaching tutorials, videos of teaching interactions, teaching objectives, data tracking and other support, allowing parents and others to help children with ASD.

Sibling Support Project
A Kindering Center program
Don Meyer, Director
6512 23rd Ave NW, #213
Seattle, WA 98117
Tel: (206) 297 6368
Email: donmeyer@siblingsupport.org
Website: http://www.siblingsupport.org/
https://www.facebook.com/SiblingSupportProject
https://www.facebook.com/groups/SibNet/

NCIA provides individual care, concern, and treatment for intellectually and emotionally disabled youth and adults and those involved in the criminal justice system.

Snip-Its (Various States)
Hairstylists
Website: http://www.snipits.com

Special Needs Alliance
Legal Service
Toll Free: (877)-572-8472
Website: http://www.specialneedsalliance.org/
https://www.facebook.com/specialneedsalliance

The Special Needs Alliance is a national network of lawyers dedicated to Disability and Public Benefits Law.

Special Needs Parents Meet-Up
Website: http://specialed.meetup.com/
Website: http://autism.meetup.com/

Special Olympics North America
3712 Benson Drive, Suite 102
Raleigh, North Carolina 27609
Office: (919) 785 0699

Contact Name: Lynn Idaszak
Manager, Internal Communications & Operations
Website: http://www.specialolympics.org/Regions/
north-america/_Region-Front/North-America.aspx/

Svetlana Masgutova Educational Institute®
PO Box 1651
Melrose, FL 32666
Website: masgutovamethod.com

For information about the Masgutova Neurosensorimotor Integration (MNRI) Method and reflex integration, and assistance in finding an MNRI certified resource.

Talk About Curing Autism (TACA)
Find your local chapter: https://www.tacanow.org/
local-chapters
Website: https://www.tacanow.org

Provides: extensive online resources, seminars/webinars/conferences and other educational events, financial scholarships, local chapter meetings, parent mentoring, Spanish language outreach, and other resources, to families affected by ASD.

TRICARE: Enhanced Access to Autism Benefits
Website: http://www.tricare.mil/autismdemo

Understanding Behavior, Inc.
Corporate Office
744 Montgomery St, Suite 400
San Francisco, CA 94111
Tel: (415) 989 5000
Email: contactubi@understandingbehavior.com

Understanding Behavior is a national professional organization of providers that specializes in individuals with developmental disabilities.

United Healthcare
UnitedHealthcare Children's Foundation
MN017-W400
PO Box 41
Minneapolis, MN 55440-0041
Toll Free: 855-MY-UHCCF
Website: http://www.uhccf.org

Wrong Planet
Website: http://www.wrongplanet.net

Wrong Planet is the web community designed for individuals (and parents of those) with Autism, Asperger's Syndrome, ADHD, PDDs, and other neurological differences. Among its features are articles, guides, blogs, and an opportunity to communicate with others on the spectrum.

INDIVIDUAL STATES

All states include the following service categories: Doctors, Clinics, Hospitals, and other Health Services; Therapy Services; Schools and Educational Services; Legal, Government & Financial Services; Community and Recreation Services.

ALABAMA

Doctors, Clinics, Hospitals, and Other Health Services

Autism Diagnostic Clinic
University of South Alabama Children's and Women's Hospital
1707 Center St. Suite 201
Mobile, AL 36604
Tel: (251) 415 8577
Contact Name: Amy Mitchell
Email: abmitchell@usouthal.edu
Website: http://www.usahealthsystem.com/autism-diagnosis

The clinic focuses on early identification and diagnosis, as well as educational outreach to families, physicians, daycare centers, churches and other organizations who serve children in the community, particularly the greater Gulf Coast area. The Clinic evaluates patients up to 5 years, 6 months of age.

Charity League Hearing & Speech Center
1600 Seventh Ave South
Birmingham, AL 35233
Tel: (205) 939 9149

Provides diagnostic and rehabilitative speech / language and audiology services for children eighteen years of age or younger.

Children's Health System
1600 S. 7th Avenue
Birmingham, AL 35233
Tel: (205) 939 9100
Website: http://www.chsys.org

Childrens Health System is an integrated child health care network dedicated to providing comprehensive pediatric expertise for the children of Childrens Hospital.

Gaie Feuerstein DC, Certified GAPS
Mobile, AL 36695
Tel: (251) 300 1335
Email: gaps@juno.com

Analysis and treatment of gastro-intestinal disorders associated with ASD. Emphasis on GAPS/SCD dietary methods, as well as other protocols.

Huntsville Hospital
101 Sivley Road
Huntsville, AL 35801
Tel: (256) 265 7952
Website: http://www.huntsvillehospital.org

Jackson Hospital
1725 Pine St.
Montgomery, AL 36106
Tel: (334) 293 8000
Website: http://jackson.org

Jackson Hospital is a community not-for-profit hospital serving Montgomery and the Alabama River Region.

Dr. Jan Mathisen
1600 7th Ave. S. CHB Ste. 314
Birmingham, AL 35243
Tel: (205) 933 5187

Lopez Family Chiropractic
401 N Section St.
Fairhope, AL 36532

Path to Wellness Clinic
240 W Laurel Ave.
Foley, AL 36535
Tel: (205) 601 2257
Contact Name: Dr J. Douglas Brown, Board Certified Neurologist
Email: Drjdouglasbrown@gmail.com
Website: http://www.drbrowncenter.com

Board Certified neurologist who specializes in the treatment of central integration disorder. Dr. Brown oversees rehabilitation protocols specific to the patient's cortical dysfunction, focusing on weak areas of the cortex and building these up results to achieve improved cognitive and behavioral function. This treatment type is highly-focused and individualized and requires good family support.

Dr. Paul Maertens
3301 Knollwood Drive
Mobile, AL 36604
Tel: (251) 344 1590

UAB Autism Clinic
Community Health Services Building 930 20th St. S
Birmingham, AL 35294
Toll Free: (800) 822 2472
Website: http://circ-uab.infomedia.com/content2.asp?id=104879

The clinic evaluates children ages 2 to 12 years of age for ASD.

Therapy Services

Alabama Psychiatric Services (APS), PC
409 2nd Ave. Northwest
Cullman, AL 35055
Tel: (256) 739 4910
Website: http://www.apsy.com

Alabama Psychological Services Center, LLC
4800 Whitesport Cir. Southwest, Suite 2
Huntsville, AL 35801
Tel: (256) 533·9393
Contact Name: Megan Crisler, Ph.D.
Website: http://www.alapsych.com/therapists_mec.php

Private psychological practice, specializing in diagnosis and therapy services for ASD. Provides individual and group services. In addition to individual therapy for all ages, social skills groups are available. Therapy approaches are based on individual needs, but typically include behavioral or cognitive strategies, Floortime, developmental and structured teaching.

The Autism Spectrum Counseling Center
821 S Perry Street
Montgomery, AL 36104-0519
Tel: (334) 868 1589
Website: http://www.autismspectrumcenter.org

The Autism Spectrum Center specializes in providing advocacy, education, intervention and community outreach programs.

Baypointe Behavioral Health
5800 Southland Drive
Mobile, AL 36693-3313

Tel: (251) 661 0153
Website: http://www.altapointe.org/baypointe.php

Behavior Analysts of Central Alabama, LLC
108 Twelve Oaks Ct
Pratville, AL 36066
Tel: (334) 595 3673
Contact Name: David F. Bicard, Ph.D., BCBA-D, LBA
Website: www.bacallc.com

Behavior Analysts of Central Alabama, LLC specializes in verbal behavior and social skill development and provides intervention services for children in Autauga, Elmore, and Montgomery Counties in Alabama under the supervision of a Doctoral level Board Certified Behavior Analyst.

Bluebird Pediatric Therapy Services, Inc.
6312 Piccadilly Square Drive Suite 3
Mobile, AL 33609
Tel: (251) 287 0378
Contact Name: Danielle Peters
Email: bluebirdtherapy@gmail.com
Website: http://www.bluebirdtherapy.com

Provides pediatric occupational therapy.

Cahaba Psychology Center (CPC)
2 Riverchase Office Plaza Suite 115
Birmingham, AL 35233
Tel: (205) 403 0955
Email: cahabaps@bellsouth.net
Website: http://www.cahabapsychology.com

Child's Play Therapy Center
3057 Lorna Road Suite 220
Birmingham, AL 35216
Tel: (205) 978 9939
Email: info@childsplaytherapycenter.com
Website: http://www.childsplaytherapycenter.com

Child's Play Therapy Center provides comprehensive pediatric therapy services, including speech therapy, physical therapy, occupational therapy, academic services, or a combination.

Dossett Clinic for People with Autism
2305 Arlington Avenue
Birmingham, AL 35205
Tel: (205) 933 5476
Contact Name: Dr. Rebecca Dossett
Email: rdossett@hiwaay.net

Dothan Behavioral Medicine Clinic
101 Medical Dr.
Dothan, AL 36303
Tel: (866) 224 2822
Contact Name: Nelson M. Handal, M.D.

Email: info@dbmclinic.com
Website: http://www.dbmclinic.com/

Dothan Behavioral Medicine Clinic specializes in pediatric behavioral medicine and its fully certified clinicians provide specialized outpatient services for mood or anxiety disorders, Obsessive Compulsive Disorder, ADHD, learning difficulties, autism spectrum disorders and more.

Glenwood Autism & Behavioral Health Center
150 Glenwood Lane
Birmingham, AL 35242
Tel: (205) 969 2880
Contact Name: Casey Coleman
Email: ccoleman@glenwood.org
Website: http://www.glenwood.org

Glenwood is a nonprofit organization educating and treating individuals diagnosed with autism, emotional disturbances, and mental illnesses.

Hand In Paw
5342 Oporto Madrid Boulevard S
Birmingham, AL 35210
Tel: (205) 591 7006
Email: handinpawinc@aol.com
Website: http://www.handinpaw.org

Hand In Paw's professionally trained teams of people and their pets motivate children with disabilities to reach therapy goals.

Helping Hands Therapy
306 Washington Street South
Livingston, AL 35470
Tel: (205) 575 1609
Contact Name: Jana Smith, Client Relations Manager
Email: info@helpinghands-therapy.com
Website: http://www.helpinghands-therapy.com

Helping Hands Therapy provides occupational therapy, physical therapy and speech therapy services throughout Alabama.

ISI Therapeutic Family Services
2206 Executive Park Drive
Opelika, AL 36801
Tel: (334) 329 9930
Contact Name: Chad Smith
Website: http://www.isitherapy.com/

ISI Therapeutic provides early intervention, school consultation and other services based on ABE principles. They also provide counseling for couples who have children with special needs.

Kids Kount Therapy Services
26420 Kensington Pl. Suite C
Daphne, AL 36526
Tel: (251) 517 0355
Email: kidskountmgmt@yahoo.com
Website: http://www.kidskounttherapy.com

Speech, occupational, and physical therapy for children ages birth to 21 years.

Magnolia Family Psychiatry and TMS Center
402 Johnston St. Southeast
Decatur, AL 35601
Tel: (256) 274 4196
Contact Name: Karis Knight, MD
Email: info@magnoliafamily.com
Website: http://www.magnoliafamily.com

Magnolia offers complete psychiatric evaluations, including testing as needed. Their methods also include family therapy, rTMS, support groups, computer based CBT, good nutrition, pharmacogenetic testing, medications and more.

Mitchell's Place
4778 Overton Road
Birmingham, AL 35210
Tel: (205) 957 0294
Contact Name: Sandy Naramore, Executive Director
Email: snaramore@mitchells-place.com

Mitchell's Place is a comprehensive treatment center for children and young adults with Autism Spectrum Disorders.

Music Together of Madison
108 Bridgefield Rd.
Madison, AL 35758
Tel: (256) 325 4718
Email: musictogetherofmadison@yahoo.com
Website: http://www.musictogether.com

Progress Center
215 Midland St
Ashford, AL 36312
Tel: (334) 899 4333
Contact Name: Angie Marshall
Email: progress@graceba.net
Website: http://www.progresscenter.us

Progress Center™ serves children and adults with a variety of challenges and specializes in a combination of programs to help with focus, attention, and listing skills, including academic tutoring, behavior therapy, cognitive therapy, speech therapy, Colored reading overlays, Dir/Floortime, Enlisten, Outreach Services, Military.

Special Equestrians
900 Woodward Drive
Pelham, AL 35124
Tel: (205) 987 9462
Website: http://www.specialequest.org/

Horseback riding program at Indian Springs School. Recreation and therapy for children or adults who are physically, mentally, or emotionally challenged.

Spectrum Center for Autism and Related Disorders
217 Graceland Drive Suite 1
Dothan, AL 36305
Tel: (334) 671 1650
Contact Email:
Email: info@spectrumdothan.org
Website: http://spectrumdothan.org

Spectrum provides comprehensive, holistic, compassionate, and affordable therapeutic interventions to children with ASD and their families.

Spoken Word Speech Language Services
29000 Hwy 98 Suite 202B
Daphne, AL 36526
Tel: (251) 786 8255
Contact Name: Melanie Waters
Email: mel.spokenword@gmail.com
Website: http://www.spokenwordspeech.com/

Speech-Language Pathology services for students with ASD.

Stepping Stone Pediatric Therapy, LLC
143 Ana Drive
Florence, AL 35630
Tel: (256) 767 1576
Contact Name: David Ainsworth, Administrator/ Manager
Email: dainsworth@steppingstonept.com
Website: http://www.steppingstonept.com

Occupational and speech therapy using a team approach with parents and doctors. Programs used include Handwriting without Tears, Sensory Integration, Interactive metronome, Therapeutic Listening, and more.

Triumph Services
2216 Tenth Court South
Birmingham, AL 35205
Tel: (205) 581 1000
Email: triumphservicesinc@gmail.com
Website: http://www.triumphservices.org

Assists those with developmental disabilities who wish to live with more independence.

Schools and Educational Services

Alabama Parent Education Center
10520 US Highway 231
Wetumpka, AL 36092

Tel: (334) 567 2252
Toll Free: (866) 532 7660
Email: apec@alabamaparentcenter.com
Website: http://www.alabamaparentcenter.com

The Alabama Parent Education Center (APEC) is a nonprofit organized by parents in central Alabama to provide parents with training and information.

Valley Haven School
6345 Fairfax Bypass P.O. Box 416
Valley, AL 36854
Tel: (334) 756 2868
Contact Name: Tony Edmondson
Email: valleyhaven@charterinternet.com
Website: http://www.valleyhavenschool.org

Valley Haven is operated to provide quality education and training programs for persons with special needs.

Bridgeway Services, LLC
3985 Parkwood Road, Suite 109-144
Bessemer, AL 35022
Tel: (866) 392 8227
Website: http://www.aascg.com

Bridgeway Services, LLC (formerly Autism Asperger Syndrome Consulting Group, LLC) is focused on intervention-based services for children, adolescents, and adults with characteristics of High Functioning Autism Spectrum Disorders in the Alabama area.

Collaborations Child Development Center
100 Jetplex Blvd
Huntsville, AL 35824
Tel: (256) 772 4400
Email: info@appliedbehavioralconcepts.net
Website: http://www.collaborationscdc.com

Collaboration Child Development Center offers a unique blending of discrete trials, inclusion and incidental teaching strategies based on findings from testing upon program intake and assessments.

High Hopes
PO Box 46
Elberta, AL 36530
Tel: (251) 986 7007
Contact Name: Rachael Mueller
Email: info@highhopes4autism.org
Website: http://highhopes4autism.org

Provides ABA therapy on an individual basis, as well as assistance in classroom integration.

The Little Tree Learning Center
P.O. Box 1368
Auburn, AL 36831
Tel: (334) 826 1847
Contact Name: Holly Rogers, Campus Director

Email: hrogers@learning-tree.org
Website: http://www.learning-tree.org

The Little Tree Learning Center is a grant funded preschool program that offers the children served a rich and nurturing environment.

May Institute

Maxwell-Gunter Air Force Base
Montgomery, AL 36112
Tel: (706) 571 7771
Contact Name: Amy Bontrager
Email: abontrager@mayinstitute.org
Website: http://www.mayinstitute.org

May Institute is committed to making services accessible to military families who have children with ASD. All May Institute services are based on ABA, the only treatment reimbursed by TRICARE's ECHO program and the Autism Demonstration Project for military families with children with ASD.

New Hope Academy

698 Silver Hills Dr
Prattville, AL 36066
Tel: (334) 361 9505
Website: http://www.newhope4kids.com/

New Hope Academy is a private school for children with learning differences, including ASD, from ages 4–18.

The Riley Behavioral and Educational Center

1900 Golf Road
Huntsville, AL 35802
Tel: (256) 882 2457
Contact Name: Melody P. Crane, Executive Director
Email: rileycenteroffice@gmail.com
Website: http://therileycenter.org

The Riley Center provides comprehensive diagnostic and treatment services throughout Northern Alabama and Southern Tennessee. Behavioral and Educational consultants provide training for parents, caregivers and professionals (teachers, therapists).

Southeast Alabama Autism Center

210 E Grubbs St Suite 1
Enterprise, AL 36330
Tel: (334) 360 1158
Contact Name: Nicole Slay MS, BCBA
Email: Info@southeastalabamaautismcenter.com
Website: http://www.southeastalabamaautismcenter.com

Center-based and in-home ABA consultation, therapy, and individualized program development. Specializing in verbal behavior therapy ABLLS-R and early intervention. Experienced school consultation and parent training (classes and 1-1).

University of Alabama ACTS Program

Tuscaloosa, AL 35487
Tel: (205) 348 0594
Contact Name: Dr. Laura Klinger
Email: lklinger@bama.ua.edu
Website: http://uanews.ua.edu/anews2007/dec07/spect121007.htm

A transition to college program for students with Asperger's Syndrome.

Legal, Government & Financial Services

Alabama Council for Developmental Disabilities (ACDD)

RSA Union Building
100 North Union Street
P.O. Box 301410
Tel: (334) 242 3973
Toll Free: (800) 232 2158
Website: http://www.acdd.org/

The mission of ACDD is to promote and support independence, advocacy, productivity and inclusion for Alabamians with developmental disabilities.

Alabama Department of Mental Health

100 North Union Street
Montgomery, AL 36130
Tel: (334) 242 3454
Toll Free: (800) 367 0955

Email: alabama.DMH@mh.alabama.gov
Website: http://www.mh.alabama.gov

Alabama Department of Rehabilitation Services (ADRS)

602 S Lawrence St.
Montgomery, AL 36104
Tel: (334) 293 7500
Toll Free: (800) 441 7607
Website: http://www.rehab.alabama.gov/

The Alabama Department of Rehabilitation Services (ADRS) serves people with disabilities from birth to old age through a "continuum of services" including: Alabama's Early Intervention (for children birth-3), Children's Rehabilitative Service (for children from birth-21), Vocational Rehabilitation Service (teens and adults), and State of Alabama Independent Living/Homebound Service.

Alabama Disabilities Advocacy Program

526 Martha Parham Hall West
The University of Alabama
Tuscaloosa, AL 35487

Tel: (205) 348 4928
Toll Free: (800) 826 1675
Contact Name: James A. Tucker, Esq., Executive
Director
Email: ADAP@adap.ua.edu
Website: http://www.adap.net

The Alabama Disabilities Advocacy Program (ADAP) is
part of the nationwide federally mandated Protection
and Advocacy (P&A) system. ADAP provides legally
based advocacy services to protect, promote, and
expand the rights of Alabamians with disabilities.

The Alabama Interagency Autism Coordinating Council

Alabama Dept. of Mental Health 100 North Union
Street, Suite 504
Montgomery, AL 36130
Tel: (334) 353 7197
Contact Name: Anna B. McConnell, LCSW, MPH
Email: anna.mcconnell@mh.alabama.gov
Website: http://www.autism.alabama.gov

The Alabama Interagency Autism Coordinating Council was created to develop and implement a statewide comprehensive, coordinated, multidisciplinary,
interagency system of care for individuals with autism
spectrum disorder and their families. The lead agency
is the Alabama Department of Mental Health. ASD.

Burke Harvey (BH), LLC

Attorneys/legal counsel
One Highland Place 2151 Highland Avenue, Suite 120
Birmingham, AL 35205
Tel: (205) 588 4057
Website: http://www.bhlongtermdisability.com

The law firm of Burke Harvey, LLC assists disabled clients across the United States to obtain long term disability benefits.

Deborah Mattison, Esq.

301 19th Street N.
Birmingham, AL 35203
Tel: (205) 314 0561
Email: dmattison@wcqp.com
Website: http://wcqp.com

Attorney specializing in legal issues concerning children and adults with developmental disabilities.

James D. Sears, Esq.

816-A Manci Avenue
Daphne, AL 36526
Tel: (251) 621 3485
Contact Email:
Email: info@searslawfirm.com

Attorney specializing in legal issues concerning children and adults with developmental disabilities.

Katherine N. Barr

305 Church Street Suite 800
Huntsville, AL 35804-8248
Contact Email:
Email: kbarr@sirote.com

Attorney specializing in legal issues concerning children and adults with developmental disabilities.

State of Alabama Client Assistance Program

2125 East South Boulevard
Montgomery, AL 36116
Tel: (334) 281 2276
Tel: (334) 288 1104
Website: http://sacap.alabama.gov

The State of Alabama Client Assistance Program provides advocacy services for Alabama Department of
Rehabilitation Services consumers and applicants for
services.

Susan Shirock DePaola

1726 West 2nd St, Suite B
Montgomery, AL 36106
Tel: (334) 262 1600
Email: specialeducationattorney@mindspring.com

Represents parents of children with disabilities in due
process proceedings in Alabama.

Wettermark & Keith, LLC

2101 Highland Ave. South #600
Birmingham, AL 35205
Tel: (334) 284 0014
Website: http://www.alabamasocialsecuritylawyer.net

Specializes in securing benefits and justice for the
physically and mentally disabled.

Community and Recreation Services

Alabama Family Ties, Inc.

Advocacy and services for people living with disabilities
400 Eastern Bypass Suite 201
Montgomery, AL 36116
Tel: (877) 834 0615
Tel: (334) 240 8437
Email: help@alfamilyties.org
Website: http://www.alfamilyties.org

Arc of Walker County

745 Russell Dairy Rd
Jasper, AL 35503

Tel: (205) 387 0562

Website: http://www.walkerarc.com

The Arc of Walker County provides services and opportunities for individuals with developmental disabilities. Programs range from Early Intervention and Early Head Start for children to Supported Employment, Residential, and Semi-Independent Living for adults.

Arts 'n Autism

2625 8th Street

Tuscaloosa, AL 35402

Tel: (205) 247 4990

Email: artsnautism@gmail.com

Website: http://www.artsnautism.org/

Arts 'n Autism is a non-profit organization providing after-school and summer camp services for children-young adults with autism. Activities include supervised visual and performing arts activities, respite for families/caregivers, music, fine motor activities, sensory integration therapy, language-rich curriculum/environment, social skills groups, field trips, karate, dance, scouting, life skills for high school graduates, vocational preparation.

Autism Gatherings at the Children's Museum of the Shoals

2810 Darby Drive

Florence, AL 35630

Tel: (256) 765 0500

Contact Name: Monica Collier

Email: monicacollier@shoalschildrensmuseum.org

Website: http://www.shoalschildrensmuseum.org

The Children's Museum of the Shoals offers Autism Gatherings for families with children with autism.

Autism Society of Alabama

4217 Dolly Ridge Rd.

Birmingham, AL 35243

Tel: (205) 951 1364

Toll Free: (877) 428 8476

Contact Name: Melanie Jones, Executive Director

Email: melanie@autism-alabama.org

Website: http://www.autism-alabama.org

State advocacy for people affected by ASD.

Easter Seals of Alabama

5960 East Shirley Lane

Montgomery, AL 36117

Tel: (334) 395 4489

Toll Free: (800) 388 7325

Email: info@al.easterseals.com

Website: http://alabama.easterseals.com

The Exceptional Foundation

1616 Oxmoor Road

Homewood, AL 35209

Tel: (205) 870 0776

Website: http://www.exceptionalfoundation.org

The Exceptional Foundation provides year-round services to individuals with special needs who have reached the age of 21 and no longer receive services from school systems.

Fred Delchamps Center and Moorer Learning Center

2424 Gordon Smith Drive

Mobile, AL 36617

Tel: (251) 665 9608

Contact Name: Flora Reiss

Email: freiss@mobilearc.org

Website: http://www.mobilearc.org

The Fred Delchamps Center and the Moorer Learning Center offer day habilitation training for adults with intellectual and developmental disabilities through in-house and community based activities.

Hoover Recreation Center

600 Municipal Drive

Hoover, AL 35216

205 444 777

Website: http://www.hooveral.org/

The EXPLORE program at the Hoover Recreation Center is designed to meet the needs of individuals with mental and physical disabilities. The program utilizes community resources in a therapeutic manner and the activities are designed and supervised by Certified Therapeutic Recreation Specialists.

Lee County Autism Resource & Advocacy (LCARA)

Opelika, AL 36801

Tel: (334) 737 6503

Contact Name: Maria Gutierrez

Email: Info@leecountyautism.com

Website: http://www.leecountyautism.com

Lee County Autism Resources and Advocacy is a non-profit organization providing resources, workshops, meetings and support.

Rainbow Omega

PO Box 740

Eastaboga, AL 36260

Tel: (256) 831 0919

Contact Email:

Email: office@rainbowomega.org

Website: http://www.rainbowomega.org

Rainbow Omega provides a Christian environment for adults with developmental disabilities providing a permanent and safe home, where their abilities and potentials are respected and nurtured in a Christian environment.

The Sensory Bus
Pell City, AL 35128
Tel: (205) 451 6268
Contact Name: Ashley Faust
Email: ashley@thesensorybus.com
Website: http://www.thesensorybus.com

The SensoryBus is a mobile sensory experience based on the Snoezelen® concept of non-directive sensory exploration.

ALASKA

Doctors, Clinics, Hospitals, and Other Health Services

Alaska Center for Pediatrics
1200 Airport Heights Drive Suite 140
Anchorage, AK 99508
Tel: (907) 777 1800
Website: http://www.akpeds.com

Bartlett Regional Hospital
3260 Hospital Drive
Juneau, AK 99801
Tel: (907) 796 8900
Website: http://www.bartletthospital.org

Children's Hospital at Providence
2401 East 42nd Avenue Suite 306
Anchorage, AK 99508
Tel: (907) 562 2211
Website: http://www.providence.org/alaska/tchap

Glacier Pediatrics
1600 Glacier Ave.
Juneau, AK 99801
Tel: (907) 586 1542
Website: http://www.glacierpediatricsllc.com

Pediatric Neurology Clinic of Alaska
2401 E 42nd Ave
Anchorage, AK 99508
Tel: (907) 562 6300

Providence Alaska Medical Center
3200 Providence Drive
Anchorage, AK 99508
Tel: (907) 562 2211
Website: http://www.providence.org/alaska

Therapy Services

Early Intervention/Infant Learning Program: Mat-Su
5000 Shennum Drive
Wasilla, AK 99654
Tel: (907) 352 1200
Email: ilp@mssca.org

The Infant Learning Program provides early intervention services to families with children from birth to age three who have delays in development.

Ghosh Psychiatric Services
9138 Arlon Street, Suite B6
Anchorage, AK
Tel: (907) 644 9927 or (907) 644 8099
Email: info@alaskamentalhealth.com
Website: http://www.alaskamentalhealth.com

Specializes in anxiety, mood, and developmental disorders, including ASD. Services provides include psychiatric assessments, individual and family therapy, consultations, medication management, teaching and training, group therapy.

Good Behavioral Beginnings, LLC
Anchorage, AK 99504
Tel: (907) 301 5471
Contact Name: Rachel L. White, PhD, BCBA-D
Email: goodbehaviorbeginnings@gmail.com
Website: http://www.rachelwhitebcba.com

Provides ABA services to families of children with autism, including assessment and program development, provider and parent training, and BCBA/BCABA supervision.

North Slope Infant Learning Program
P.O. Box 169
Barrow, AK 99723
Tel: (907) 852 9676
Email: asaganna@nvbarrow.net

An early intervention program serving families with infants and toddlers who experience a developmental delay or disability. Services include developmental screening; multidisciplinary team developmental assessment; and home-based early intervention services. Group, parent, and child sessions are also offered.

Programs for Infants and Children
3330 Arctic Blvd. Suite 101
Anchorage, AK 99503
Tel: (907) 561 8060
Email: mridges@picak.org
Website: http://www.picak.org

Programs for Infants and Children, Inc. provides early intervention services for children ages 0 - 3 with developmental delays or disabilities.

STRIDE: Southcentral Therapeutic Riding, Inc.
P.O. Box 671828
Chugiak, AK 99567
Tel: (907) 929 7876
Email: stride@gci.net

STRIDE provides supervised therapeutic equestrian activities.

Schools and Educational Services

Bright Beginnings Early Learning Center
12228 Lake St
Eagle River, AK 99577
Tel: (907) 694 4910
Website: http://www.brightbeginningselc.com

Lighthouse Community Christian School
1524 Westwood Way
Fairbanks, AK 99709
Tel: (907) 457 5227

Special Education Service Agency
3501 Denali Street Suite 101
Anchorage, AK 99503
Tel: (907) 334 1300
Toll Free: (877) 890 9269
Website: http://www.sesa.org/content/autism-impairment

University of Alaska - Anchorage
3211 Providence Drive
Anchorage, AK 99508
Tel: (907) 264 6229
Contact Name: Karen Ward
Email: afkmw@uaa.alaska.edu
Website: http://www.uaa.alaska.edu/dss

Whaley School
2220 Nichols St.
Anchorage, AK 99508
Tel: (907) 742 2350
Contact Name: Ed Scherer, President
Email: scherer_ed@asdk12.org

Legal, Government & Financial Services

Alaska Autism Resource Center
3501 Denali Street Suite 101
Anchorage, AK 99503
Tel: (907) 334 1300
Contact Name: Krist James

Email: kjames@sesa.org
Website: http://www.alaskaarc.org

The AARC provides state wide services, including in person and online educational presentations and classes, resources for parents, caregivers, educators, grandparents and first responders, referral services and a weekly telephone support group.

Department of Housing and Urban Development
3000 C. Street Suite 401
Anchorage, AK 99503
Tel: (907) 677 9800
Email: AK_webmanager@hud.gov
Website: http://www.hud.gov/local/index.cfm?state=ak&topic=offices

Disability Law Center of Alaska
Anchorage Office
3330 Arctic Blvd. Suite 103
Anchorage, AK 99503
Tel: (907) 344 1002
Toll Free: (800) 478 1234
Email: Disablaw@anc.ak.net
Website: http://www.dlcak.org

Disability Law Center is an independent non-profit organization providing legal advocacy services for people with disabilities in Alaska.

Division of Vocational Rehabilitation
801 West 10th Street Suite A
Juneau, AK 99801
Tel: (907) 465 2814
Contact Name: Cheryl Walsh
Email: dol.dvr.info@alaska.gov
Website: http://labor.alaska.gov/dvr/

Assisting individuals with disabilities to obtain and maintain employment.

Law Office of Ernest M. Schlereth, LLC
225 East Fireweed Lane Suite 301
Anchorage, AK 99503
Tel: (907) 272 5549
Email: ernie@ernieattorney.com
Website: http://www.ernieattorney.com

Ernest M. Schlereth is a member of the Special Needs Alliance (SNA), a national network of lawyers dedicated to Disability and Public Benefits Law.

Sonja D. Kerr, Esq.
Sonja D. Kerr, Esq.
1114 Covington Court
Anchorage, AK 99503
Tel: (907) 222 9994
Email: nalaof608@yahoo.com

Provides legal representation for children with disabilities.

Stone Soup Group

Parent Training and Information Center
307 E. Northern Lights Boulevard Suite 100
Anchorage, AK 99503
Tel: (907) 561 3701
Toll Free: (877) 786 7327
Contact Name: Annette Blanas
Email: ssg@stonesoupgroup.org
Website: http://www.stonesoupgroup.org

A statewide non-profit organization based in Anchorage, Alaska that provides support and assistance to families caring for children with special needs.

Community and Recreation Services

Adam's Camp

Anchorage, AK 99501
Tel: (303) 690 4402
Contact Name: Bob Horney, Director of Outreach
Website: http://www.adamscamp.org

Adam's Camp is a nonprofit organization offering a variety of intensive, personalized and integrated therapeutic programs for children with special needs and their families as well as recreational programs for youth and young adults with moderate developmental disabilities.

Alaska Youth & Family Network

Alaska Chapter of the National Federation of Families for Children's Mental Health
AYFN's Offices are located throughout the state.
AK
Toll free: (888) 770 4979
Website: http://www.ayfn.org

Alaska Youth and Family Network advocates for families and children with social / emotional / behavioral challenges and related disabilities to be included as equal partners with professionals in developing policies, programs and ensuring adequate mental health and substance abuse services, prevention and information for Alaskan children and youth.

Alpine Assisted Living Home

Alpine Assisted Living Home
3811 Gardner St.
Anchorage, AK 99508
Tel: (907) 333 2542
Email: alpine38@acsalaska.net

Alpine home is an assisted living home that provides personal care services and assistance with activities of daily living to the elderly and adults with disabilities.

Center for Community

700 Katlian, Suite B
Sitka, AK 99835
Tel: (907) 747 6960
Toll Free: (800) 478 6970
Website: http://www.ptialaska.net/~cfcsitka

CFC is a state-wide provider of home and community-based services for people with disabilities, the elderly and others who experience barriers to community living in Alaska.

Central Peninsula Independent Living Center

47255 Princeton Avenue
Soldotna, AK 99669
Tel: (907) 262 6333
Contact Name: Joyanna Geisler
Email: ilc@xyz.net
Website: http://peninsulailc.org

Community Connections

201 Deermount St.
Ketchikan, AK 99901
Tel: (907) 225 7825
Toll Free: (800) 478 7825
Email: bclark@comconnections.org
Website: http://www.comconnections.org

Focus, Inc.

18606 Old Glenn Hwy. P.O. Box 671750
Chugiak, AK 99567
Tel: (907) 688 0282
Email: info@focusoutreach.org
Website: http://www.focusoutreach.org

FOCUS is a community-based non-profit agency serving families in both Chugiak and Eagle River as well as in Anchorage and Palmer. The agency serves families with early intervention/infant learning and developmental disabilities services.

Hope Community Resources

540 W. International Airport Rd.
Ancorhage, AK 99518
Tel: (907) 561 5335
Website: http://www.hopealaska.org

Hope Community Resources, Inc., provides services and supports requested and designed by individuals and families with disabilities, emphasizing choice, control, family preservation and community inclusion.

Kenai Peninsula Independent Living Center

P.O. Box 2474
Homer, AK 99603
Tel: (907) 235 7911

Toll Free: (800) 770 7911
Contact Name: Joyanna Geisler
Email: ilc@xyz.net
Website: http://peninsulailc.org

Rainbow Connection
PO Box 240663
Anchorage, AK 99524
Tel: (907) 566 8768
Email: ride@therainbowconnection.org
Website: http://www.therainbowconnection.org

Providing physically, mentally and emotionally challenged individuals an opportunity for emotional and
physical growth through horsemanship.

ARIZONA

Doctors, Clinics, Hospitals, and Other Health Services

Melmed Center
4848 East Cactus Road Suite 940
Scottsdale, AZ 85254
Tel: (480) 443 0050
Email: Contact.us@melmedcenter.com
Website: http://www.melmedcenter.com

Southwest Behavioural Health Services
3450 N. 3rd Street
Phoenix, AZ 85012
Tel: (602) 265 8338
Email: info@sbhservices.org

Southwest Behavioral Health Services provides day
treatment, inpatient crisis, outpatient and residential
care.

Bee Well Kidz
14300 N. Northsight Blvd. Suite 207
Scottsdale, AZ 85260
Tel: (480) 650 0729
Email: info@beewell.com

Bee Well provides holistic healthcare services, products and information.

Focus For Life Naturopathic Medical Center
10405 N. Scottsdale Rd Suite 5
Gilbert, AZ 85253
Tel: (480) 553 5200
Email: support@naturopathscottsdale.com
Website: http://www.naturopathscottsdale.com

Offers both traditional medical approaches and alternative healing practices.

Southwest Human Development
2850 North 24th Street
Phoenix, AZ 85008
Tel: (602) 266 5976
Website: http://www.swhd.org/programs/disabilities-
services/autism-services

Using a relationship-based approach, SWHD specializes in working with children ages birth to five, providing assessment, diagnosis, and intervention.

Reconnective Healing
8117 N. 11th Place
Phoenix, AZ 85020
Tel: (602) 943 4399
Contact Name: Kathy Scioscia
Email: Kathy@ReconnectiveHealing-AZ.com
Website: http://TheReconnection.com

Working with individuals and their families through
frequency healing based on Eric Pearl's book, "The
Reconnection: Healing Others, Healing Yourself."

Barrow Neurological Institute at Phoenix Children's Hospital
1919 East Thomas Road Ambulatory Building, 3rd
Floor
Phoenix, AZ 85016
Tel: (602) 933 0970
Contact Name: Nancy Quay, RN, Clinical Manager
Email: nquay@phoenixchildrens.com
Website: http://www.phoenixchildrens.org/

Barrow Neurological Institute at Phoenix Children's
Hospital offers evaluation, diagnosis, and multidisciplinary programs that provide services for children with
learning and/or behavior problems.

Infinite Healing Arts Center
6 East Palo Verde Suite 12
Gilbert, AZ 85296
Tel: (480) 558 1560

Website: http://www.infinitehealingarts.com
Chiropractic.

Phoenix Pediatrics
4434 N 12th Street
Phoenix, AZ 85014
Tel: (602) 242 5121
Website: http://www.phoenixpediatrics.com

Alternative Intervention Research Clinic (AIRC)
5410 S. Lakeshore Dr. #104
Tempe, AZ 85283
Tel: (608) 770 7221 or (602) 361 5355

Contact Name: Debbie Crews
Email: Debbie@aircaz.org
Website: http://www.aircaz.org

AIRC provides alternative therapies as non-drug alternatives or to complement drug therapy.

Anna DeOcampo, M.D.
4848 East Cactus Road Suite 940
Scottsdale, AZ 85254
Tel: (480) 443 0050
Website: http://www.melmedcenter.com

Developmental pediatrician.

Debra A. Davis, Ph.D.
4600 N 16th Street
Phoenix, AZ 85020
Tel: (602) 625 4273
Email: debra@doctordavis.org
Website: http://www.doctordavis.org

Provides diagnostic, psycho-educational, and behavioral assessment and intervention.

Janet Chao, EdD
4848 East Cactus Road Suite 940
Scottsdale, AZ 85254
Tel: (480) 443 0050
Website: http://www.melmedcenter.com
Psychologist.

Shabana Jessani, M.D.
4848 East Cactus Road Suite 940
Scottsdale, AZ 85254
Tel: (480) 443 0050
Website: http://www.melmedcenter.com

Developmental pediatrician.

Banner Good Samaritan Medical Center
925 E. McDowell, 4th Floor
Phoenix, AZ 85006
Tel: (602) 839 6800
Website: https://www.bannerhealth.com/Locations/

Evaluates and treats essentially all mental illnesses as well as the psychological aspects of complicated physical issues.

Friendship Community Mental Health Center
730 E Highland Avenue
Phoenix, AZ 85014
Tel: (602)-241-6656 or (602)-241-7506
Contact Name: Adam Saxton
Email: asaxton@friendshipcmhc.org
Website: http://www.friendshipcmhc.org

Friendship CMHC provides comprehensive and integrated services tailored to the specific needs of patients.

The Guidance Center
2695 E Industrial Dr
Flagstaff, AZ 86004-6106
Tel: (928) 527 1899
Website: http://www.tgcaz.org

The Guidance Center is a Community Mental Health Center that offers a full continuum of Behavioral Health programs and services for children, adolescents, adults and families.

Affiliated Children's Dental Specialists
6320A W. Union Hills Drive Suite 280
Glendale, AZ 85308
Tel: (623) 362 1150
Email: info@kidsteethandbraces.com
Website: http://www.kidsteethandbraces.com

Arizona Dental Association & Arizona Dental Foundation
Scottsdale, AZ 85251
Tel: (480) 344 5777
Website: http://www.azda.org
Website: http://www.findadentist4.me

The Arizona Dental Association Find-a-Dentist program allows you to search for dentists in your neighborhood that treat individuals with special needs.

Cardon Children's Medical Center
1400 S. Dobson Road
Mesa, AZ 85202
480 512 KIDS (5437)
Website: http://www.bannerhealth.com/Locations/Arizona/Cardon+Childrens+Medical+Center

Services including developmental pediatrician.

Daniel B. Kessler, M.D. & Associates
Southwest Human Development 2850 N. 24th Street
Phoenix, AZ 85008
Tel: (602) 633 8811
Website: http://www.swhd.org/drkessler

Developmental and behavioral pediatricians.

Diamond Children's
The University of Arizona Medical Center
1501 N Campbell Ave.
Tucson, AZ 85724
Tel: (520) 626 6615

Website: http://www.uahealth.com/diamondchildrens/services/developmental-behavioral

Developmental and behavioral services

Phoenix Children's Hospital Developmental Pediatrics
1919 E Thomas Rd
Phoenix, AZ 85016
(602) 933 0970

Board Certified Developmental-Behavioral Pediatrician

North Scottsdale Pediatric Associates, P.C.
10200 N. 92nd Street Suite 150
Scottsdale, AZ 85258
Tel: (480) 860 8488
Website: http://www.nspeds.com

Arizona Center for Young Children, PLLC
17505 N. 79th Ave. Ste. 211-G
Glendale, AZ 85308
Tel: (623) 986 8069
Contact Name: Dr. Lori Brill
Email: Lori@azyoungchildren.com

The Arizona Center for Young Children provides psychological assessments and treatment for young children aged one to seven.

Arrowhead Neruopsychology
Bell Plaza North Building 10451 W. Palmeras Dr., Ste. 126C
Sun City, AZ 85373
Tel: (623) 810 5501
Contact Name: Karla Mueller, Ph.D.
Email: info@arrowheadneuropsychology.com
Website: http://www.arrowheadneuropsychology.com

Comprehensive diagnostic, developmental, and neurocognitive evaluations for children ages 18 months and older.

North Valley Clinical Services
10575 N. 114th Street, Suite 109
Scottsdale, AZ 85259
Tel: (480) 661 1075
Contact Name: Jennifer Ader
Email: jader@youthetc.org
Website: http://www.northvalleyclinicalservices.org

North Valley Clinical Services is a non-profit that has Licensed Professional Counselors and Board Certified Behavior Analysts (BCBA) on staff who diagnose Autism Spectrum Disorders. Develops individualized treatment plans with a variety of options.

Gentry Pediatric Behavioral Services
7600 N. 16th St Suite 218
Phoenix, AZ 85020
Tel: (602) 904 3405
Website: http://www.gentrypbs.com

Specializes in autism spectrum disorder evaluations for children and adolescents aged 2–21 years.

Patricia Beldotti, PsyD
1102 W Ina Rd. Suite 4
Tucson, AZ 85704
Tel: (520) 404 7553
Contact Name: Patricia Beldotti, PsyD
Email: drbeldotti@aol.com
Website: http://www.drbeldotti.com

Specializes in assessments of children (age 3+) and adults with challenges including ASD.

Therapy Services

Arizona Horseriding Adventures
14629 W. Peoria
Waddell, AZ 85355
Tel: (623) 640 3814
Contact Name: Anita Norton
Email: no1cowgirl@rocketmail.com
Website: http://ArizonaHorseridingAdventures.com

Provides regular and therapeutic horse riding instruction for ages 3 to 75 with an emphasis on specialized children's programs for children and adults with special needs.

Behavioral Consultation Services of Northern Arizona (BCSNA), LLC
906 W. University Avenue Suite 120
Flagstaff, AZ 86001
Tel: (928)522 3780
Contact Name: Andrew Gardner
Email: Services@BehaviorAZ.com
Website: http://www.behavioraz.com

BCSNA provides a variety of services including diagnosis, functional behavior assessments, in-home curriculum planning, and center-based ABA therapy.

CPES
4825 North Sabino Canyon Road
Tucson, AZ 85750
Tel: (520) 884 7954
Website: http://www.cpes.com

Provides coordinated service for individuals with developmental disabilities. They focus on integrated models of care.

Desert Valley Pediatric Therapy
16815 S. Desert Foothills Pkwy. Suite 126
Phoenix, AZ 85048
(480) 704 5954
Contact Name: Julie Sorrick
Email: julie@dvpediatrictherapy.com
Website: http://www.dvpediatrictherapy.com
Website: https://www.facebook.com/
DesertValleyPediatricTherapy

Desert Valley Pediatric Therapy provides a variety of services and programs to children with developmental delays including occupational, speech, and physical therapy.

Horses Help
P.O. Box 71005
Phoenix, AZ 85050
Tel: (602) 569 6056
Contact Name: Nyluh or Denise
Website: http://www.horseshelp.org

Horses Help is an accredited therapeutic and recreational agency that serves the special needs population.

Hunkapi Horse Programs
12051 North 96th Street
Scottsdale, AZ 85260
Tel: (480) 393 0870
Contact Name: Terra Schaad
Email: terra@hunkapi.org
Website: http://www.hunkapi.org

Hunkapi offers a vast range of services including riding programs, corporate teambuilding, equine therapy and parties.

Marc Center
924 N Country Club Drive
Mesa, AZ 85201
Tel: (480) 969 3800
President and CEO, Randy Gray
Email: randy.gray@marcr.com
Website: http://www.marccenter.com

Marc Center is a private not-for-profit organization providing educational, therapeutic, rehabilitation and social services to children and adults with developmental and physical disabilities and behavioral health challenges.

Mental & Martial Enrichment Program
7830 E. Redfield Rd. Ste 12
Scottsdale, AZ 85260
(480) 200 1187
(480) 330 2066
Contact Name: Tiffany Richards

Email: info@peacefulwarriorphx.com
Website: http://www.peacefulwarriorphx.com/
specialty/adhd-program.html
Website: http://www.peacefulwarriorphx.com/media.
html

Milestone Pediatrics
600 W Ray Rd. Suite D-1
Chandler, AZ 85225
Tel: (480) 322 1927 or (480) 322 1928 (español)
Contact Name: Lyndsey Steele, Co-Founder, Client Coordinator
Email: Lyndsey@milestoneAz.com
Website: http://www.MilestoneAz.com

Provides in-home early intervention and therapeutic services to promote growth in the areas of cognition, language, gross and fine motor, as well as social and self-help skills to the Spanish and English speaking disabled and special needs community.

Nicole C. Yule, M.A., CCC-SLP
7331 East 16th street Suite A-120
Phoenix, AZ 85020
Tel: (602) 349 2078
Contact Name: Nicole Yule
Email: NCYule@gmail.com

Licensed speech-language pathologist providing evaluation and treatment of speech, language and pragmatics (social skills) abilities for children ages 2 to school aged.

Pediatric Speech and Language Specialists
6865 East Becker Lane Suite 101
Scottsdale, AZ 85254
Tel: (480) 991 6560
Website: http://www.pediatricspeech.net

Provides evaluation and treatment to children and adolescents with speech, language, and communication difficulties.

Silver Lining Riding Program
@Dale Creek Equestrian Village 13424 W Camelback Rd
Litchfield Park, AZ 85340
(623) 262 1307
Contact Name: Amanda Adams
Email: amanda@silverliningriding.org
Website: http://www.silverliningriding.org

Silver Lining Riding Program is a non-profit, therapeutic horseback riding organization.

Dr. Sue Lerner, Ph.D.
8300 North Hayden Road, Suite A207
Scottsdale, AZ 85258
Tel: (480) 348 6899
Email: drsuelerner@cox.net
Website: http://www.drsuelerner.com

A licensed psychologist & social disorders specialist providing diagnostic, therapy, and consultation for individuals with ASD and disorders of social functioning. Uses ABA and cognitive behavioral therapy as guides for therapy as well as "Social Thinking" curriculum.

Therapeutic Riders of Tuscon
8920 East Woodland Road
Tuscon, AZ 85749
Tel: (520) 749 2360
Email: info@trotarizona.org
Website: http://www.trotarizona.org

Therapeutic equine programs.

United Cerebral Palsy of Arizona
1802 W. Parkside Lane
Phoenix, AZ 85027
Tel: (602) 943 5472
Toll Free: (888) 943 5472
Contact Name: Kimberly Phillips
Email: kphillips@ucpofaz.org
Website: http://www.ucpofcentralaz.org

Provides early intervention, day treatment and training, childcare, occupational therapy, physical therapy, speech therapy, assistive technology, attendant care, habilitation, respite care and vocational training.

United Cerebral Palsy of Southern Arizona
2451 S Avenue A Suite 20
Yuma, AZ 85364
Tel: (928) 317 8800
Contact Name: Abbie Lechler
Email: alechler@ucpsa.org
Website: http://www.ucpsayuma.org

UCPSA offers Music Therapy services along with habilitation and respite services to children with developmental disabilities, including autism.

Arizona Autism United
5025 E Washington St Suite 212
Phoenix, AZ 85034
Tel: (602) 773 5773
Contact Name: Aaron Blocker-Rubin
Email: info@azunited.org
Website: http://www.azunited.org

Provides customized services and supports that enhance quality of life for all individuals with autism and their families.

Peaks Arc
1050 West Beal Road
Flagstaff, AZ 86001
Contact Name: Cindy McClung

Santa Cruz County Arc
P.O. Box 972
Nogales, AZ 85648
Tel: (520) 287 6271
Contact Name: Christopher Causey
Email: fsctpinc@theriver.com

Behavioral Consultation Services of Northern Arizona (BCSNA), LLC
906 W. University Avenue Suite 120
Flagstaff, AZ 86001
Tel: (928) 522 3780
Contact Name: Andrew Gardner
Email: Services@BehaviorAZ.com
Website: http://www.behavioraz.com

Provides a variety of services including diagnosis, functional behavior assessments, in-home curriculum planning, and afterschool center-based ABA therapy.

Head 2 Toe Therapy
5314 North 7th Street
Phoenix, AZ 85014
(602) 277 5006
Contact Name: Danielle Hunt
Email: Danielle@headtotoeinc.com
Website: http://www.headtotoeinc.com

Services include Physical, Occupations, Speech, Music and Feeding therapies; as well as Respite and Habilitation Services. They also offer Before and After School Programs (DTT), and a Summer Program (DTS) at our satellite locations. We are here to provide care and assistance to all of our kiddos and their families!!

TEAM Ed
2040 S. Alma School Road Suite 1, PMB 500
Chandler, AZ 85286
Tel: (602) 323 0894
Tel: (602) 373 0365
Contact Name: Alice Schnepf
Email: contactus@teamed.net
Website: http://www.teamed.net

Provides therapy in homes and school districts in Arizona. They also help schools find and apply for grants.

Trumpet Behavioural Health
82 W. Ray Rd. Suite 104
Gilbert, AZ 85249

Tel: (480) 812 4789
Contact Name: Dr. Paige Raetz, BCBA-D
Email: praetz@tbh.com
Website: http://www.tbh.com

Provides behavior treatment services for children and adults with ASD based on ABA.

The Center for Preventative & Restorative Health
Scottsdale, AZ
Tel: (480) 255 1650
Contact Name: Tiffany Kuehn
Email: tiffany@tcprh.com
Website: http://www.tcprh.com

Offers services including in-home services for adults and children living with autism; including cranial sacral therapy, therapeutic exercise and medical nutritional therapy.

Autism Development and Parent Training (ADAPT)
Phoenix, AZ 85003
Tel: (562) 665 6226
Contact Name: Denise Larkin
Email: Denise@adaptaba.com
Website: http://www.adaptaba.com

Provides ABA services to children, teens, and adults with ASD.

Asperger Parent Network of Arizona
15821 S. 35th Way
Phoenix, AZ 85048
Tel: (480) 759 6329
Contact Name: Carolyn Warden, President
Website: http://apnarizona.com/

The Asperger Parent Network of Arizona serves families raising children affected by Asperger Syndrome and related autism spectrum disorders.

Touchstone Behavioral Health Family Centered Autism Program
15648 N. 35th Ave
Phoenix, AZ 85054
(602) 732 4950
Contact Name: Elizabeth Rinaldo
Email: elizabeth.rinaldo@touchstonebh.org
Website: http://www.touchstonebh.org

FCAP emphasizes a family-based intervention protocol and provides services in the most natural environment for the child.

Tucson Alliance for Autism
1002 N. Country Club
Tucson, AZ 85716

Tel: (520) 319 5857
Contact Name: Kim Crooks
Email: kcrooks1@aol.com
Website: http://www.tucsonallianceforautism.org

Promotes community awareness, provides diagnostic and therapeutic services for individuals with ASD, educates and supports professionals and families; provides resources for families.

Jim Clear, MS/LMT
2339 Mabel St.
Tucson, AZ 85719-4348
See map: Google Maps
520.396.4670
Contact Name: Jim Clear
Email: jimclear@ymail.com

Adult and Children's Integrative Massage and Bodywork.

Beginners Edge Sports Training (BEST), LLC
7000 East Shea Blvd Suites 1830 & 1840
Scottsdale, AZ 85254
Tel: (623) 748 9453
Tel: (602) 301 6171
Contact Name: Mitchell Goldberg, Director
Email: info@thebestinaz.com
Website: http://thebestinaz.com

MetroCare
Gilbert, AZ 85234
Tel: (480) 507 8831
Email: info@metrocareaz.com
Website: http://www.metrocareaz.com

Provides nonmedical, in-home healthcare services.

Northeastern Pinal County Arc
Kearny, AZ 85237
Tel: (520) 363 5581

Above & Beyond Therapy Services
3233 W. Peoria Ave Suite 224
Phoenix, AZ 85029
Tel: (602) 866 2231

and

21321 E. Ocotillo Rd Bldg. H Suite 119
Queen Creek, AZ 85242
Tel: (480) 987 1870
Email: info@aboveandbeyondtherapy.com
Website: http://www.aboveandbeyondtherapy.com

Center for Autism and Related Disorders (CARD), Inc.
1620 N 48th St.
Phoenix, AZ 85008

Tel: (602) 325 2485
Tel: (855) 345 2273
Email: info@centerforautism.com
Website: http://www.centerforautism.com

Provides ABA treatment.

The BISTA Center

10231 N 35th Ave Suite 113
Phoenix, AZ 85051
Tel: (602) 926 7200
Tel: (602) 995 7366
Contact Name: Don Stenhoff
Email: bista@accel.org
Website: http://www.thebistacenter.org

Provides therapy based on ABA, Discrete Trial and Pivotal Response Training, Verbal Behavior, and early intensive behavioral intervention. Provides clinical and in-home services.

The Clubhouse Inovative Therapy Centers

4600 East Shea Boulavard, Suite 101
Phoenix, AZ 85028
Tel: (602) 368 8601
Contact Name: Susan Raad
Email: Susan@theclubhousecenters.com
Website: http://www.theclubhousecenters.com

ABA Therapy & Gymstar Gymnastics

9494 E Redfield Road # 2062
Scottsdale, AZ 85260
Tel: (480) 391 3074
Contact Name: Jennifer Montouri
Email: jmontouri@yahoo.com
Website: http://www.scottsdalegymnastics.com

Behavioral Consultation Services of Northern Arizona (BCSNA), LLC

906 W. University Avenue Suite 120
Flagstaff, AZ 86001
Tel: (928) 522 3780
Contact Name: Andrew Gardner
Email: Services@BehaviorAZ.com
Website: http://www.behavioraz.com

Provides a variety of services including, but not limited to, diagnosis, functional behavior assessments, in-home curriculum planning, and afterschool center-based ABA therapy.

Exceptional Expectations

2500 S. Power Road Building 8, Suite 119
Mesa, AZ 85209
Tel: (480) 209 4357
Email: exceptionalexpectations@yahoo.com

Website: http://www.exceptionalexpectations.com

Offer a range of services including Applied Behavior Analysis.

H.O.P.E. Group

4530 E Muirwood Dr. Suite 103
Phoenix, AZ 85048
Tel: (480) 610 6981
Contact Name: Ann Monahan, Director of Operations
Email: amonahan@hopegroupaz.com
Website: http://www.hopegroupaz.com

Offers services including ABA.

SKILLS

1620 N. 48th St.
Phoenix, AZ 85008
 (877) 975 4559
(602) 325 2485 (CARD)
Email: info@centerforautism.com
Website: http://www.skillsforautism.com/
Website: http://phoenix.centerforautism.com/

Offer a range of services including Applied Behaviour Analysis.

The Play Project

Child & Family Resources, Inc. 700 W. Campbell, Ste. 3
Phoenix, AZ 85013
Tel: (602) 903 0948
Contact Name: Dr. Lori Lichte-Brill
Email: llichte-brill@cfraz.org
Website: http://www.childfamilyresources.org

Psychological testing for ASD for toddlers, preschoolers, and young school-aged children. The Play Project program is an intensive, in-home, developmental treatment program for children aged 15 months to seven years of age, and is based on the floortime/DIR model.

Listening Ears

1815 E. Queen Creek Rd. Suite 1
Chandler, AZ 85286
Tel: (480) 219 3953
Contact Name: Lynn Carahaly, MA,CCC-SLP
Website: http://www.listening-ears.com

Offer a range of services including speech and language therapy.

Massage Therapy

1025 E. Orange St.
Tempe, AZ 85281
Tel: (480) 381 2901
Contact Name: Casey Lee Jones

Email: Casey@ReleaseMyotherapy.com
Website: http://www.ReleaseMyotherapy.com

Massage Therapist in Tempe who works with those on the spectrum providing deep pressure massage and also with parents who would like to learn a massage protocol to use at home as part of the nightly bedtime routine.

Nelson Pediatric Therapy
1930 E Southern Ave.
Tempe, AZ 85282
Tel: (480) 456 0719
Website: http://www.nelsonpediatric.com

Provides in-home and clinic-based therapy.

Envision Therapeutic Horsemanship, Inc.
Phoenix, AZ 85046
Tel: (480) 262 3434
Email: info@envisiontherapy.org
Website: http://envisiontherapy.org

Offering therapeutic riding and driving and equine-facilitated mental health programs.

Hoofbeats with Heart
43491 North Coyote Road
San Tan Valley, AZ 85140
Tel: (602) 421 7718
Contact Name: Kelley Hullihen
Email: Kelley@hoofbeatswithheart.org
Website: http://www.hoofbeatswithheart.org

Arizona Music Therapy Services (AMTS)
Chandler, AZ 85286
Tel: (480) 329 3155
Contact Name: Scott Tonkinson, MM, MT-BC
Email: info@arizonamusictherapy.com
Website: http://www.arizonamusictherapy.com

Arizona Music Therapy Services provides music therapy to children and adults with special needs, including ASD, with board-certified music therapists.

Heart & Soul Music Therapy
1000 N Beeline Hwy, Suite 103
Payson, AZ 85541
Tel: (928) 478 8680
Contact Name: Cynthia Sambrano, MT-BC
Email: cysambrano@gmail.com
Website: http://www.heartandsoulmusictherapy.com

Provider of Music Therapy services in Payson, Arizona. Ages 0 to adult.

Music Therapy with Jackie Berger
1200 N. El Dorado Pl.
Tucson, AZ 85715
(520) 406 9848
Contact Name: Jackie Berger, MT-BC
Email: jackiebergermt@gmail.com
Website: http://www.azmusictherapy.com/

Jackie Berger, MT-BC, offers private one-on-one music therapy sessions, sibling/pair music therapy sessions, group music therapy sessions, and traditional/adapted instrumental lessons. Goals are individualized.

Neurologic Music Therapy Services of Arizona (NMTSA)
2702 N. 3rd St. Suite 1000
Phoenix, AZ 85004
Tel: (602) 840 6410
Email: info@nmtsa.org
Website: http://www.nmtsa.org

Provides preventative and rehabilitative neurologic music therapy.

Advanced Therapy Solutions
312 N. Alma School Rd Suite 14
Chandler, AZ 85224
Tel: (480) 820 6366
Email: ats@atsaz.net
Website: http://www.atsaz.net

Offering services including occupational therapy and physical therapy.

Arcadia Therapy Services
455 North Third Street Suite 200
Phoenix, AZ 85004
Tel: (602) 528 3450
Toll Free: (800) 277 0823
Contact Name: Annie Zimmerman, Clinical Director
Email: arcadiatherapy@juno.com
Website: http://www.arcadiatherapy.com

Home-based occupational therapy, physical therapy and speech and language therapy.

Baio Enterprises
1745 S. Alma School Rd Suite 145
Mesa, AZ 85210
Tel: (480) 963 3634
Email: info@baioenterprises.com
Website: http://www.baioenterprises.com

Provides speech, language, occupational, and physical therapy to children and their families.

Fiesta Pediatric Therapy
1641 E. Osborn Rd. Suite 1
Phoenix, AZ 85016
Tel: (602) 265 4124

Scottsdale Fiesta Pediatric Therapy
5040 E. Shea Blvd. Suite 168
Scottsdale, AZ 85254
Tel: (480) 483 1025

Email: phx@fiestapeds.com
Website: http://www.fiestapeds.com
Offering services including occupational therapy and physical therapy.

Henry OT Services
500 N. Estrella Pkwy Suite B2-454
Goodyear, AZ 85338
Tel: (623) 882 8812
Contact Name: Diana or Carla
Email: chenryot@aol.com
Website: http://www.henryot.com
Offering services including occupational therapy and sensory integration therapy.

Piller Child Development, LLC – Ahwatukee
10631 S. 51st Street #8
Phoenix, AZ 85044
(480) 398 4280
Email: office.staff@pillerchilddevelopment.com
Website: http://www.PillerChildDevelopment.com
Pediatric occupational therapy and sensory integration therapy. Sensory integration certified therapists on staff.

Progressive Therapy LLC
17958 W Brown Street
Waddell, AZ 85355
Tel: (623) 535 5741
Contact Name: Sarah Slack
Email: sslack@progressivetherapyaz.com
Website: http://www.progressivetherapyaz.com

Southwest Speech Services
12409 West Indian School Road Suite C
Avondale, AZ 85323
Tel: (623) 935 6040
Offering services including occupational therapy and speech and language therapy.

Therapy One
110 West University Drive
Mesa, AZ 85201
Tel: (480) 668 1917

Email: office@therapyone.com
Website: http://www.therapyone.com
Provides home-based, school-based, and clinic-based therapy services throughout Arizona.

Wee Care Corporation
12409 W. Indian School #C306
Avondale, AZ 85392
Tel: (623) 935 6040
Contact Name: Amy Donnel
Email: amydonnel.weecarecorp@yahoo.com
Website: http://www.weecarecorp.com
Wee Care Corporation offers pediatric therapy for children with a wide range of conditions, including ASD.

Behavioral Consultation Services of Northern Arizona (BCSNA), LLC
Tel: (928) 522 3780
Contact Name: Andrew Gardner
Email: Services@BehaviorAZ.com
Website: http://www.behavioraz.com
BCSNA provides a variety of services including, but not limited to, diagnosis, functional behavior assessments, in-home curriculum planning, and afterschool center-based ABA therapy.

Communication Skills Center
8356 E San Rafael Drive
Scottsdale, AZ 85258
Tel: (480) 951 9707
Contact Name: Mirla G. Raz
Email: mirlag@communicationskillscenter.com
Website: http://www.communicationskillscenter.com
State-licensed speech pathologist certified by the American Speech-Language Association. Coaches and consults parents to help maximize their children's speech and language skills.

Ther-a-dog Services
6331 W Cheryl Dr
Glendale, AZ 85302
Tel: (602) 647 0133
Contact Name: Cindy Ferrante
Email: ther-a-dog@cox.net
Website: http://www.ther-a-dog.com
Ther-a-dog provides animal assisted therapy and activities to children living with autism. They incorporate the use of an AKC, professionally trained therapy dog and a swimming pool (seasonally).

Arizona Goldens LLC
P.O. Box 40776
Mesa, AZ 85274-0776

Tel: (480) 205 6810
Contact Name: Brian Daugherty
Email: azgoldensllc@cox.net
Website: http://www.AzGoldensLLC.com/autism.php

Arizona Goldens LLC is a company that raises, trains, and places highly trained service dogs with adults and children with disabilities.

Schools and Educational Services

AFH/Casa Grande Rehabilitation Center
208 West Main Street
Casa Grande, AZ 85222
Tel: (520) 836 9798
Website: http://www.azafh.com

AFH's mission is to teach eligible adults the skills they need to become employable and independent, and place them in meaningful jobs or further education.

AFH/Perry Rehabilitation Center
3146 E. Windsor Avenue
Phoenix, AZ 85008
See map: Google Maps
Tel: (602) 956 0400
Email: perrycenter@qwest.net
Website: http://www.azafh.com

Phoenix branch of AFH

Gompers Center
6601 North 27th Avenue
Phoenix, AZ 85017
Tel: (602) 336 0061
Tel: (877) 687 2656
Website: http://www.gomperscenter.org

Gompers Center describes its mission as 'developing innovative opportunities for people with disabilities.'

One Step Beyond, Inc.
9299 West Olive Ave. Suite 311
Peoria, AZ 85345
Tel: (623) 266 7490
Tel: (623) 215 2449
Contact Name: Justin Watson
Email: justinwatson@osbi.org
Website: http://www.osbi.org

Provides programs to empower individuals with developmental disability to achieve optimal independence, meaningful employment, significant social relationships, and full participation in the community.

STARS Transition Program
11130 E. Cholla St
Scottsdale, AZ 85215

Tel: (480) 371 2342 or (480) 607 1301
Contact Name: Krista Anderson
Email: kanderson@starsaz.org
Website: http://www.starsaz.org/

This program is designed to foster vocational skills in a fun, interactive environment. Activities include art classes, cooking classes, community outings and recreational activities.

Arizona Centers for Comprehensive Education and Life Skills (ACCEL)
1430 E Baseline Rd
Tempe, AZ 85283
Tel: (602) 926 7200
Contact Name: Bryan Davey, PhD, BCBA-D
Email: bdavey@accel.org
Website: http://www.accel.org

Provides educational, behavioral, therapeutic, and vocational programs to individuals with special needs.

Southwest Autism Research & Resource Center
300 N 18th Street
Phoenix, AZ 85006
Tel: (602) 340 8717
Contact Name: Janet Kirwan
Email: jkirwan@autismcenter.org
Website: http://www.autismcenter.org

SAARC provides clinical services, educational services, and a Vocational/Life Skills Academy.

Spectrum College Transition Program
Scottsdale, AZ 85258
Tel: (480) 443 7331
Email: spectrumtransition@gmail.com
Website: http://www.spectrumcollegetransition.org

Provides a supportive, residential, post-secondary program for young men with Aspergers Syndrome and High Functioning Autism, who need assistance academically, socially, and emotionally.

University of Arizona Tucson
AZ 85721
See map: Google Maps
Tel: (520) 621 5165
Contact Name: Stephanie Z. C. MacFarland
Email: szm@email.arizona.edu
Website: http://drc.arizona.edu

Wide-ranging resources for disabled students.

Pieceful Solutions
Apache Junction, AZ 85117
Tel: (480) 309 4792
Email: piecefulsolutions@yahoo.com

Website: http://www.piecefulsolutions.com

Offers children with autism and other developmental disabilities comprehensive schooling with individualized curriculums. Staff ratio is 2:1 and 1:1 during all learning. Department of Education approved.

Specializing in the Education of Exceptional Kids (S.E.E.K)
1830 S Alma School Road Suite 130
Mesa, AZ 85210
Tel: (480) 902 0771
Contact Name: Jessica Irwin
Email: Info@SEEKArizona.org
Website: http://www.SEEKArizona.org

S.E.E.K. Arizona provides services and therapies with an ABA focus to children and young adults with ASD.

Play ABA
600 E Baseline Rd. Suite B-6
Tempe, AZ 85283
Tel: (480) 839 6000
PA: Tel: (480) 838 9797
Contact Name: Parents Association: De Freedman
Email: play.aba@gmail.com
Website: http://www.play-aba.com

Private year-round school approved by AZ Department of Education. All staff are ABA certified.

Arizona State University Infant Child Research Programs
P.O Box 1908
Tempe, AZ 85287
Tel: (480) 965 9396
Email: kathiesm@asu.edu
Website: http://www.asu.edu/clas/icrp

Casa Niños School of Montessori, Inc.
1 W Orange Grove Rd.
Tuscon, AZ 85704
Tel: (520) 297 3898
Contact Name: Rebecca Cotton, Office Manager
Email: info@casaninos.org
Website: http://www.casaninos.org

Children's Center for Neurodevelopmental Studies
5430 West Glenn Drive
Glendale, AZ 85301
Tel: (623) 915 0345
Email: Info@thechildrenscenteraz.org
Website: http://www.thechildrenscenteraz.org

Kyrene Preschool
Kyrene School District

8700 S Kyrene Road
Tempe, AZ 85284
Tel: (480) 783 4156
Website: http://www.kyrene.org

Small (approximately 7 typical students and 7–9 special needs students) classes with a certified teacher, a speech/language pathologist, and a teaching assistant. Classes are 2.5 hours per day, AM or PM, 3–4 days per week.

Mesa Montessori
2830 S Carriage Ln.
Mesa, AZ 85202
Tel: (480) 839 7661
Email: mesamontessori@gmail.com

Montessori Academy
6050 N Invergordon Rd.
Paradise Valley, AZ 85253
Tel: (480) 945 1121
Contact Name: Juli Newman, Executive Director/Principal
Email: jlewis@azma.org

Montessori of Surprise
18540 Parkview Pl.
Surprise, AZ 85374
Tel: (623) 760 7548
Website: http://www.montessoriofsurprise.com

St. Dominic Savio Academy
1230 E. Guadalupe Rd.
Tempe, AZ 85282
Tel: (480) 659 5456
Contact Name: Corinna Siegler-Ndolo
Email: info@stdomsavio.com
Website: http://www.stdomsavio.com

Programs for children preschool through 6th grade. With a 2:1 ratio and an ABA based program model. A Department of Education approved private day school.

Valle Del Encanto Learning Center
400 N. Cesar Chavez Ave.
Somerton, AZ 85364
Tel: (928) 341 6700
Contact Name: Norma Villegas
Email: nvillegas@ssd11.org
Website: http://www.ssd11.org/elc/ELC

Foundations Developmental House, LLC
1815 E. Queen Creek Rd. Suite 1
Chandler, AZ 85286
Tel: (480) 219 3953

Contact Name: Lynn Carahaly, MA,CCC-SLP
Email: lynn@listening-ears.com
Website: http://www.fdhkids.com

A supplementary preschool program focusing on social skills for children needing extra support.

Arizona Autism Charter School, Inc.
4433 N. 7th Street
Phoenix, AZ 85014
Tel: (602) 822 5544
Email: info@autismcharter.org
Website: http://www.autismcharter.org

Arizona Autism Charter School is a public charter school focused on children with ASD.

ASCEND
6741 Corsair Ave.
Prescott, AZ 86301
Tel: (928) 443 9290
Contact Name: Angela Levin, BA ED., Director

Autism Academy for Education & Development
1540 North Burk Street
Gilbert, AZ 85234
Tel: (480) 240 9255
Contact Name: Shannon Henley, M.Ed, Director
Email: shenley@autismacademyed.com
Website: http://www.autismacademyed.com

Specializes in educating students with ASD grades K–8. Low teacher/student ratios and services include speech, OT, art, PE, music, social skills, life skills, and more.

Devereux Arizona
11000 N. Scottsdale Road
Scottsdale, AZ 85254
Tel: (480) 998 2920
Website: http://www.devereuxaz.org

Devereux Arizona provides treatment programs & community services to children, adults, and families experiencing behavioral challenges.

Gateway Academy
9659 N Hayden Rd.
Scottsdale, AZ 85258
Tel: (480) 998 1071
Contact Name: O. Robin Sweet, Executive Director & CEO
Email: gatewayacademy@cox.net
Website: http://www.gatewayacademy.us

K-12th Grade Private Day School for students with Asperger's Syndrome. Class size 6:1.

Hi-Star Center for Children
5807 North 43rd Avenue
Phoenix, AZ 85019
Tel: (602) 548 3038
Email: info@histarcenter.com
Website: http://www.histarcenter.com

The Hi-Star Center for Children is a private academically based special education day school (K–12), serving students with severe language/communication, learning and behavioral needs.

Life Development Institute
18001 N. 79th Ave. Suite E-71
Glendale, AZ 85308
Tel: (623) 773 2774
Website: http://www.lifedevelopmentinstitute.org

Offers residential and fully-accredited high school, college and career-focused programs for young adults with Learning Disabilities, ASD, and similar conditions.

Sierra Academy of Scottsdale
17800 N. Perimeter Dr. #110
Scottsdale, AZ 85255
Tel: (480) 767 8659
Contact Name: Debra Watland, School Director
Email: dwatland@sierra-school.com
Website: http://www.sesi-schools.com/schools/sierra-academy-of-scottsdale-az

The Abbie School
5780 East 14th Street
Tucson, AZ 85711
Tel: (520) 747 5280
Tel: (520) 243 3203
Contact Name: Zak Cushing
Email: zak.cushing@abbieschool.org
Website: http://www.abbieschool.org

Provides individualized learning in small class settings specifically crafted for students with Autism Spectrum Disorders and other developmental and social struggles.

Arizona Department of Education Exceptional Student Services
AZ
Tel: (602) 542 4013
Website: http://www.azed.gov/special-education/

Transition from School Age Services to Adult Services
Department of Economic Security
3221 N. 16th Street Phoenix, AZ 85016 Suite 200
Tel: (602) 266 6752
Contact Name: David Berns, Director

Website: http://www.ade.state.az.us/ess/
SpecialProjects/transition

Coordinator for Transition Services.

Kids of the King Tutoring Service
Tucson, AZ 85748
Tel: (520) 790 5904
Contact Name: Vanessa Southard
Email: kids_of_the_king@hotmail.com
Website: http://kidsofthekingtutoring.weebly.com

Specialized one-to-one tutoring.

Legal, Government & Financial Services

Amy Langerman, Esq. (licensed in Arizona only)
Amy Langerman, PC
951 Coronado Ave.
Coronado, CA 92118
Email: info@amylangerman.com
Website: www.amylangerman.com

Special education law.

Arizona Department of Economic Security
Tel: (602) 542 3332
Email: AZRSA@mail.de.state.az.us
Website: https://www.azdes.gov/main.aspx?id=3320

Information and support on a wide range of issues
affecting disabled citizens.

Arizona Rehabilitation Services
103 West Highland Avenue Suite 202
Phoenix, AZ 85013
(602) 274 0132
Email: AZRSA@azdes.gov
Website: https://www.azdes.gov/rsa/

Department of Housing and Urban Development
1 N. Central Ave Suite 600
Phoenix, AZ 85004
Tel: (603) 379 7100

And

6245 E. Broadway Blvd Suite 350
Tucson, AZ 85711
(520) 308 3007
Contact Name: William Shaw
Email: AZ_Webmanager@hud.gov
Website: http://www.hud.gov/local/index.
cfm?state=az&topic=offices

Arizona Department of Health Services
150 N. 18th Avenue, 2nd Floor
Phoenix, AZ 85007
(602) 364 4558
(602) 364 4570
Email: dbhsinfo@azdhs.gov
Website: http://www.azdhs.gov/bhs/index.htm

ADHS/DBHS provides behavioral health services
through Child and Family Team (CFT) practice to children, adolescents and young adults with intellectual
and developmental disabilities.

Arizona Health Care Cost Containment System
801 E. Jefferson Street MD 4100
Phoenix, AZ 85034
(602) 417 4000
1-(800) 654 8713
Website: http://www.azahcccs.gov/

Arizona Health Care Cost Containment System
(AHCCCS) is Arizona's Medicaid agency that offers
health care programs to serve Arizona residents. Individuals must meet certain income and other requirements to obtain services.

Arizona Ombudsman – Citizen's Aide
3737 N. 7th Street Suite 209
Phoenix, AZ 85014
Tel: (602) 277 7292
Toll Free: (800) 872 2879
Website: http://www.azleg.state.az.us/ombudsman

For help and advice.

ABIL
Central Avenue Office 2400 N. Central Ave.
Phoenix, AZ 85004
Tel: (602) 296 0551 or (602) 256 0184
Email: boardofdirectors@abil.org
Website: http://www.abil.org

ABIL – Arizona Bridge to Independent Living.

Advocates of Northern Arizona
Flagstaff, AZ 86004
Tel: (928) 221 7864
Contact Name: Kathleen Temple
Email: advocatesofnorthernarizona@gmail.com
Website: http://advocatesofnorthernarizona.weebly.com

Professional advocates to assist in IEP, 504 Plan, or
IFSP processes.

Arizona Advocates
Glendale, AZ 85304
(602) 471 0346
Contact Name: Kim Yamamoto

Email: Kimyamamoto@me.com
Website: http://Www.azvice.com

Special education and 504 advocacy, assisting families in the IEP and 504 process.

Arizona Autism Coalition
300 N 18th St
Phoenix, AZ 85006
Tel: (480) 268 1453
Contact Name: Jessica Lewis
Email: jessica@azautism.org
Website: http://www.azautism.org

Improves the lives of individuals with ASD. Provides resources and advocacy.

Arizona Center For Disability Law
100 North Stone Ave. Suite 305
Tucson, AZ 85701
Tel: (520) 327 9547
Toll Free: (800) 922 1447

And

3839 N. Third St. Suite 209
Phoenix, AZ 85012
Tel: (602) 274 6287
Toll Free: (800) 927 2260
Email: center@azdisabilitylaw.org
Website: http://www.acdl.com

AZ Transitions Chandler, AZ
Tel: (480) 274 4541
Contact Name: Kelly McGuire
Email: Info@kellymcguireadvocate.com
Website: http://www.kellymcguireadvocate.com

Assists families and individuals with disabilities; from k-12 advocacy to college and employment search and preparations.

Cates & Sargeant Law Group, PLLC
1747 E. Morten Suite 202
Phoenix, AZ 85020
Tel: (602) 296 3434
Contact Name: Dwane Cates
Email: dwanecateslaw@gmail.com
Website: http://www.criminallawyer4u.com

The Cates & Sargeant Law Group, PLLC is a criminal defense law firm specializing and offering individuals with disabilities free legal consultations.

Kirsch-Goodwin & Kirsch, PLLC
8900 East Pinnacle Peak Rd. Suite 250
Scottsdale, AZ 85255
Tel: (480) 585 0600
Contact Name: Lori Kirsch-Goodwin, Esq.
Email: lkg@kgklaw.com
Website: http://www.azwpecialeducationlawyers.com

Special Education attorneys.

Academy of Special Needs Answers AZ
Website: http://www.specialneedsanswers.com

Frazer, Ryan, Goldberg & Arnold LLP
3101 N Central Avenue Suite 1600
Phoenix, AZ 85012
Tel: (602) 277 2010
Website: http://www.frgaglaw.com

Specialize in special needs particularly special needs trusts.

Phoenix Injury Lawyer
101 W Commonwealth Ave
Chandler, AZ 85225
Tel: (480) 634 7480
Contact Name: Christy Thompson
Email: christymthompson11@gmail.com
Website: http://www.phxinjurylaw.com

Focuses on personal injury law, including assisting families with adults and children with ASD addressing ongoing medical law needs.

Bart Stevens Special Needs Planning, LLC
4121 E. Palo Brea Ln.
Cave Creek, AZ 85331
Tel: (480) 991 0909
Toll Free: (888) 447 2525
Contact Name: Bart Stevens, ChLAP

Gabrielle M. Luoma, CPA, PLLC
7225 N. Mona Lisa Rd. Ste 210
Tucson, AZ 85742
 (520) 572 1248
Contact Name: Levon Lamy
Email: llamy@gmlcpa.com
Website: http://www.gmlcpa.com

Tax and accounting services.

Northwestern Mutual
1760 E River Rd. Suite 427
Tucson, AZ 85718
Tel: (520) 481 9730
Contact Name: Cailen McDonagh, Financial Representative
Email: Cailen.McDonagh@nm.com

Special needs financial planning.

Special Needs Planning
1640 S. Stapley Dr. Suite 209
Mesa, AZ 85204
Tel: (480) 641 1315
Contact Name: Wendy Kenney
Email: wkenney@metlife.com

SpecialCareSM
MassMutual Financial Group 17550 N. Perimeter Dr., #450
Scottsdale, AZ 85255
Tel: (480) 538 2950
Contact Name: Karen Starbowski, SpecialCare Planner
Email: SpecialCareAZ@massmutual.com
Website: http://www.massmutual.com/specialcare
Special needs financial planning.

Arizona Fiduciaries Association
Scottsdale, AZ 85267
Tel: (480) 220 1766
Email: charity@azfid.org
Website: http://www.azfid.org
Website: http://www.guardianship.org
Provides help with guardianship issues.

KidsCare – Arizona's Children's Health Insurance Program (CHIP)
701 E Jefferson St
Phoenix, AZ 85034
Tel: (602) 417 5437
Email: ApplicationHelp@azahcccs.gov
Website: http://www.azahcccs.gov/applicants/categories/KidsCare.aspx

Northern Arizona Chapter of the Autism Society of America
Flagstaff, AZ 86011
Tel: (928) 523 4870
Email: info@nazasa.org
Provides resources to those with ASD, families, medical professionals, educators, and all those with an interest in helping individuals with ASD.

STOMP Central Regional Office
Sierra Vista, AZ 85650
Tel: (520) 458 7911
Email: amartinez@washingtonpave.com
Website: http://www.stompproject.org
Federally funded Parent Training and Information Center established to assist military families who have children with special education or health needs.

Arizona Early Intervention Program (AzEIP)
801A-6 3839 North Third Street
Phoenix, AZ 85012
Tel: (602) 532 9960
Toll Free: (888) 439 5609 (in AZ)
Contact Name: Molly Dries Bright, DES/AzEIP Executive Director
Email: mdries@azdes.gov
Website: http://www.azdes.gov/azeip

Community and Recreation Services

AIRES
824 E. Ft. Lowell Rd.
Tucson, AZ 85719
Tel: (520) 623 0962
District director: Kimberly Huffman
Website: http://www.aires.org

American Focus Care
14620 North Cave Creek Road Ste#6
Phoenix, AZ 85022
Tel: (602)-595-4677
Contact Name: American Focus Care Team
Email: afcinquiry@yahoo.com
Website: http://www.americanfocuscare.com

Arion Care Solutions, LLC.
1405 N Dobson Rd Suite 3
Chandler, AZ 85224
Tel: (480) 722 1300
Website: http://www.arioncaresolutions.com
Arion Care Solutions LLC is contracted statewide to provide 7Attendant Care, Habilitation, Respite, Housekeeping and Individually Designed Living Arrangements.

Arizona Care Poviders, LLC.
2432 W Peoria Ave. Suite 1048
Phoenix, AZ 85029
Tel: (602) 635 4220
Email: admin@azcareproviders.com
Website: http://www.azcareproviders.com

Best Buddies Arizona
1940 E Camelback Rd. Suite 205
Phoenix, AZ 85016
Tel: (602) 954 3877
Contact Name: Deona Cole
Email: DeonaCole@bestbuddies.org
Website: http://www.bestbuddiesarizona.org
Creates opportunities for one-to-one friendships, integrated employment and leadership development for people with intellectual and developmental disabilities.

Bethany Ranch Home, Inc.
6130 N 16th St
Phoenix, AZ 85016
Tel: (602) 279 5448
Website: http://www.bethanyranchhome.org

Bethany Ranch Home is a long-term care agency for the developmentally disabled with a holistic approach to meeting their needs.

Chapel Haven West
1701 N Park Ave.
Tucson, AZ 85719
Tel: (877) 824 9378
Contact Name: Kenneth Hosto, director.
Email: khosto@chapelhaven.org
Website: http://www.chapelhaven.org/west

Provides residential transition and lifelong supports for adults 18+ with mild developmental disabilities and ASD.

Echoing Hope Ranch
PO Box 4471
Bisbee, AZ 85603
Contact Name: Marla Guerrero, President
Email: info@echoinghoperanch.org
Website: http://www.echoinghoperanch.org

Fenix Group
919 North Dysart Rd. Suite V
Avondale, AZ 85323
Tel: (602) 377 6759 or (623) 882 2016
Contact Name: Kim Dorshaw
Email: kdorshaw@fenixgroup.co
Website: http://www.fenixgroup.co

Provides day program and respite services and supportive programs.

Good Neighbor Support Services
15655 W. Roosevelt St. #213
Goodyear, AZ 85338
Tel: (623) 932 4878
Contact Name: Operations Supervisor
Email: support@gncares.com
Website: http://www.gncares.com

In-home non-medical care services for the elderly and individuals with developmental disabilities.

Inteli-Care, LLC
1345 E. Main St #110
Mesa, AZ 85203
Tel: (480) 969 5480
Contact Name: Brian
Email: intelicare@yahoo.com
Website: http://www.inteli-care.com

Inteli-Care provides HCBS services (respite, habilitation, attendant care, housekeeping) and Day Programs for individuals with developmental disabilities of all ages.

Gryphen Specialty Products and Services
1301 E. University Drive, Suite 130
Tempe, AZ 85281
Tel: (480) 966 9500
Contact Name: Jill Houtchens
Email: jhoutchens@gryphensps.com
Website: http://www.gryphensps.com

Provides a variety of day options to individuals with developmental disabilities, with a goal of independence to the best of an individual's ability.

Guthrie Mainstream Services
3200 N. Dobson Bldg. E
Chandler, AZ 85224
Tel: (480) 491 5553
Contact Name: Terry Guthrie (CEO)
Email: terryg@gmsaz.org
Website: http://www.guthriemainstream.org

Adaptive Recreation Services
1946 West Morningside Drive
Phoenix, AZ 85023
Tel: (602) 262 4543
Website: https://www.phoenix.gov/parks/adaptive-recreation

A range of adaptive services offered by Phoenix parks and recreation.

Glendale- Peoria YMCA – Special Needs Swim Instruction
14711 N. 59th Avenue
Glendale, AZ 85306
See map: Google Maps
Tel: (602) 588 9622
Contact Name: Shelly Smith
Email: slbrown@vosymca.org
Website: http://www.glendale-peoriaymca.org

Ott Family YMCA – Special Needs Swim Instruction
401 S. Prudence Road
Tuscon, AZ 85710
See map: Google Maps
Tel: (520) 885 2317
Contact Name: Kate Saavedra
Email: kates@tucsonymca.org
Website: http://www.tucsonymca.org/selectionSwimSportsPlay.cfm

Tucson branch of YMCA offering swim instruction.

Blue Sky Fitness
2509 N Campbell Ave.
Tuscon, AZ 85719
Tel: (520) 323 3146
Tel: (520) 247 8160 Cell
Contact Name: Robert Chris Rooney, Director
Email: crooney@blueskyfitrec.com
Website: http://blueskyfitrec.com

Fitness and recreation program for children and adults with a developmental, emotional and/or psychiatric disability.

Gilbert Parks and Recreation
Gilbert Community Services 90 E Civic Center Dr
Gilbert, AZ 85296
Tel: (480) 503 6200

Gilbert offers a wide variety of activities and programs for residents with Special Needs. Activities include dances, bowling, karaoke, cheerleading, movies and more.

KEEN Phoenix
PO Box 45186
Phoenix, AZ 85028
Tel: (602) 508 3939
Contact Name: Johanna Bookbinder
Email: jbookbinder@keenphoenix.org
Website: http://www.keenphoenix.org

KEEN is a national, nonprofit volunteer-led organization that provides one-to-one recreational opportunities for children and young adults with developmental and physical disabilities at no cost to their families and caregivers.

Noel's Barn
Tuscon, AZ 85740
Tel: (520) 975 9103

Horseback riding and equestrian sports.

One Step Beyond, Inc.
9299 West Olive Ave. Suite 311
Peoria, AZ 85345
Tel: (623) 266 7490
Tel: (623) 215 2449
Contact Name: Justin Watson
Email: justinwatson@osbi.org
Website: http://www.osbi.org

Provides programs to empower individuals with developmental disability to achieve optimal independence, meaningful employment, significant social relationships, and full participation in the community.

Penny Pulz Golf Program for Autistic Kids
Sun City Country Club 9433 N 107th Ave
Sun City, AZ 85351
Tel: (623) 298 2781
Email: Academy@PennyPulzGolf.com
Website: http://www.pennypulzgolf.com/autistic_golf_program.asp

Penny Pulz, 2 time LPGA Champion and LPGA Top 50 Teacher 2008 and 2004, works with children and adults who have mental disabilities.

Phoenix Public Library
1221 N. Central Ave.
Phoenix, AZ 85004
Tel: (602) 261 8690
Email: specialneeds@phxlib.org.
Website: http://www.phoenixpubliclibrary.org

Library services for those with special needs.

ResCare HomeCare Arizona
(866) 737 2273
Contact Name: Cathy Shiroda
Email: cshiroda@rescare.com
Website: http://rescarehomecare.com

Provides habilitation and respite services, as well as a variety of other supports, to people living in their own homes.

Rusty's Morningstar Ranch
PO Box 759
Cornville, AZ 86325
Tel: (928) 634 4784
Contact Name: Marla Guerrero, Executive Director - Cornville, Arizona
Email: marla@rmr.org
Website: http://www.rmr.org

A home for adults with autism on a 10-acre ranch where residents take part in work program therapies and traditional therapies.

STARS Transition Program
11130 E. Cholla St
Scottsdale, AZ 85215
4803712342
(480) 607 1301
Contact Name: Krista Anderson
Email: kanderson@starsaz.org
Website: http://www.starsaz.org/

This program is designed to foster vocational skills in a fun, interactive environment. Activities include art classes, cooking classes, community outings and recreational activities.

T.E.A.M. Habilitation & Respite
12625 N. Saguaro Blvd. Suite 116
Fountain Hills, AZ 85268
Tel: (480) 816 1866
Contact Name: Donna M. Barelski, PhD.
Email: donnabarelski@teamhabilitation.com
Website: http://www.teamhabilitation.com

Provides daily in-home Habilitation and Respite care to persons with ASD and other developmental delays.

The Madasun Lee Foundation
1470 E Hammer
Fort Mohave, AZ 86426
Tel: (928) 716 2767
Contact Name: Mallorie Rich
Email: richmn720@gmail.com

Offers family support groups, family meet ups, and trying to bring more resources and activities to Mohave County, AZ.

The Tungland Corporation
240 Jennifer Lane Suite 201
Cottonwood, AZ 86326
Tel: (928) 649 9305
Website: http://www.tungland.com

The Tungland Corporation (TTC) offers support services for children, adolescents, adults and elders, including day treatment programs, in-home respite, habilitation and attendant care, to specialized living arrangements, foster or host homes, counseling, consulting, and employment/vocational support services.

Tuscon Branch
5049 E. Broadway Suite 114
Tucson, AZ 85711
Tel: (520) 745 8777
Website: http://www.tungland.com
Tucson branch of the Tungland Corporation.

Youth Evaluation and Treatment Centers (YETC)
4414 N. 19th Ave
Phoenix, AZ 85015
Tel: (602) 285 5550
Website: http://www.yetc.org

Dedicated to partnering with youth and families to provide knowledge, skills, independence and stability.

AZ ASSIST
Tempe, AZ 85202
Tel: (480) 779 0899
Contact Name: Debbie Weidinger, Executive Director
Email: info@azassist.com
Website: http://www.azassist.com

AZ ASSIST provides information to families of teens and young adults with ASD about public and private services and opportunities to promote independent living and access to a variety of employment options, post-secondary education, and social opportunities.

East Valley Autism Network
2068 S. Sailors Court
Gilbert, AZ 85295
Tel: (480) 231 4214
Contact Name: Melissa van Hook
Email: melissavanhook@hotmail.com
Website: http://eastvalleyautismnetwork.blogspot.com

Parent-led support group providing hope, resources, information, and support for families with children with ASD.

Grupo De Apoya Para Latinos Con Autismo
P.O Box 13425
Tempe, AZ 85284
Tel: (480) 772 7961 or (480) 967 4256
Contact Name: Lorena Palacios Gomez
Email: lorena@arizongala.org
Website: http://www.arizonagala.org

Serves and supports minority individuals with developmental disabilities and their families. GALA's main focus is on the Hispanic/Latino autism community in Arizona and provides resources and services in Spanish.

P.A.C.T. Parenting Autism Challenges Together
Kingman, AZ 86401
Tel: (928) 757 2288
Contact Name: Crystal D. Miller
Email: pact_of_kingman@yahoo.com
Website: http://www.pactaz.com

A support group providing resources, workshops, and topics to assist parents; it services a large area of Mohave and La Paz county.

Child Care Resource and Referral
Association for Supportive Child Care 3910 South Rural Road
Tempe, AZ 85282
Tel: (602) 244 2678
Email: becky@arizonachildcare.org
Website: http://www.arizonachildcare.org
Website: http://www.asccaz.org

Dads 4 Special Kids, Inc.
PO Box 73182
Phoenix, AZ 85050
Tel: (602) 909 5463
Contact Name: Ray Morris

Email: ray@dads4specialkids.com
Website: http://www.dads4specialkids.org

Dads 4 Special Kids is an organization for men that have a child with special needs in their lives.

Phoenix High Functioning Autism/Asperger Family Network
4512 E Juniper Avenue
Phoenix, AZ 85032
Tel: (602) 492 8033
Email: hfautism@cox.net
Website: http://www.phoenixautism.com

Pilot Parents of Southern Arizona
2600 North Wyatt Drive
Tucson, AZ 85712
Tel: (520) 324 3150
Email: ppsa@pilotparents.org
Website: http://www.pilotparents.org

PVPAG
Coco's 4514 E Cactus Rd
Phoenix, AZ 85032
Tel: (480) 585 9312
Contact Name: Cynthia Macluskie
Email: cynthia.marksmom@cox.net

This group is all parents of children with autism spectrum disorders.

West Valley Autism Parent Support Group
New Life Community Church 8155 W Thunderbird Road
Peoria, AZ 85381
Tel: (623) 572 5289

Yuma Autism Support Group
399 West 32nd Street
Yuma, AZ 85364
Contact Name: Gwen Conner
Email: autismyuma@yahoo.com
Website: http://autismyuma.cfsites.org

S-Club
Glendale, AZ 85304
(602) 471 0346
Contact Name: Kim Yamamoto
Email: Kimyamamoto@me.com

Promotes and teaches social skills, language, and real world situations.

Raising Special Kids
5025 E. Washington St #204
Phoenix, AZ 85034

Tel: (602) 242 4366
Toll Free: (800) 237 3007
Email: info@raisingspecialkids.org
Website: http://www.raisingspecialkids.org

Providing support, training, information, and individual assistance so families of individuals from birth to age 26 can become effective advocates.

Recovering Our Kids Biomedical Organization
5042 E. Lucia Drive
Cave Creek, AZ 85331
Tel: (480) 563 8215
Contact Name: Cynthia McCluskie
Email: cynthia.marksmom@cox.net
Website: http://www.vsan.org/rok-az

Kris' Camp
3925 E. Devonshire Ave
Phoenix, AZ 85018
Tel: (602) 366 5867
Contact Name: Camp Director: Michelle Hardy, MT-BC, NMT
Email: michelle@kriscamp.org
Website: http://www.kriscamp.org

The Kris' Camp Arizona therapy camp focuses on children with ASD ages 4–15.

Desert Dragons Kenpo Karate
9836 W Yearling Rd. Bldg "F", Ste 1360
Peoria, AZ 85383
(623) 670 7979
Contact Name: Julie Gonzalez
Email: Julie@Desertdragonsaz.com
Website: http://www.Desertdragonsaz.com

Desert Dragons Kenpo Karate offers an Adaptive Martial arts program for children with developmental disabilities.

Stable Influence Charity Programs
P.O. Box 54006
Phoenix, AZ 85078
Tel: (623) 465 0637
Email: stableinfl@aol.com
Website: http://www.stableinfluence.org

WEDCO Employment and Training Center
Phoenix, AZ
Tel: (602)-274-2605 or (520) 584 8648
Email: jims@wedco.net
Website: http://www.wedco.net/

Provides comprehensive rehabilitative and employment support services in a partnership with all stakeholders, including individuals, businesses, and other institutions.

ARKANSAS

Doctors, Clinics, Hospitals, and Other Health Services

Arkansas Autism Alliance
Website: arkansasautismalliance.org
A collaboration of researchers and clinicians researching autism causes and treatments and providing care to children with ASD. The site offers information on research, clinical care and other information for parents.

Ascent Children's Health Services
806 Glendale St
Jonesboro, AR 72401
Tel: (870) 933.9528
Email: info@ascentchs.com
Website: http://www.ascentchs.com/

Provides developmental early intervention day treatment services and outpatient therapeutic and mental health services to children, adolescents, and families throughout central, northeast, and southern Arkansas.

Arkansas Children's Hospital
Neuroscience Center, South Wing, 2nd Floor 1
Children's Way Little Rock, AR 72202-3591
Tel: (501) 364 4000, Enter Option 5 for Pod 5

The clinic provides multi-specialty treatment services for children formally diagnosed with ASD. Treatments include Gastroenterology, Nutrition, Genetics and Genetic Counseling, Neurology and Sleep Disorders.

Autism Treatment Network Clinic
James L. Dennis Developmental Center
1301 Wolfe Street
Little Rock, AR 72202
Tel: (501) 364 1830

Offers diagnosis and evaluation by developmental pediatricians.

Lowell Pharmacy
114 Harrison Avenue
Lowell, AR 72745
Tel: (479) 770 0111
Contact Name: Sumer Brandon
Email: info@c-rx.com
Website: http://www.c-rx.com

Compounding pharmacy for special medication needs.

Pediatric Dentistry of Eastern Arkansas (PDEA)
4850 N Washington St.
Forrest City, AR 72335
Tel: (870) 630 1500
Website: http://www.pdeakids.com

Provides dental services for children with ASD from infancy to teens.

UT Medical Group
Pediatric Neurology
Crittenden County Memorial Hospital 200 West Tyler Avenue
West Memphis, AR 72301
Tel: (870) 735 1500
Toll Free: (866) 278 4966
Website: http://www.utmedicalgroup.com

Therapy Services

ACCESS Group Inc.
10618 Breckenridge Drive
Little Rock, AR 72211
Tel: (501) 217 8600
Contact Name: Beth Rice
Email: info@accessgroupinc.org
Website: http://www.accessgroupinc.org

ACCESS Group Inc. offers comprehensive resources and services for children with language learning disabilities.

First Step Arkansas
407 Carson Street PO Box 2440
Hot Springs, AR 71914
Tel: (501) 624 6468
Website: http://firststeparkansas.com

First Step offers programs and services to individuals with developmental disabilities and delays.

Jonesboro Human Development Center
4701 Colony Drive
Jonesboro, AR 72404
Tel: (870) 932 5230
Contact Name: Forrest Steele, Superintendent
Email: Forrest.Steele@arkansas.gov
Website: http://humanservices.arkansas.gov/ddds/Pages/JonesboroHDC.aspx

The center emphasizes individualized services focusing on dignity, respect, training, and support for people who reside there.

Bost Human Development Services
PO Box 11495
Fort Smith, AR 72917
Tel: (479) 478 5596

Contact Name: Jeff Lambert, Assistant Executive Director
Email: jlambert@bost.org
Website: http://www.bost.org

Bost is a community-based, not-for-profit agency dedicated to developing services for and providing services to individuals with developmental disabilities in Western Arkansas and adjacent regions.

Pathfinder, Inc.
Various Facilities
Jacksonville, AR 72076
Email: icfmr@pathfinderinc.org
Website: www.pathfinderinc.org

Provides an array of services for individuals with disabilities, like ASD, living in Arkansas.

Helping Hand Children's Center
4901 Northshore Dr.
North Little Rock, AR 72118
Tel: (Tel: (501)) 791 3331
Email: info@helpinghandcc.com
Website: http://www.helpinghandcc.com

Schools and Educational Services

Forrester-Davis Development Center
1000 Buchanan Street
Clarksville, AR 72830
Tel: (479) 754 6210
Website: http://www.forresterdavis.com

Provides a wide range of services to individuals with disabilities age 6 weeks through adults.

Autism Support Program at the University of Arkansas
117 Peabody University of Arkansas
Fayetteville, AR 72701
Tel: (479) 595 6071
Contact Name: Aleza Greene
Email: asgreene@uark.edu
Website: http://coehp.uark.edu/10656.php

Program provides comprehensive services to students in the areas of academics, social skills and transitioning to independent adult roles.

College for Living
5200 South Thompson Avenue
Springdale, AR 72764
Tel: (479) 713 1171
Website: http://www.lifestylesinc.org/cfl.php

College for Living (CFL) is the educational arm of Life Styles. Classes and activities are designed to go beyond the basics and offer individuals enrichment programs such as Money Management, Rights and Responsibilities, Relationships, Safety and Voter Education, along with recreational classes and activities.

Grow Learning Centre
5 Remington Cove
Little Rock, AR 72207
Tel: (501) 850 8788
Toll Free: (800) 556 GROW (4769)
Contact Name: Lindsey Berardi
Email: lindsey@growlearningcentre.com
Website: http://www.growlearningcentre.com

Grow Learning Centre is a comprehensive day treatment program for children ages 6 weeks through 6 years with developmental challenges. Individualized treatment plans utilize the SCERTS model.

The Jones Learning Center at University of the Ozarks
415 North College Ave.
Clarksville, AR 72830
Tel: (479) 979 1403
Contact Name: Julia Frost
Email: jfrost@ozarks.edu
Website: http://www.ozarks.edu/jlc

Provides support that emphasizes social thinking skills for college students with ASD, with specific training in social and life skills as well as comprehensive academic support.

Legal, Government & Financial Services

Department of Housing and Urban Development
425 West Capitol Avenue Suite 1000
Little Rock, AR 72201
Tel: (501) 918 5700
Contact Name:
Alice Rufus
Email: AR_Webmanager@hud.gov

Arkansas Division of Medical Services
Donaghey Plaza South P.O. Box 1437, Slot S401
Little Rock, AR 72203
Toll Free: (800) 482 8988
https://www.medicaid.state.ar.us/

The Department of Human Services (DHS) runs the Medicaid program in Arkansas.

Arkansas Advocates for Children and Families
1400 W Markham St. Suite 306
Little Rock, AR 72201

Tel: (501) 371 9678
Email: connect@aradvocates.org
Website: http://www.aradvocates.org

Protects and promotes through research, education and advocacy the rights and well-being of Arkansas children and their families.

Arkansas Rehabilitation Services

3 Capitol Mall
Little Rock, AR 72201
Toll Free: (800) 330 0632
Website: http://ace.arkansas.gov/arRehabServices/Pages/default.aspx

Provides a variety of training and career preparation programs.

Disability Rights Center

Evergreen Place Suite 201
Little Rock, AR 72207
Tel: (501) 296 1775
Website: http://www.arkdisabilityrights.org

Disability Rights Arkansas (DRA) is the independent, private, nonprofit organization designated by the governor of Arkansas to implement the federally funded and authorized protection and advocacy systems throughout the state.

Law Office of Thomas G. Buchanan

217 W. Second Street Suite 115
Little Rock, AR 72201
Tel: (501) 296 9820
Contact Name: Thomas Buchanan
Email: thomasbuchananlaw@yahoo.com
Website: http://www.thomasbuchananlaw.com

Disability injury, accident, and medical malpractice attorneys. These disability and injury attorneys offer free legal consultations to anyone in need of expert legal counsel or representation in the state of Arkansas.

Arkansas Special Education Law Firm

10515 W. Markham Street Suite H-9
Little Rock, AR 72205
Tel: (501) 823 0550
Website: http://www.arkspedlaw.com

Hilburn, Calhood, Harper, Pruniski & Calhoun, Ltd.

US Bank Building One Riverfront Place, Eighth Floor,
PO Box 5551
North Little Rock, AR 72114
Tel: (501) 372 0110
Contact Name: Sam Hilburn
Email: shilburn@hilburnlawfirm.com

Website: http://www.hilburnlawfirm.com

Kieklak Law Firm

1 E Center St. #140
Fayetteville, AR 72701
Tel: (479) 251 7767
Contact Name: Ken Kieklak, Attorney at Law
Email: kieklaklawfirm@gmail.com
Website: http://www.kieklaklawfirm.com

Arkansas Social Security Disability lawyers handling claims for adults and children with ASD and processing Supplemental Security Income specifically designed for children diagnosed with ASD.

Raymond B. Harvey, Esq.

650 S. Shackleford Rd. Suite 400
Little Rock, AR 72211
Tel: (501) 221 3416
Email: rharvey@arkansaselderlaw.com
Website: http://www.arkansaselderlaw.com

NWA Autism Support Group

1200 W. Walnut Street
Bentonville, AR 72756
Tel: (479) 925 4044 or (479) 925 4044
Contact Name: Traci Sickels
Email: traci@nwaautismsupport.com
Website: http://www.nwaautismsupport.com

Northwestern Mutual

650 S. Shackleford #300
Little Rock, AR 72211
Tel: (501) 228 9300
Contact Name: Matt Hall
Email: matt.hall@nm.com
Website: http://matthall.nm.com/

Provides special needs financial planning.

Community and Recreation Services

Civitan Services

121 Cox
Benton, AR 72015
Tel: (501) 776 0691
Contact Name: Carrie Schatz
Email: cschatz@civitanservices.com
Website: http://www.civitanservices.com

Civitan Services provides quality educational and life skills training for people with developmental disabilities.

DaySpring Behavioral Health Services of Arkansas

20 Locations throughout the State
AR

Tel: (479) 872 5580
Email: arinfo@dayspringbhs.com
Website: http://www.dayspringbhs.com

Delta Resource Independent Living Center
1514 South Poplar
Pine Bluff, AR 71601
Toll Free: (800) 824 0009
Website: http://www.ar-ilc.org/drc.htm

Provides services, support and advocacy, enabling people with severe disabilities to live as independently as possible.

Elizabeth Richardson Center
3917 S. Old Missouri Rd.
Springdale, AR 72764
Tel: (479) 872 1Toll Free: (800)
Email: admin@ercinc.org
Website: http://www.richardsoncenter.org/adultServices

The Elizabeth Richardson Center provides services to adults ages 18 and over in a wide variety of programs including Skills for Life training, Job Placement, Contract Work, and Residential services.

Independent Living Services
PO Box 1070
Conway, AR 72032
Tel: (501) 327 5234
Website: http://indliving.org/services/residential

Millcreek of Arkansas
PO Box 727
Fordyce, AR 71742
Tel: (Tel: (870)) 352 8203
Email: info.mc-ar@yfcs.com
Website: http://www.millcreekofarkansas.com

Arkansas Support Network (ASN)
6836 Isaac Orchard's Rd.
Springdale, AR 72762
Tel: (479) 927 4100
Toll Free: (800) 748 9768
Contact Name: Keith Vire, CEO
Email: kvire@supports.org
Website: http://www.supports.org

Independent Case Management (ICM)
13310 Kanis Road
Little Rock, AR 72211
Tel: (501) 412 1768

ICM is a (501)(c)(3) non-profit organization. Provides support to individuals with developmental disabilities.

Focus Adult Development Programs
410 East Hale
Osceola, AR 72370
Tel: (870) 563 0012
Contact Name: Annette Thomas
Email: focus31945@sbc-global.net

And

904 Speedway
Trumann, AR 72472
Tel: (870) 483 7942
Contact Name: Ruth Dunn
Email: focus5@cebridge.net

And

70 Church Road
Paragrould, AR 72450
Tel: (870) 586 8100
Contact Name: Tina Chapple
Email: focusparagould@bscn.com
Website: http://www.focusinconline.org

Friendship Community Care, Inc
920 North University
Russellville, AR 72802
Tel: (479) 967 2322
Website: http://www.friendshipcommunitycare.org

Friendship Community Care, Inc. is a nonprofit organization working to build care-based communities for children, adults, and seniors with disabilities.

Life Styles, Inc.
2471 West Sycamore Street
Fayetteville, AR 72703
Tel: (479) 521 3581
Website: http://www.lifestylesinc.org

Life Styles supports individuals with developmental disabilities in reaching their full potential as contributing members of the community.

Ozark Regional Transit
2423 E. Robinson Ave
Springdale, AR 72764
(Tel: (479)) 756 5901
Website: http://www.ozark.org/index.php/en/riding-ort/ada-paratransit

The paratransit service is a "safety net", and is only for those persons who do not have the functional capability to access the fixed route bus system.

CALIFORNIA

Doctors, Clinics, Hospitals, and Other Health Services

All Kids Dental Surgery Center
2525 Eye Street suite 100
Bakersfield, CA 93301
Tel: (661) 325 5437
Contact Name: Vickie Kasprzyk
Email: kasgilnursing@sbcglobal.net

Behavioral/Neuro-Optometrist
17524 Yorba Linda Blvd
Yorba Linda, CA 92886
Tel: (714) 996 6210
Contact Name: K. Sharieff
Email: kvsharieff@gmail.com

Calabasas Pediatric Dentistry
23695 Calabasas Road
Calabasas, CA 91302
Tel: (818) 222 4543
Contact Name: Elena Rumack, DDS
Email: calabasaspediatricdentistry@hotmail.com
Website: http://www.calabasaspediatricdentistry.com

California Pacific Medical Center
California West Campus 3700 California Street
San Francisco, CA 94118
Tel: (415) 600 6200
Website: http://www.cpmc.org/advanced/pediatrics/
services/child_development.html

Provides comprehensive developmental assessment and treatment programs for infants, preschoolers, school-age children, and families.

Cindy Schneider, MD
5949 Lankershim Boulevard
North Hollywood, CA 91601
Tel: (323) 850 7177
Website: www.center4autism.com

The Children's Dental Health Center
4655 Hoen Ave Suite #1
Santa Rosa, CA 95405
Tel: (707) 546 5437
Contact Name: Shana Berger Van Cleave, DDS
Email: nokandy@gmail.com
Website: http://nokandy.com

Dan Rossignol, MD FAAFP, FMAPS
Rossignol Medical Center
16251 Laguna Canyon Road
Suite 175

Irvine, CA 92618-3623
Tel: (949) 428 8878
Website: www.rossignolmedicalcenter.com/
Provides comprehensive biomedical treatments to children with ASD and other conditions.

Daniel and Davis Optometry
3144 El Camino Real Suite 202
Carlsbad, CA 92008
Tel: (760) 434 3314
Website: http://www.optometrists.org/Carlsbad

Donna Ruiz, MD
1601 El Camino Real
Suite 101
Belmont, CA 94002
Tel: (650) 595 KIDS
Website: www.wholechildwellness.com

Elisa Song, MD
1601 El Camino Real
Suite 101
Belmont, CA 94002
Tel: (650) 595 KIDS
Website: www.wholechildwellness.com

Eric Sletten, MD
64 North Brent Street
Suite A
Ventura, CA 93003
Tel: (805) 643 7902
Website: www.slettenwellness.com

Happy Kids Dental Planet
Pediatric Dentist & Orthodontist
11980 San Vincente Blvd. Suite 901
Los Angeles, CA 90049
Tel: (310) 826 6075
Contact Name: Dr. Shahrzad Sami
Email: drsherrysami@gmail.com
Website: http://www.Happykidsdentalplanet.com

A dual specialized pediatric dentist and orthodontist with extensive training in ASD.

Hela Kammoun Bali, MNRI Core Specialist
Brain Reconnection
14271 Jeffrey Road #2541929
Main Street #103
Irvine, CA 92620
Tel: (949) 307 6914
Website: www.brainreconnection.com

Hirani Medical Wellness Center
Karima Hirani, MD
9736 Venice Boulevard
Los Angeles, CA 90066

Tel: (310) 559 6634
Website: www.drhirani.com

A comprehensive alternative treatment center offering many different treatment modalities to customize care.

Ingels Family Health
Darin Ingels, ND
5150 El Camino Real, Suite B14
Los Altos, CA 94022
Tel: (203) 254 9957
Email: info@ingelsfamilyhealth.com
Website: www.ingelsfamilyhealth.com

Dr. Ingels uses a variety of modalities to treat, among others, those with ASD and his practice emphasizes treatment of chronic immune dysfunction, including allergies, asthma, recurrent or persistent infections and other genetic or acquired immune problems.

Itani Dental San Francisco
450 Sutter St. Suite 2318
San Francisco, CA 94108
Tel: (415) 685 0011
Contact Name: Theresa Nguyen, RDA
Email: mail@itanidental.com
Website: http://www.SFOdentist.com or http://www.itanidental.com

Jerry Kartzinel, MD
Kartzinel Wellness Center
16263 Laguna Canyon Rd., Suite 150
Irvine CA 92618
Tel: (949) 398 7654
Website: www.drjerryk.com

Dr. Kartzinel is a board-certified pediatrician practicing Translational Medicine (translating diverse scientific findings into treatments for patients).

Julie Matthews CNC
Nourishing Hope
PO Box 170061
San Francisco, CA 94117
Tel: (415) 235 2960
Email: Appointments@NourishingHope.com
Website: www.nourishinghope.com

Based in Northern California, Julie Matthews consults with families around the country on individualized diet and nutrition programs to address a variety of health concerns, including ASD.

Karima Hirani, MD
9736 Venice Boulevard
Los Angeles, CA 90066
Tel: (310) 559 6634
Website: www.drhirani.com

Lollipop Pediatric Dentistry
1041 E Yorba Linda Blvd Suite 206
Placentia, CA 92870
Tel: (714) 528 8252
Contact Name: Dr. Mary Pham
Email: lollipopdental@gmail.com

Specially trained in introducing children with ASD.

Mobile Dental Hygiene Services
Mobile Dental Hygiene Services Folsom, CA 95758
Tel: (916) 717 7436
Contact Name: Jennifer Geier
Email: jennifer@thehappyhyjennist.com
Website: http://www.thehappyhyjennist.com

Provides oral evaluations and dental hygiene services for patients with special needs and homebound individuals.

Nancy Mullan, MD
2829 West Burbank Boulevard
Suite 202
Burbank, CA 91505
Tel: (818) 954 9267
Email: NancyMullanMD@aol.com
Website: www.nancymullanmd.com

Dr. Mullan provides an integrative approach to healthcare including nutrition and genetics-based supplementation to treat chronic health conditions, including ASD.

Pacific Palisades Pediatric Dentistry
881 Alma Real Drive Suite 315
Pacific Palisades, CA 90272
Tel: (310) 459 3088
Contact Name: Eddie Surger, D.D.S.
Email: info@PaliKidSmiles.com
Website: http://www.PaliKidSmiles.com

Peninsula Children's Dentistry
Purvi Zavery, DDS, MS, Pediatric Dentist
1390 El Camino Real Suite 150
San Carlos, CA 94070
Tel: (650) 394 4200
Email: info@PeninsulaKidsDDS.com
Website: http://www.PeninsulaKidsDDS.com

Rachel West, OD
1454 Cloverfield Blvd #200
Santa Monica, CA 90404
Tel: (310) 450 8959
Website: www.drrachelwest.com

Robert Sears, MD, FAAP
Sears Family Pediatrics
26933 Camino De La Estrella

Suite A
Capistrano Beach, CA 92624
Tel: (949) 493 5437
Website: www.AskDrSears.com

Sikka Dental Corporation
150 N Jackson Ave. Suite 203
San Jose, CA 95116
Tel: (408) 259 1280
Email: info@sikkadental.com
Website: http://www.sikkadental.com

Suzanne Goh, MD
Pediatric Neurology Therapeutics
3636 5th Avenue
San Diego, CA 92103

and

3530 Camino del Rio North, Suite 107
San Diego, CA 92108

and

11512 El Camino Real, Suite 350
San Diego, CA 92130
Tel: (858) 304 6440
Website: www.gohmd.org

Dr. Goh is board-certified pediatric neurologist with expertise in the evaluation and treatment of children with ASD and other neurological conditions. Dr. Goh uses a variety of approaches in assessing and treating patients, including biomedical interventions, and among other things, assesses patients for underlying metabolic and mitochondrial conditions.

Valley Mountain Regional Center (VMRC)
704 Mountain Ranch Rd. Suite 203
San Andreas, CA 95249
Tel: (209) 754 1871
Website: http://www.vmrc.net

Serves children and adults with developmental disabilities in San Joaquin, Stanislaus, Amador, Calaveras and Tuolumne counties. Free diagnosis and assessment services and ongoing services for qualifying individuals.

Wedieman Pediatric Denistry and Orthodontics
7916 Pebble Beach Dr. Suite 101
Citrus Heights, CA 95610
Tel: (916) 962 0577
Contact Name: Allison, Colleen or Karla
Email: khweideman@sbcglobal.net
Website: http://www.SacChildrensDentist.com

Wellness Integrative Naturopathic Center, Inc.
Jessica Tran, ND
Darin Ingels, ND
14795 Jeffrey Road, Suite 101
Irvine, CA 92618

Tel: (949) 551 8751
Fax: (949) 551 1272
Email: admin@wellnessintegrative.com
Website: www.wellnessintegrative.com

Treating children with ASD and others with a variety of health conditions using natural, integrative modalities.

Whole Family Wellness
Suruchi Chandra, MD
1601 El Camino Real
Suite 101
Belmont, CA 94002
Tel: (650) 595 5437
Website: www.wholefamilywellness.org

Integrative health care family practice for treatment of current conditions as well as preventative medicine.

Therapy Services

BIG FUN Therapy and Recreational Services
464 E. Walnut St.
Pasadena, CA 91101
Tel: (310) 837 7849
Toll Free: (877) BIG FUN8
Email: info@bigfungymnastics.com
Website: http://www.bigfungymnastics.com

Offers families throughout southern California occupational therapy services, gymnastics, swimming, after-school enrichment programs, social skills, camps, and more.

Bridges to Recovery
P.O. Box 1493
Pacific Palisades, CA 90272
Tel: (877) 586 5931
Email: info@bridgestorecovery.com
Website: http://www.bridgestorecovery.com

Bridges to Recovery offers individualized treatment programs including music therapy, art therapy, yoga, physical fitness and nutrition counseling.

Creative Solutions for Hope
3152 Red Hill, Ave, Suite #100
Costa Mesa, CA 92626
Tel: (714) 582 5936 or (714) 881 0427, ext. 1706
Contact Name: Asha Bhakta
Email: abhakta@cs4hope.com
Website: http://www.cs4hope.com

Creative Solutions for Hope uses ABA principles to create individualized instruction and strategies.

Early Childhood Treatment Center
3524 Torrance Blvd Suite 104
Torrance, CA 90503

Tel: (310) 540 1603
Contact Name: Christy Hovsepian; JeNae Waterfield
Email: jenae.w@pediatricminds.com

Hoofprints on the Heart Adaptive Riding Center
455 Olivina Avenue
Livermre, CA 94551
Tel: (925) 449 9090
Contact Name: Gina Rutigliano
Email: office@hoofprintsontheheart.com
Website: http://www.hotharc.org
Therapeutic riding program.

Joan M. Pagan
24564 Hawthorne Blvd. Suite 209
Torrance, CA 90505
Tel: (310) 465 6138
Contact Name: Joan Marie Pagan
Email: SouthBayTherapy@gmail.com

Offers psychotherapy for children and adolescents with ASD and works with families with children with developmental disabilities.

Leaf Wing Center
7149 Woodley Ave.
Van Nuys, CA 91406
Tel: (818) 442 0921 or (714) 634 8500
Contact Name: John Lubbers
Email: jlubbers@leafwingcenter.org
Website: http://www.leafwingcenter.org
ABA programs for children with ASD.

Learning Dynamics, Inc.
22837 Ventura Blvd. Suite 200
Woodland Hills, CA 91364
Tel: (310) 855 3276
Contact Name: Nicole Brown, Psy.D., Founder and Executive Director
Email: info@learningdynamicsinc.org
Website: http://www.learningdynamicsinc.org

Provides services for high-functioning individuals with Autism, ADHD, learning disabilities, and other difficulties. Offers psychoeducational, neuropsychological, and diagnostic testing.

Meli Music
Sun Valley, CA 91353
Tel: (818) 394 0649 or (818) 397 5170
Contact Name: Melissa St. John, MM, MT-BC
Email: Melissa@MeliMusicLA.com
Website: http://www.MeliMusicLA.com

Meli Music provides music therapy (individual & group) and music lessons (traditional & adapted) to children, adolescents, and adults of all ages & abilities. Specialized training in Neurologic Music Therapy and DIR/Floortime.

Mewsic Moves
Agoura Hills, CA 91301
Tel: (818) 877 6797
Contact Name: John Mews, MA, MTA
Email: john@mewsicmoves.com
Website: http://www.mewsicmoves.com

Incorporates music therapy elements into specifically designed programs to improve a whole range of challenges for individuals with ASD including social, communication, learning, memory, behavioral, emotional, and self-regulation.

Monterey Bay Horsemanship & Therapeutic Center
783 San Andreas Road
La Selva Beach, CA 95076
Tel: (831) 251 0777
Contact Name: Gail Wright
Email: info@mbhorsecenter.com
Website: http://www.mbhorsecenter.com

Monterey Bay Horsemanship & Therapeutic Center is a fully inclusive, nonprofit, horse ranch organization.

Dr. Raymond Jones
Aspen Counseling Center
541 S Glendora Ave.
Glendora, CA 91741
Tel: (626) 914 1456
Email: raymond@aspencenter.org

A psychotherapist working with adults with Asperger's Syndrome.

Salisbury Farms
13036 Willow Road
Lakeside, CA 92040
Tel: (619) 723 6202
Contact Name: Amy Oleson
Email: janespurs@hotmail.com
Website: http://www.salisburyfarms.net

Salisbury Farms offers psychotherapy, experiential learning, and horseback riding lessons for children, youth, and adults with ASD.

Shadow Hills Riding Center
10263 La Canada Way
Shadow Hills, CA 91040
Tel: (310) 508 1589 or (213) 761 0549
Contact Name: Andrew Mikiel or Johnny Higginson
Email: andrew@shadowhillsridingclub.org
Website: http://www.shadowhillsridingclub.org

A PATH International premier accredited Equine Assisted Therapeutic riding program serving all children and adults with physical, mental and emotional disabilities.

The Shape of Behavior
10623 Riverside Drive
Burbank, CA 91602
Tel: (832) 358 2655
Toll Free: (866) 437 2165
Website: http://www.shapeofbehavior.com

Provides ABA, HBI, Behavior Medicine, EEG Biofeedback, Behavioral Services and Autism Therapy.

Schools and Educational Services

Achievekids
Palo Alto
3860 Middlefield Road
Palo Alto, CA 94303
Tel: (650) 494 1200
Website: http://www.achievekids.org

With two locations in Palo Alto and East San Jose, AchieveKids serves Bay Area children, aged 5 to 22, with emotional and/or developmental disabilities including mental retardation, autistic spectrum disorder, mood, disruptive behavior, anxiety, and psychotic disorders.

Actors for Autism Vocational Training Program
121 W. Lexington Drive, Suite L600
Glendale, CA 91203
(818) 705 1600
Contact Name: Alisa Wolf
Email: actorsforautism@aol.com
Website: http://www.actorsforautism.org or http://www.vocationalacademy.net

Vocational training in Film, Television, Animation, and Video Game Design for adults with ASD.

Balboa City School
525 Hawthorn Street
San Diego, CA 92101
Tel: (619) 298 2990
Contact Name: Monica Studevent
Website: http://www.balboaschool.com

Balboa City School (BCS) is an accredited, K-12 private school in San Diego offering college preparatory curriculum in smaller classes.

California State University - Fresno
California State University - Fresno Fresnco, CA 93740
Tel: (559) 278 0325
Contact Name: Charles Arokiasamy
Email: charlesa@csufresno.edu

Website: http://www.csufresno.edu/ssd

California State University East Bay Hayward
CSU East Bay autism center. 29000 Hesperian Blvd.
Hayward, CA 94545
Contact Name: Michael Bernick
Website: http://www.sfgate.com/cgi-bin/article.cgi?f=/c/a/2009/08/03/EDPN193F67.DTL

Carousel School
7899 La Tijera Blvd.
Los Angeles, CA 90045
Tel: (310) 645 9222
Website: http://www.carouselschool.com

Provides Early Childhood Education programs to young children and their families, including infant and preschool classes, Early Intervention instruction, Non-Public School for Elementary through High School students, After-School Programs for children with special needs or disabilities, and an Adult Program for adults 18 to 55 years old.

College Internship Program (CIP) Berkeley
2070 Allston Rd. Suite 101
Berkeley, CA 94704
Tel: (510) 704 4476, X104
Contact Name: Marjorie Paul, JD, Admissions Director
Email: mpaul@cipberkeley.org
Website: http://www.cipberkeley.com

CIP's full-year postsecondary programs provide young adults with ASD, ADHD, Nonverbal and other Learning Differences with the social, academic, career and life skills.

Coryell Autism Center
Coryell Autism Center
111 Errett Circle
Santa Cruz, CA 95060
Tel: (831) 713 5186
Contact Name: Lisa Hyde
Email: lhyde@coryellautismcenter.org
Website: http://www.CoryellAutismCenter.org

Coryell Autism Center is a nonpublic school providing educational services to young people with autism ages 14 to 22. In addition, the Center offers Supportive Living Services (SLS).

CSULB Disabled Student Services
1250 Bellflower Blvd Brotman Hall 270
Long Beach, CA 90840
Tel: (562) 985 1675
Contact Name: Nicole Smith, Autism Services Coordinator
Email: Nicole.smith@csulb.edu

Website: http://www.csulb.edu/divisions/students/dss

California State University, Long Beach offers comprehensive services to enrolled, qualifying students with disabilities including Autism.

Excelsior Academy
7202 Princess View Drive
San Diego, CA 92120
Tel: (619) 583 6762
Email: nmacnamara@excelsioracademy.com
Website: http://www.excelsioracademy.com

Exceptional Minds
13400 Riverside Drive, Suite #211
Sherman Oaks, CA 91423
Tel: (818) 387 8811
Contact Name: Yudi Bennett
Email: info@exceptionalmindsstudio.org
Website: http://www.ExceptionalMindsStudio.org/

Exceptional Minds provides visually-gifted young adults with ASD with customized instruction in animation, computer graphics, and visual effects.

Hidden Wings
P.O. Box 1912
Santa Ynez, CA 93460
Tel: (805) 705 3918
Email: jim@hiddenwings.org
Website: http://www.hiddenwings.org
FB: http://www.facebook.com/hiddenwingscollege

Dedicated to nurturing the gifts of young adults with autism so that they might have full and productive lives in society.

Kayne Eras Center
Exceptional Children's Foundation
8740 Washington Blvd.
Culver City, CA 90232
Tel: (310) 204 3300
Website: http://www.ecf.net/programs/kayne-eras-center

Marinia Academy Alternative Christian Education Center
15118 Clark Ave.
Bellflower, CA 90706
Tel: (310) 692 1598
Contact Name: Shani Sambrano, M.Ed.
Email: ShaniSambrano@MariniaAcademy.org
Website: http://www.mariniaacademy.org/

Marinia Academy provides alternative education and intervention for children and youth with academic or behavior challenges.

Opportunity Acres (OA), Inc.
7315 S. Shingle Road
Shingle Springs, CA 95682
Tel: (916) 216 8680 or (530) 672 9462
Contact Name: Michelle Wenell, CEO
Email: mwenell@oppacres.com
Website: http://www.oppacres.com

Opportunity Acres has an ABA-based adult day program and high school on a working horse ranch.

Pathway at UCLA Extension
10995 LeConte Avenue Suite 639
Los Angeles, CA 90024
Tel: (310) 794 1235
Contact Name: Eric Latham
Email: pathway@uclaextension.edu
Website: http://uclaextension.edu/pathway

Postsecondary education program for young adults with intellectual and other developmental disabilities.

Taft College Transition to Independent Living Program
29 Emmons Park Drive
Taft, CA 93268
Tel: (661) 763 7775
Email: intake@taftcollege.edu
Website: http://www.taftcollege.edu/tcwp/til/

The Transition to Independent Living Program provides an educational experience that focuses on acquisition of skills necessary for independent living.

University of California - Oakland
University of California - Oakland Oakland, CA 94610
Tel: (310) 794 1235
Contact Name: Carlos O. Cortez
Email: pathway@uclaextension.edu
Website: http://www.universityofcalifornia.edu/admissions/campuses/special-populations

Upendo Learning Center (ULC)
14545 Victory Blvd. #504
Van Nuys, CA 91411
Tel: (818) 426 7239 or (818) 720 7059
Contact Name: Letty Chavez
Email: lettychavezph@hotmail.com
Website: http://upendolearningcenter.com/enrichment-program.html

Wayfinders at California State University, Fresno
5005 North Maple Avenue Kremen Education Room 151; M/S ED301
Fresno, CA 93740
Tel: (559) 278 0390

Email: wayfinders@mail.fresnostate.edu
Website: http://www.csufresno.edu/kremen/wayfinders/index.html

The Wayfinders Program is an inclusive postsecondary education and residential program for students with intellectual disabilities.

West Kern Community College District - Taft College
Taft, CA 93268
Tel: (661) 763 7776
Contact Name: Jeffrey G. Ross
Email: jross@taft.org
Website: http://www.taftcollege.edu/newtc/StudentServices/SSS

Legal, Government & Financial Services

A2Z Educational Advocates
881 Alma Real Drive Suite 309
Pacific Palisades, CA 90272
Tel: (310) 573 1430
Toll Free: (888) IDEA ADA
Email: inquiry@a2zedad.com
Website: http://a2zedad.com

A2Z helps parents obtain special education services for their children.

Abilities United
525 East Charleston Road
Palo Alto, CA 94306
Tel: (650) 494 0550
Email: info@abilitiesunited.org
Website: http://www.abilitiesunited.org

Adams ESQ
449 Fifteenth St. Suite 101
Oakland, CA 94612
Tel: (510) 832 6000
Email: oaklandadmin@adamsesq.com
Website: http://www.adamsesq.com
Special education law.

Amy Langerman
Amy Langerman, PC
951 Coronado Ave.
Coronado, CA 92118
Email: info@amylangerman.com
Website: www.amylangerman.com

Special education consulting services provided in California. Licensed to practice law in Arizona only.

California Department of Mental Health
1600 9th Street, Rm. 151
Sacramento, CA 95814
Tel: (800) 896 4042
Email: dmh.dmh@dmh.ca.gov

California Special Needs Law Group
1901 Newport Blvd.
Costa Mesa, CA 92627
Tel: (888) 900 0744
Contact Name: Richard Isaacs
Email: risaacs@csnlg.com
Website: http://www.csnlg.com

Department of Rehabilitation Services
San Francisco County Offices 301 Howard St. Suite 700
San Francisco, CA 94105
Tel: (415) 904 7100
Website: http://www.rehab.cahwnet.gov

DOR assists people with disabilities obtain and retain employment and maximize their ability to live independently in their communities.

Disability Rights Education & Defense Fund (DREDF)
3075 Adeline St. Suite 210
Berkeley, CA 94703
Tel: (510) 644 2555
Email: info@dredf.org
Website: http://www.dredf.org

Advances the civil and human rights of people with disabilities through legal advocacy, training, education, and public policy and legislative development.

DLD Ed Consulting
Los Angeles, CA 90012
Tel: (323) 377 8356
Contact Name: Damien Danielly
Email: dldedconsulting@gmail.com
Website: http://www.dldedconsulting.com

An academic consulting company that services families in California and nationwide.

Estey & Bomberger, LLP
2869 India St.
San Diego, CA 92103
Toll Free: (800) 925 0723
Contact Name: Stephen Estey
Email: esteybombergercmv@yahoo.com
Website: http://www.childmolestationvictims.com

Inner City Law Center at the Weingart Access Center
Serving Los Angeles' Skid Row
506 S Main St.
Los Angeles, CA 90013
Tel: (213) 891 2880

Email: info@innercitylaw.org
Website: http://www.innercitylaw.org

Marin Center for Independent Living
710 4th Street
San Rafael, CA 94901
Tel: (415) 459 6245
Contact Name: Bob Roberts, Executive Director
Website: http://www.marincil.org

Marin Center for Independent Living is a community based 501 (c) 3 non-profit organization that provides advocacy and services for older adults and persons with disabilities.

Public Counsel for Childrens Rights Project
(For Minors Only)
610 South Ardmore Avenue
Los Angeles, CA 90005
Tel: (213) 385 2977, ex. 500
Website: http://www.publiccounsel.org/overview/crp.html

Special Education Attorneys Sherman & Ziegler
20301 Ventura Blvd. Suite 338
Woodland Hills, CA 91364
Tel: (415) 924 1300
Contact Name: Stan Ziegler
Email: info@saritlaw.com
Website: http://www.saritlaw.com

Special Education Law Firm
5206 Montair Ave
Lakewood, CA 90712
Tel: (562) 735 4111
Contact Name: Jennifer Guze Campbell
Email: Jennifer@selfapc.com
Website: http://www.selfapc.com

State of California Department of Developmental Disabilities–Regional Centers
Website: www.dds.ca.gov/RC/Home.cfm

California has 21 regional centers serving individuals with ASD and other developmental disabilities and their families. These centers contract with the State of California to provide and/or coordinate services and supports for individuals with developmental disabilities.

Timothy A. Adams & Associates, APLC
Timothy Adams, Esq.
1930 Old Tustin Ave., Ste. A
Santa Ana, CA 92705
Tel: (714) 698 0239
Website: www.californiaspecialedlaw.com

Law firm specializing in special education.

United Advocates for Children of California (UACC)
1401 El Camino Ave Suite 340
Sacramento, CA 95815
Tel: (916) 643 1530
Toll Free: (866) 643 1530
Email: information@uacc4families.org
Website: http://www.php.com/united-advocates-children-california-uacc

Community and Recreation Services

Ability First
Pasadena
1300 Green St.
Pasadena, CA 91106
Tel: (626) 396 1010
Email: contactus@abilityfirst.org
http://www.abilityfirst.org

Through 25 locations across Southern California, AbilityFirst provides programs for children and adults with disabilities and special needs including employment, recreational and socialization special needs programs and operate 12 accessible residential housing complexes.

Advance LA
15600 Mulholland Drive
Los Angeles, CA 90077
Tel: (310) 440 0201 or (818) 779 5198
Website: http://www.advancela.org

Provides resources, support, and training to teens and young adults with a wide range of special needs.

Advocacy for Respect and Choice-Long Beach, Inc.
4519 E. Stearns Street
Long Beach, CA 90815
Tel: (562) 597 4396 or (562) 597 7716
Contact Name: Yasmine Malayeri, Intake Coordinator
Email: ymalayeri@gmail.com
Website: http://www.hillsideenterprises.org

The Artist In Me
1085 E Herndon Ave #108 United States
Fresno, CA 93720
Tel: (559) 299 2935
Contact Name: Teresa L Mathias
Email: teresamathias@hotmail.com
Website: http://theartistinme.us

Autism Center for Young Adults
Fresno, CA 93722
Tel: (559) 301 6946
Contact Name: Wendi Vartabedian

Adult day program for young adults with autism with a focus on self-help, job skills, life skills, recreation, social activities, and technology.

Autism Social Connection
Autism Network for Global Education and Lifelong Support
1020 Sullivan Ave
Daly City, CA 94015
Tel: (650) 755 7558
Email: info@autismsocialconnection.org
Website: http://www.autismsocialconnection.org

The Autism Social Connection offers opportunities for socialization with typical peers.

BETA
P.O. Box 225129
San Francisco, CA 94122
Tel: (415) 564 7830
Toll Free: (800) 368 2382
Email: info@aintmisbehavin.com
Website: http://www.aintmisbehavin.com

The mission of BETA: Behavior Education Training Associates is to assist people considered disabled to maximize their participation and involvement in all areas of life.

Build Rehabilitation Industries
1323 Truman St.
San Fernando, CA 91340
Tel: (818) 898 0200
Website: http://www.buildindustries.com

California Autism Foundation
4075 Lakeside Drive
Richmond, CA 94806
Tel: (510) 758 0433
Email: contactcaf@calautism.org
Website: http://www.calautism.org

The mission of the California Autism Foundation is to provide people with autism and other developmental disabilities the best possible opportunities for lifetime support, training and assistance in helping them reach their highest potential for independence, productivity and fulfillment.

California Mentor
4085 Long Beach Blvd.
Long Beach, CA 90808
Tel: (855) 636 8672
Website: http://www.ca-mentor.com

California MENTOR's services and supports specializes in creating individualized programs that combine personal choice and community integration with professional oversight, family involvement, and stability.

California Pools of Hope
6801 Long Beach Blvd.
Long Beach, CA 90805
Tel: (310) 537 2224
Email: capoolsofhope@aol.com
Website: http://www.californiapoolsofhope.org

The mission of California Pools of Hope is to promote wellness and improve the quality of life for individuals with health needs in an accessible, warm-water aquatic facility.

Camping Unlimited
Boulder Creek, CA 95006
Tel: (510) 222 6662
Email: campkrem@campingunlimited.com
Website http://www.campingunlimited.com

Camping Unlimited is a non-profit organization providing special needs children and adults a full program of recreation, education, fun and adventure.

Center for Adaptive Learning
3227 Clayton Rd.
Concord, CA 94519
Tel: (925) 827 3863
Contact Name: Jana Scrivens
Email: jscrivens@c4al.org
Website: http://www.c4al.org

Provides comprehensive services designed to meet the emotional, social, vocational and functional needs of clients.

Community Resources for Independent Living
439 'A' Street
Hayward, CA 94541
Tel: (510) 881 5743
Email: info@cril-online.org
Website: http://www.cril-online.org

Danny's Farm
South Pasadena, CA 91030
Tel: (213) 607 4432
Contact Name: Jenny Sukys, Office Manager
Email: dannysfarm@yahoo.com
Website: http://www.dannysfarm.org

Disabled Sports Eastern Sierra
P.O. Box 7275
Mammoth Lakes, CA 93546
Tel: (760) 934 0791
Email: kcopeland@disabledsportseasternsierra.org
Website: http://www.disabledsportseasternsierra.org

Esperanza Services
1000 S. Fremont Ave. Suite 1110
Alhambra, CA 91803
(626) 457 5242
Contact Name: Shellyn Aguirre
Email: saguirre@esperanzaservices.com
Website: http://www.esperanzaservices.com

Provides supportive services to adults with ASD and other developmental disabilities. Services include assistance with daily life skills and sustained support to help those who choose to live independently.

Farming Independence
Agoura Hills, CA 91301
Tel: (818) 865 1418
Contact Name: Sheila Mayfield
Email: info@farmingindependence.org
Website: http://www.farmingindependence.org

Fred Finch Youth Center
3800 Coolidge Avenue
Oakland, CA 94602
Tel: (510) 482 2244
Website: http://www.fredfinch.org

Services are available in several configurations and many locations including residential treatment, public school, non-public school, homes, community settings, specialized independent and shared housing.

Greenacres Homes
7590 Atkinson Road
Sebastopol, CA 95472
Tel: (707) 823 8722
Email: GAH@GreenacreHomes.org
Website: http://www.greenacrehomes.org

A private non-profit California corporation, operates five (5) residential treatment programs and a special education school.

Hacienda Oaks Estates
2175 Agate Ct.
Simi Valley, CA 93065
Tel: (805) 302 7167
Contact Name: Cynthia Conway
Email: haciendaoaks@gmail.com
Website: http://www.haciendaoaksestates.org

Promoting green living, education, life skills, vocational opportunities for those with ASD and other special needs.

Hand in Hand Family and Child Development Center
17200 Ventura Boulevard Suite 112
Encino, CA 91316
Contact Name: Connie Carter
Email: connie@handinhandonline.org

Heart of Sailing
Dana Point
Dana Point Yacht Club PO Box 4073
Dana Point, CA 92629
Tel: (812) 935 7245
Email: uschildren@heartofsailing.org
Website: http://www.heartofsailing.org

Heart of Sailing introduces sailing to special needs children and adults as a form of education and recreational therapy.

Kid Quest
704 North Plymouth St.
Santa Cruz, CA 95060
Tel: (831) 421 9159
Contact Name: Nichole Griffin OR Colleen Russell
Email: kid_quest@sbcglobal.net
Website: http://www.balance4kids.org

Kid Quest is a non-profit social center for children and young adults with special needs.

Learning Light Foundation
Adult Developmental Program
1212 East Lincoln Ave.
Anaheim, CA 92805
Tel: (714) 533 2314
Website: http://www.learninglight.net

Provides day program services to adults with developmental disabilities.

Mayfair Community Center
City of San Jose Department of Parks, Recreation and Neighborhood Services
2039 Kammerer Ave
San Jose, CA 95116
Tel: (408) 794 1060
Contact Name: Liz Best
Email: liz.best@sanjoseca.gov
Website: http://www.sanjoseca.gov/prns

Providing recreation and fitness opportunities for people with disabilities ages 5 and up.

Mountain Shadows Support Group
970 Los Vallecitos Blvd. Suite 240
San Marcos, CA 92069
Tel: (760) 736 898, X201
Contact Name: Wade Wilde, Executive Director/CEO
Email: wwilde@mtnshadows.org
Website: http://www.mtnshadows.org

North County Quality of Life Center
P.O. Box 230150
Encinitas, CA 92023
Tel: (760) 473 2683
Email: info@ncqualityoflife.com
Website: http://www.ncqualityoflife.com

Specializes in transition services for young adults, including limited conservatorship issues, employment, post-secondary education, independent living skills, self-advocacy, and long-term planning.

Peppermint Ridge
825 Magnolia Avenue
Corona, CA 92879
Tel: (951) 273 7324 or (951) 273 7320
Contact Name: Rev. Audrey Turner, Executive Director
Email: aturner@peppermintridge
Website: http://www.peppermintridge.org

Peppermint Ridge, an intentional community, is comprised of 11 homes for adults age 18 and over. Services are also provided to those who live independently in the area. Peppermint Ridge is a faith-based non-profit organization.

Rose Bowl Aquatics Center
360 North Arroyo Blvd
Pasadena, CA 91103
Tel: (626) 564 0330
Contact Name: Kathy Schmitt
Email: kschmittt@rosebowlaquatics.org
Website: http://www.rosebowlaquatics.org

Sacramento Valley Region Care Coalition
Champion Special Needs Program
Sacramento Valley Region Care Coalition Sacramento, CA 95817
Tel: (916) 856 5605
Website: http://www.sacvalleycares.org

SAILS
16662 Hale Ave
Irvine, CA 92606
Tel: (949) 250 5730
Contact Name: Ihab Shahawi
Email: ceo@sailsgroup.com
Website: http://www.sailsgroup.com

Develops and operates service programs and facilities across California for behaviorally challenging children and adults.

South Bay Workforce Investment Board
11539 Hawthorne Boulevard Suite 500
Hawthorne, CA 90250
Tel: (310) 970 7700 or (910) 970 7774
Contact Name: Catherine Blaylock
Email: cblaylock@sbwib.org
Website: http://www.sbwib.org

Teen Recreation Integration Program
Lifehouse 100 Smith Ranch Rd., Suite 309
San Rafael, CA 94903
Tel: (415) 472 2373
Contact Name: Michael Sus
Email: msus@lifehouseagency.org

Provides recreational opportunities for individuals ages 13-22 with ASD.

Valley Achievement Center
1300 Stine Rd
Bakersfield, CA 93309
Tel: (661) 617 6040
Contact Name: Melvin Thomas
Email: mthomas@autism-vac.org
Website: http://www.autism-vac.org

Provides educational programs, life skills training, and supported employment and supported living services.

Unlimited Possibilities Martial Arts
3170 W.Lincoln Ave Ste 102
Anaheim, CA 92801
Tel: (562) 756 0709
Contact Name: Kristen
Email: info@up-ma.com
Website: http://www.up-ma.com

Valley Village
20830 Sherman Way
Winnetka, CA 91306
Tel: (818) 587 9450
Contact Name: Debra Donovan
Email: Debra@vvc.org
Website: http://www.ValleyVillage.org

Valley Village has day and residential programs for developmentally disabled adults.

YMCA Community Services- New Horizons
13821 Newport Ave, Suite 200
Tustin, CA 92780
Tel: (714) 508 7635 or (714) 508 7654
Contact Name: Tiffany Lockshaw
Email: newhorizons@ymcaoc.org
Website: http://www.ymcaoc.org/about-community-services/new-horizons

Yoga For The Special Child
3329 Yonge St.
San Diego, CA 92106
Tel: (619) 223 3611
Contact Name: Michelle Frandsen
Email: michelle.frandsen@gmail.com
Website: http://www.myyogaworld.net

Yoga For The Special Child is a registered yoga program designed for children with special needs.

Willie Ross Foundation
6621 Van Nuys Blvd
Van Nuys, CA 91405
Tel: (818) 786 7677
Contact Name: Tim Boydstun
Email: tim@willieross.org
Website: http://www.willierossfoundation.org/

The Willie Ross Foundation operates two group homes in L.A.'s San Fernando Valley and provides a day program for adults with developmental disabilities. Uses ABA principles to improve social skills and overall functioning.

COLORADO

Doctors, Clinics, Hospitals, and Other Health Services

Avista Adventist Hospital
100 Health Park Drive
Louisville, CO 80027
Tel: (303) 673 1000 or (303) 673 1247
Website: http://www.avistahospital.org

Boulder Community Hospital
Several campuses and free standing locations in Boulder County to better serve you.
Boulder, CO 80301
Tel: (303) 440 2273
Email: pr@bch.org
Website: http://www.bch.org

Carpenter Pediatric Dentistry
25521 East Smoky Hill Rd.
Aurora, CO 80016
Tel: (303) 617 5437
Contact Name: Jenny
Email: info@cpedo.com
Website: http://www.carpenterpediatricdentistry.com

Cedar Springs Hospital
2135 Southgate Road
Colorado Springs, CO 80906
Tel: (719) 633 4114 or (719) 578 0857
Website: http://www.cedarspringsbhs.com/

Provides a full continuum of care, including outpatient, case management, residential, and continuing care services.

Centennial Peaks Hospital
2255 S. 88th Street
Louisville, CO 80027
Tel: (303) 673 9990 or (303) 673 9703
Website: http://www.centennialpeaks.com

Centennial Peaks Hospital is dedicated to providing a full range of mental health services to the state of Colorado.

Children's Dentistry
5150 West 80th Avenue
Westminster, CO 80030

Tel: (303) 427 1951
Email: info@ddschild.com
Website: http://www.ddschild.com

The Children's Hospital
13123 East 16th Avenue
Aurora, CO 80045
Tel: (720) 777 1234
Contact Name: Robin Gabriels
Website: http://www.childrenscolorado.org

Cynthia Maguire, ND, CTN, CBS
716 N. Tejon St. #9
Colorado Springs, CO 80903
Tel: (719) 635 2879 or (719) 209 3592
Email: drcynthia@natural-doctor.org
Website: http://natural-doctor.org

A board-certified Traditional Naturopath treating using kinesiology and the L.I.F.E. biofeedback system. Cleansing and balancing of the body is provided by herbal remedies and essential oils and L.I.F.E. biofeedback sessions.

Debby Hamilton, MD MSPH
Holistic Pediatric Consulting
455 South Hudson Street
Suite 103
Denver, CO 80246
Tel: (303) 835 9130
Website: www.holisticpediatric.com

Provides comprehensive care to children with ASD and others and seeks to determine and treat causes, not just treat symptoms.

Foothills Pediatric Dentistry
1120 W South Boulder Rd Suite 204
Lafayette, CO 80026
Tel: (303) 604 9500
Website: http://www.foothillspediatricdentistry.com

Neuroscience Center of the Rockies
2500 Rocky Mountain Ave Suite #310
Loveland, CO 80538
Tel: (970) 619 6000
Contact Name: Dr. Terry Mark Himes

Diagnosis and management of ASD.

North Park Vision Center
Dr. Marcy Rose
10359 Federal Blvd. Suite 100
Westminster, CO 80260
Tel: (303) 469 7770
Email: office@northparkvision.com
Website: http://www.northparkvision.com

University of Colorado Denver School of Medicine
Department of Pediatrics
13123 East 16th Ave. B065
Aurora, CO 80045
Tel: (720) 777 2715 or (720) 777 6602
Contact Name: Autism Treatment Network
Email: atn@autismspeaks.org
Website: http://www.ucdenver.edu/academics/colleges/
medicalschool/departments/pediatrics/Pages/Pediatrics.
aspx

Wholeness Center
2620 E Prospect Rd Suite 190
Fort Collins, CO 80525
Tel: (970) 221 1106
Contact Name: Dr. Rondeau
Email: info@wholeness.com
Website: http://www.wholeness.com

Integrative medical practice providing a wide variety of collaborative services from diagnosis to treatment and family support for people with autism spectrum disorders and other developmental disorders.

Therapy Services

Colorado Therapies and Aquatic Center
5412 Idylwild Trail
Boulder, CO 80301
Tel: (303) 530 1503
Website: http://www.coloradotherapies.com

Colorado Therapies & Aquatic Center, LLC consists of independent practitioners who offer a complete array of services in traditional and complimentary health fields.

Dream Catcher Therapy Center
Dream Catcher Therapy Center Olathe, CO 81425
Tel: (970) 323 5400
Email: khamm@dctc.org
Website: http://dctc.org

Specializing in Equine Assisted Therapy

Equinox Counseling & Wellness Center
2480 W. 26th Ave Suite B-330
Denver, CO 80211
Tel: (303) 861 1916
Website: http://www.equinoxcounseling.com

Equinox Counseling and Wellness Center is a comprehensive community based counseling and treatment center treating, among others, youth with Aspergers and High Functioning Autism.

Music Therapy Rocks
P.O. Box 1205
Monument, CO 80132
Tel: (719) 360 8420

Contact Name: Cathy
Email: jacksonranchmt@q.com
Website: http://musictherapyrocks.net

NeuroRhythm Music Therapy Services, LLC
1255 Lake Plaza Dr #269
Colorado Springs, CO 80906
Tel: (719) 213 4330
Contact Name: Kate St. John, MT-BC, NMT
Email: KateStJohn@NeuroRhythm.com
Website: http://www.NeuroRhythm.com

Specializes in neurologic and developmental disabilities including ASD, cerebral palsy, down syndrome, sensory processing disorder, and other cognitive, speech/language and motor delays. Integrates neurologic music therapy (NMT) with sensory integration and ABA.

Pikes Peak Therapeutic Riding Center
13620 Halleluiah Trail
Elbert, CO 80106
Tel: (719) 495 3908
Website: http://www.pptrc.org

Provides therapeutic horseback riding.

The Right Step, Inc.
7990 South Santa Fe Drive
Littleton, CO 80120
Tel: (303) 731 9057 or (303) 904 7261
Contact Name: Sheryl Clossen
Email: xsap@aol.com
Website: http://www.therightstepinc.org

A therapeutic riding program.

Rocky Mountain Autism Center
8600 Park Meadows Dr. Suite 800
Lone Tree, CO 80124
Tel: (303) 985 1133
Contact Name: Elizabeth Rydell
Email: elizabeth@rockymountainautismcenter.com
Website: http://www.rockymountainautismcenter.com

Dr. Patrick Rydell, founder of RMAC, is the co-author of the nationally recognized SCERTS® Model and developer of the Learning Style Profile. These two approaches, along with other evidence-based practices, are used.

Spectra Autism Center, Inc.
1200 Wadsworth Blvd.
Lakewood, CO 80232
Tel: (303) 665 6800
Email: info@spectracenter.org
Website: http://www.spectracenter.org

Summit Music Therapy Services
Fort Collins, CO 80524
Tel: (970) 372 9956
Contact Name: Blythe LaGasse, Ph.D., MT-BC
Email: blythel@summitmusictherapy.com
Website: http://www.summitmusictherapy.com

Thrive Autism Collaborative
1728 Downing Street
Denver, CO 80218
Email: info@thriveautismcollaborative.com
Website: http://www.thriveautismcollaborative.com/

Provides intervention to children and adults with autism and related disorders from 12 months on, incorporating principles of ABA and the Early Start Denver Model.

Schools and Educational Services

Aspire Autism, LLC
14 Garden Center
Broomfield, CO 80020
Tel: (720) 379 3812 or (720) 379 3812
Contact Name: Jeremy Blower
Email: jeremy.blower@aspireautism.org
Website: http://www.aspireautism.org

Bal Swan Children's Center
Bal Swan Children's Center
1145 E. 13th Ave.
Broomfield, CO 80020
Tel: (303) 466 6308
Contact Name: Brian Conly, Executive Director
Email: info@balswan.org
Website: http://www.balswan.org

Bal Swan individualizes preschool and/or therapy services to help prepare children for kindergarten.

Breckenridge Outdoor Education Center
P.O. Box 697
Breckenridge, CO 80424
Tel: (970) 453 6422
Email: boec@boec.org
Website: http://www.boec.org

Colorado Institute of Autism
Box 50254
Colorado Springs, CO 80949
Tel: (719) 593 7334

Colorado State University
Colorado State University Fort Collins, CO 80523
Tel: (970) 491 0225
Contact Name: Catherine L Schelly
Email: catherine.schelly@colostate.edu
Website: http://rds.colostate.edu

Provides support and help for students with both permanent and temporary limitations and health conditions (physical and mental health).

Eastern Colorado Services for the Developmentally Disabled
P. O. Box 1682 617 South 10th Avenue
Sterling, CO 80751
Website: http://www.easterncoloradoservices.org

Programs include Infant/Toddler including Early Intervention and Part C, Adult Supported Employment services, Supported Community Connections, Pre-Vocational services, Personal and Social Skills training, Residential Placement services, Supported Living Services and the Family Services and Support Program.

Fisher Early Learning Center
Fisher Early Learning Center
1899 E Evans Ave.
Denver, CO 80208
Tel: (303) 871 2723
Website: http://www.du.edu/fisher

Gold Star Learning Options
15387 E. 99th Place
Commerce City, CO 80022
Tel: (720) 979 4309
Contact Name: Katie Burpo
Email: GoldstarLearningoptions.@gmail.com
Website: http://www.goldstarlearning.webs.com

Offers support at home, at school, and in the community, to families of children with and without developmental disabilities, and who are affected by ASD.

The Joshua School (TJS)
2303 E. Dartmouth Ave.
Englewood, CO 80113
Tel: (303) 758 7171
Contact Name: Kristin Buchanan, Education Director
Email: kbuchanan@joshuaschool.org
Website: http://www.joshuaschool.org

The Joshua School is a private, non-profit school and resource center for individuals with autism, Asperge syndrome, or other special needs, and their families.

Little Indians Preschool
709 West 3rd Avenue
Yuma, CO 80759
Tel: (970) 848 4572
Website: http://www.yumaschools.org/LIPS/lipsindex.htm

Legal, Government & Financial Services

Community Centered Boards
Website: www.colorado.gov/cs/Satellite/CDHS-VetDis/CBON/1251586997819

Community Centered Boards are the single entry point into the long-term service and support system for persons with developmental disabilities. The State contracts with twenty Community Centered Boards to deliver community-based services.

Cypers Law, PC
700 N. Colorado Blvd. #232
Denver, CO 80206
Tel: (720) 663 9859
Contact Name: Elizabeth Cypers
Email: elizabeth@cyperslaw.com
Website: http://www.cyperslaw.com or http://www.elizabethcyperslaw.com

Estate planning for families of individuals with special needs.

Division Of Vocational Rehabilitation
1574 Sherman Avenue 4th Floor
Denver, CO 80203
Tel: (303) 866 4150
Email: voc.rehab@state.co.us
Website: http://www.colorado.gov/cs/Satellite/CDHS-SelfSuff/CBON/1251580884712

Family Voices
c/o CP of Colorado
2200 S. Jasmine Street
Denver, CO 80222
Tel: (303) 447 8447
Toll Free: (800) 881 8272
Website: http://www.familyvoicesco.org

Information for parents of children with health challenges.

Imagine!
Boulder County CCB
1400 Dixon Street
Lafayette, CO 80026
Tel: (303) 665 7789
Contact Name: John Taylor, Ph.D., Executive Director
Website: http://www.imaginecolorado.org

Point of entry into local, state and federally funded programs for people with developmental disabilities in the community. Also provides educational and therapeutic services, job training and placement, recreation and leisure activities, opportunities for community living, behavioral health services, technology solutions and support for families.

Legal Center for People with Disabilities
455 Sherman Street Suite 130
Denver, CO 80203
Toll Free: (800) 288 1376
Contact Name: Mary Anne Harvey
Email: hn6282@handsnet.org
Website: http://www.thelegalcenter.org

Mountain Valley Developmental Services
PO Box 338
Glenwood Springs, CO 81602
Tel: (970) 945 2306
Email: info@mtnvalley.org
Website: http://www.mtnvalley.org

Community and Recreation Services

A Place 4 Me, LLP
11651 W. 64th Ave. A-4
Arvada, CO 80004
Tel: (720) 771 1295
Website: http://www.aplace4me.net

A Place 4 Me is an appointment-based recreational place for parents of children with ASD and their families.

Adam's Camp
6767 South Spruce St. Suite 102
Centennial, CO 80112
Tel: (303) 563 2890
Website: http://www.adamscamp.org

Adams Camp is a Colorado-based nonprofit organization providing intensive, personalized and integrated therapeutic programs for children with special needs and their families as well as recreational programs for youth and young adults with moderate developmental disabilities.

Adaptive Sports Center
PO Box 1639
Crested Butte, CO 81224
Tel: (970) 349 2296
Toll Free: (866) 349 2296
Email: info@adaptivesports.org
Website: http://www.adaptivesports.org

African American Autism Center
5511 Xanadu Street
Denver, CO 80239
Tel: (303) 335 5207
Contact Name: Vicki L Clark, Director
Email: africanamerautism@gmail.com
Website: http://www.africanamerautism.com

Art Reach
3400 W. 38th Avenue Suite 200
Denver, CO 80211
Tel: (303) 433 2882
Email: info@artreachdenver.org
Website: http://www.artreachdenver.org
Supporting access to arts and culture.

Ascendigo
520 South 3rd Street #29
Carbondale, CO 81623
Tel: (970) 927 3143
Email: info@extremesportscamp.org
Website: www.ascendigo.org
Provides supervised outdoor opportunities for individuals ages 5 and up with ASD.

Challenge Autism
Snowmass Village Mall #309 PO Box 6639
Snowmass Village, CO 81623
Tel: (970) 923 0578
Contact Name: Brett Coleman
Email: brett@challengeaspen.com
Website: http://www.challengeaspen.org
Highly recreational, educational, and cultural activities, including adapted skiing, snowboarding, white water rafting, fishing, climbing, ropes course, horseback riding.

Chestor House
1831 Boston Ave Suite 100
Longmont, CO 80501
Tel: (303) 926 8840
Email: info@chestorhouse.org
Website: http://www.chestorhouse.org
Provides support services in managed residential settings.

Colorado Bluesky Enterprises (CBE)
115 W. 2nd Street
Pueblo, CO 81003
Tel: (719) 546 0572
Website: http://www.coloradobluesky.org

Community Options, Inc.
336 S. 10th Street PO Box 31
Montrose, CO 81402
Tel: (970) 249 1412
Email: info@communityoptionsinc.org
Website: http://www.communityoptionsinc.org
Community Options, Inc. provides and coordinated services and supports to people with developmental disabilities.

Foothills Gateway
301 W. Skyway Drive
Fort Collins, CO 80525
Tel: (970) 226 2345
Email: info@foothillsgateway.org
Website: http://www.foothillsgateway.org
Advocates for and empowers individuals with disabilities to lead lives of their choice.

Hope Farms Project
47200 CR 29
Elizabeth, CO 80107
Tel: (720) 217 2959
Contact Name: Lisa Kramer
Email: lisa@hopefarmsproject.org
Website: http://www.hopefarmsproject.org

Independent Living Experience (ILE)
1045 Lincoln Street Suite 109
Denver, CO 80203
Tel: (855) 664 9333
Email: info@independentlivingexperience.com
A customized support service for adults desiring a life of independence.

Peak Parent Center
611 North Weber St. Suite 200
Colorado Springs, CO 80903
Tel: (719) 531 9400, X100
Toll Free: (800) 284 0251
Contact Name: Elizabeth Paine
Email: epaine@peakparent.org
Website: http://www.peakparent.org
Provides training, information and technical assistance to equip families of children birth through twenty-six including all disability conditions with advocacy strategies.

Pinyon Ranch Inc.
7087 S. Madison Way
Centennial, CO 80122
Tel: (303) 229 2331
Website: http://www.pinyonranch.org
Pinyon Ranch, Inc. is a 501(c)(3) not-for-profit organization dedicated to providing a sustainable day community for adults with neurodevelopmental disabilities.

The Resource Exchange
418 S. Weber St.
Colorado Springs, CO 80903
Tel: (719) 380 1100
Email: info@tre.org
Website: http://www.tre.org

Spectrum Foundation of Colorado
803 Beauprez Ave
Lafayette, CO 80026
Tel: (303) 548 7173
Contact Name: Cynthia Shaffer
Email: SpectrumFoundation.Colorado@Gmail.com
Website: http://www.spectrumfoundationofcolorado.org/

CONNECTICUT

Doctors, Clinics, Hospitals, and Other Health Services

Advance Biomedical Treatment Center
Eileen Comia, MD
35 Jolley Drive
Suite 102
Bloomfield, CT 06002
Tel: (860) 242 2200
Website: www.advbiomedtx.com

Ailene Tisser, PT
Angelfish Therapy
78 Federal Road
Danbury, CT 06810
Tel: (203) 545 0024
Website: www.angelfishtherapy.com

Ayelet Connell-Giammatteo, PhD PT IMT C
Integrative Wellness and Physical Therapy
34 Jerome Avenue
Suite 305
Bloomfield, CT 06002
Tel: (860) 519 1916
Website: www.integrativewellnessandpt.com

Barbara Greenspan, MS OTR
Kidworks of Westport
6 East Main Street
Westport, CT 06880
Tel: (203) 858 8490
Website: www.kidworksofwestport.com

Brian Henninger, ND
1305 Post Road
Suite 301
Fairfield, CT 06824
Tel: (203) 255 4325
Website: www.brianhenningernd.com

Center for Integrative Health
Nancy O'Hara, MD
Gail Szakacs, MD
3 Hollyhock Lane

Wilton, CT 06897
Tel: (203) 834 2813
Website: www.ihealthnow.org

Providing integrative biomedical treatments for ASD and other health conditions.

Cindy Freedman, MOTR CTRS OTR
Angelfish Therapy
78 Federal Road
Danbury, CT 06810
Tel: (203) 545 0024
Website: www.angelfishtherapy.com

Center for Children with Special Needs
2213 Main Street
Glastonbury, CT 6033
Tel: (860) 430 1762
Contact Name: Eliza Ferzacca
Website: http://www.autismct.com

The Center for Children with Special Needs & The Center for Independence is an interdisciplinary clinic specializing in the diagnosis, evaluation, and treatment of children and adolescents with complex developmental disabilities.

Connecticut Children's Medical Center
282 Washington Street
Hartford, CT 6106
Tel: (860) 545 7493 x 4
Website: http://www.ccmckids.org

CornerStone Integrative Care
Lauren Lee Stone, PhD
3 Hollyhock Lane
Wilton, CT 06897
Tel: (203) 794 9700
Email: lauren@cornerstoneicare.com
Website: www.cornerstoneintegrativecare.com

Advanced BioSet practitioner and Homotoxicologist.

Enhanced Health Coaching (EHC)
2 Greenwich Office Park
Greenwich, CT 06831
Tel: (914) 607 6904
Website: http://www.enhancedhealthcoaching.com

Helps parents understand how food and lifestyle choices affect health and provides personalized care focusing on valid, evidence-based resources to improve health.

Gail Szakacs, MD Center for Integrative Health
3 Hollyhock Lane
Tel: (203) 834 2813
Website: www.ihealthnow.org

Greenwich Hospital
5 Perryridge Road
Greenwich, CT 6830
Tel: (203) 863 3000
Website: http://www.greenhosp.org

Holcare Nutrition
Victoria Kobliner, MS RD
3 Hollyhock Lane
Wilton, CT 06897
Tel: (203) 834 9949
Website: www.holcarenutrition.com

Ingels Family Health

Darin Ingels, ND
2425 Post Road, Suite 100
Southport, CT 06890
Tel: (203) 254 9957
Email: info@ingelsfamilyhealth.com
Website: www.ingelsfamilyhealth.com

Dr. Ingels uses a variety of modalities to treat, among others, those with ASD and his practice emphasizes treatment of chronic immune dysfunction, including allergies, asthma, recurrent or persistent infections and other genetic or acquired immune problems.

Jared Skowron, ND Harvest Park Naturopathic Medicine
101 North Plains Industrial Road
Building #1B
Wallingford, CT 06492
Tel: (203) 500 5532
Website: www.naturopathicanswer.com

Jennifer Boyd
85 Turkey Hill South
Westport, CT 06880
Tel: (203) 981 3757
Website: www.boydwellness.com

Lighthouse Psycho-educational Services
867 Pequot Ave.
New London, CT 6320
Tel: (860) 442 1133
Contact Name: Maureen F. Shea
Email: moshea867@ct.metrocast.net
Website: http://www.lighthousepsyched.com

Psycho-educational assessments, advocacy, coaching, tutoring, consulting, age 3-21, parent education, workshop presentations, brain-based neuropsychological approach.

Lynn Williamson, RN
45 Notch Road

Bolton, CT 06043
Tel: (860) 649 9130

Mark Goldenberg, DC
Brain Balance Center of Norwalk
15 Cross Street
Norwalk, CT 06851
Tel: (203) 847 3000
Website: www.brainbalancecenters.com/locations/norwalk

Nancy O'Hara, MD
Center for Integrative Health
3 Hollyhock LaneWilton, CT 06897
Tel: (203) 834 2813
Website: www.ihealthnow.org

Natura Medica - The Center for Natural Medicine
12 Roosevelt Ave.
Mystic, CT 6355
Tel: (860) 572 9566
Contact Name: Deirdre O'Connor, ND
Website: http://www.naturamedicamystic.com

Natura Medica is a primary care medical practice integrating therapeutic nutrition, homeopathic medicine, botanical medicine, acupuncture, and lifestyle counseling with conventional therapies for the treatment of both acute and chronic illnesses as well as prevention of disease.

Natural Pediatric Medicine, LLC Robin Russell, MD
176 Ashley Falls Road
Canaan, CT 06018
Tel: (860) 453 4090
Contact Name: Dr. Robin Russell
Website: http://www.naturalpediatricmedicinellc.com

Pediatric Dental Associates of Southbury
One Pomperaug Office Park, Suite 206
Southbury, CT 06488
Tel: (203) 264 1497
Contact Name: Dr. Mimi
Email: Adelessio@aol.com
Website: http://www.kidstoothcare.com

Randy Schulman, OD MS FCOVD
Southport Eyecare Associates
2600 Post Road
Southport, CT, 06890
Tel: (203) 255 4005

Center for Integrated Vision of Norwalk
139 Main Street
Norwalk, CT 06851
Tel: (203) 840 1991

Trumbull Eyecare Associates
6515 Main Street
Trumbull, CT, 06611
Tel: (203) 374 2020
Email: office@cteyecareassociates.com
Website: www.cteyecareassociates.com

Dr. Schulman offers vision therapy among other vision and eyecare services.

Sheila Reed, LCSW CHHP BEP
12 Old Boston Post Road
Old Saybrook, CT 06475
Tel: (860) 577 0419
Website: www.essentialhealingsolutions.net

A holistic healthcare practitioner, Ms. Reed is a LCSW and board-certified Holistic Healthcare practitioner and BioEnergetic practitioner specializing in Homotoxicology for children and adults.

The Southfield Center for Development
85 Old Kings Highway North
Darien, CT 06820
Tel: (203) 202 7654
Email: info@southfieldcenter.com
Website: http://www.southfieldcenter.com

Specializes in the diagnosis and treatment of autism and other neurodevelopmental disorders in children, from the ages of 2 through 7.

Todd Stelik, OTR/L CHHP
88 Norwich New London Turnpike
Suite 1
Uncasville, CT 06382
Tel: (860) 848 9157
Website: www.communitytherapeutix.com

Yale-New Haven Children's Hospital
20 York St.
New Haven, CT 6510
Tel: (877) 611 KIDS
Website: http://www.ynhh.org/ynhch/ynhch.html

Therapy Services

Ahlbin Centers for Rehabilitation
226 Mill Hill Avenue
Bridgeport, CT 06610
Tel: (203) 336 7338
Website: http://www.bridgeporthospital.org/ahlbin/default.aspx

Provides a full range of adult and pediatric rehabilitation services, including physical, speech and language, and occupational therapy, Childhood Early Intervention Program, cranial sacral therapy, hearing services, sensory integration, feeding disorders, and ADHD and ADD.

Angelfish Therapy
Tel: (203) 545 0024
Fax: (203) 321 2138
Email: Info@AngelfishTherapy.com
Website: www.angelfishtherapy.com

Aquatic therapy, swim lesson and summer camps with many locations in Connecticut, Massachusetts, New York, and New Jersey.

Baron Therapy Services
15 Research Dr.
Woodbridge, CT 6525
Tel: (203) 387 1401
Contact Name: Lisa Baron
Email: lisabaron@barontherapy.com
Website: http://www.barontherapy.com

Provides speech-language therapy, occupational therapy, physical therapy, behavioral intervention, therapeutic day programs, extended day programs, tutoring, and animal assisted therapy to children of all ages who have special needs.

Beacon Services of Connecticut
160 West Street, Suites F & G
Cromwell, CT 6416
Tel: (860) 613 9930
Contact Name: Christine Eichelberger
Email: ceichelberger@beaconct.org
Website: http://www.beaconct.org

Provides intensive behavioral/instructional services to individuals with disabilities.

Branches of Hope, Inc.
335 Post Road West
Westport, CT 06880
Tel: (203) 227 3383
Contact Name: Justin Burke
Email: justin@branchesofhope.org
Website: http://www.branchesofhope.org

The Center for Growth & Development, Inc.
84 Danbury Road
Wilton, CT 06897
Tel: (203) 563 9360
Contact Name: Lynn Hartigan
Email: TheCenter_ABA@yahoo.com
Website: http://thecenteraba.com

Provides verbal behavior based ABA services to children with ASD and related disorders. On-site services are available in our Wilton, CT location. In home services are available throughout the tri-state area.

Center for Social Enrichment and Educational Development, LLC
30 Buxton Farm Road, Suite 105
Stamford, CT 6905
Tel: (203) 674 8200
Contact Name: Evan Schermer
Email: info@seedautismcenter.com
Website: http://seedautismcenter.com

Offers services such as ABA, speech and language therapy, occupational therapy, social skill development, family training, assessment and testing, counseling, advocacy, home programming and professional development.

Children's Therapy and Learning Center (CTLC)
2228 Black Rock Turnpike Suite 201
Fairfield, CT 06825
Tel: (203) 908 4433
Contact Name: Stefanie Seanor, OTR/L
Email: stefanie.ctlc@optimum.net
Website: http://www.childtherapycenter.com

Services include occupational therapy, speech and language therapy, tutoring and support, IEP review, psychological testing and counseling, behavior management, handwriting and social skills groups and summer learning camps. Age-appropriate services are available for infants through adults.

Communication Foundations, LLC
42 Ashwell Drive
Plantsville, CT 06479
(860) 853 0205
Contact Name: Meredith Bandish, MA/CCC-SLP
Email: meredith@communicationfoundations.com
Website: http://www.communicationfoundations.com

Speech therapy incorporating, as appropriate, principles of ABA and PROMPT techniques.

Connec-to-Talk, LLC
1011 High Ridge Rd. 2nd Floor
Stamford, CT 06905
Tel: (203) 200 7256
Website: http://www.connec-to-talk.com

Provides speech, occupational, and ABA therapy.

High Hopes Therapeutic Riding
36 Town Woods Road
Old Lyme, CT 6371
Tel: (860) 434 1974
Email: hhinfo@highhopestr.org
Website: http://www.highhopestr.org

High Hopes uses an interdisciplinary team approach that includes the applied practices of both the Therapeutic Riding Instructor and licensed Therapists in the areas of Physical, Occupational, Speech and Language and Expressive Therapies.

Integrative Wellness and Physical Therapy
34 Jerome Avenue
Suite 305
Bloomfield, CT 06002
Tel: (860) 519 1916
Website: www.IntegrativeWellnessandPT.com

Holistic physical therapy, Integrative Manual Therapy, and other treatments, including nutritional treatments.

Interim Health of Eastern Connecticut, Inc.
12 Case Street, Suite 215
Norwich, CT 6060
Tel: (860) 889 3388
Website: http://www.interimhealthcare.com/norwichct

Speech/language, occupational therapy, physical therapy, social workers, respite care, home health care. Provides services to individuals and organizations in New London, Tolland, Middlesex, and Windham counties.

Just Breathe Connecticut, LLC
24 Battle Street, Suite 2A
Somers, CT 06071
Tel: (860) 265 3122
Contact Name: Kerry L. Tuttle, LCSW
Email: admin@JustBreatheCT.com
Website: http://www.JustBreatheCT.com

A therapeutic wellness center providing services to individuals, couples and families and offering a variety of services for youth, adults, and families challenged by ASD.

Kelley Hopkins-Alvarez, MS, MSED, NCC
158 Danbury Rd. Suite 7
Ridgefield, CT 6877
Tel: (203) 948 0938
Email: kellda@charter.net
Website: http://www.KelleyHopkinsAlvarez.com

Group for Young Adults Living with Aspergers & other disabilities. Focuses on social skills, self-advocacy and appropriate assertiveness.

King's Speech & Learning Center
225 Hopmeadow St. Suite 500
Simsbury, CT 06089
Tel: (860) 217 0098
Website: http://www.kingsspeechandlearning.com

King's Speech and Learning Center offers speech and occupational therapists, counselors, educators, and tutors to meet individual needs.

Lori Coda, MS SpEd
3 Hollyhock Lane
Wilton, CT 06897
Tel: (203) 414 0834
Email: loricoda@gmail.com
Website: www.loricoda.com

Providing Neurofeedback, QEEG, Social Skills Training, and Social Cognitive Therapy

PAWSitive Animal Therapy LLC
56 Eddy Rd.
Barkhamsted, CT 06063
Tel: (860) 379 1138
Contact Name: Maryann
Email: pbeachene@sbcglobal.net
Website: http://pawsitiveanimaltherapy.com

Reilly and Associates LLC
Tel: (860) 560 6773
Contact Name: Linda Reilly-Blue M.H.S.A.
Email: lreillyblue@reillyandassociatesllc.com
Website: http://reillyandassociatesllc.com

Provides in-home training and support to parents to assess and design effective parenting interventions for challenging situations.

St. Vincent's Behavioral Services
1 Lois Street
Norwalk, CT 06851
Tel: (203) 221 8899

St. Vincent's Outpatient Behavioral Health Services in Norwalk offers the following programs: Intensive day and evening programs for adults with mental health and substance abuse disorders. Intensive afterschool treatment program for adolescents with emotional/behavioral and psychological needs.

TherapyWorks Pediatrics, LLC
19 Halls Road, Suite 204
Old Lyme, CT 6420
Tel: (860) 434 5524
Contact Name: Debra Dickson
Email: deb@therapyworksct.com
Website: http://www.therapyworksct.com

Occupational therapy: physical therapy; registered dietitian; evaluations; continuing therapy; groups; play; sensory integration; school observation.

Tracey Taylor, MSW
Wilton, CT
Tel: (203) 357 1370

Offers parent support groups and one on one counseling with children, siblings and older children with ASD and other challenges.

United Services Center for Autism
303 Putnam Rd.
Wauregan, CT 06387
Tel: (860) 412 8686 or 1-(800) 953 0295
Contact Name: Debora Moyer
Email: dmoyer@usmhs.org
Website: http://www.UnitedServicesCT.org/autism

Services include assessments, ABA therapy, social thinking and social skills groups, vocational groups, parent training, and parent, grandparent and sibling support groups.

Victoria Shaw, PhD LPC
3 Hollyhock Lane
Wilton, CT 06897
Tel: (203) 210 5700
Email: vfshawphd@gmail.com.
Website: www.victoriashawpsychotherapy.com

Provides holistic psychotherapy to children and teens and others using many different approaches, allowing for highly individualized therapy.

Schools and Educational Services

AspergersCollegeBound
8 Lunar Drive
Woodbridge, CT 6525
Tel: (203) 397 5001
Contact Name: Barbara Ravski or Nancy Walls
Email: aspergerscollegebound@gmail.com

A family based program to prepare students with Asperger's, NVLD, PDD-NOS for college.

The Bentsen Learning Center
Mitchell College
437 Pequot Avenue
New London, CT 06320
Tel: (860) 701 5000
Contact name: Jason Ebbeling
Email: ebbeling_j@mitchell.edu
Website: http://community.mitchell.edu/blc

Provides a comprehensive academic support program for students with learning disabilities and attention deficit disorders, focusing on the teaching and application of learning strategies and career readiness skills.

Capitol Region Education Council
111 Charter Oak Avenue
Hartford, CT 06106
Tel: (860) 247 2732
Website: http://www.crec.org/index.php

Children's Academy
Stamford, CT 06907
Tel: (914) 374 2601

Contact Name: Rachel Albone
Email: ralbone@childrensacademyct.com
Website: http://www.childrensacademyct.com

Offers a birth to nine, home and community based early intervention program.

Cooperative Educational Services
25 Oakview Drive
Trumbull, CT 6611
Tel: (203) 365 8840
Contact Name: Anthony Maida
Email: maidat@ces.k12.ct.us
Website: http://www.ces.k12.ct.us

Offers highly specialized regional programs and services for students with ASD from birth to age 21 with school year and extended year services.

Glen Ridge College and Employment Coaching Program
77 New Milford Turnpike
New Preston, CT 6777
Tel: (860) 868 7377
Contact Name: Kathi Fitzherbert, Admissions Director
Email: kfitzher@devereux.org
Website: http://www.glenridgeprogram.org

Glen Ridge is a post secondary program for young adults with learning disabilities and Asperger's Syndrome.

Glenholme School
81 Sabbaday Lane
Washington, CT 06793
Tel: (860) 868 7377
Website: www.glenholme.org/podium

The Grove School
175 Copse Rd.
Madison, CT 06443
Tel: (203) 245 2778
Contact Name: Kelly Webster
Email: kelly@groveschool.org
Website: http://www.groveschool.org

The Grove School program is a co-educational, therapeutic boarding school.

Learn: Partners for Autism
44 Hatchett's Hill Rd.
East Lyme, CT 6371
Tel: (860) 434 4800
Contact Name: Pip Fritzsche
Email: pfritzsche@learn.k12.ct.us
Website: http://www.learn.k12.ct.us

LEARN Special Education offers both a center-based program and a school district based program based on ABA principles.

The Learning Clinic
Route 169, PO Box 324
Brooklyn, CT 6234
Tel: (860) 774 5619
Website: http://www.thelearningclinic.org

The Learning Clinic offers highly individualized educational programs in a friendly, rural setting.

Lighthouse Voc-Ed Center
P.O. Box 271
Old Mystic, CT 06372
46 Plaza Court,
Groton, CT 06340
Tel: (860) 445 7626
Email: info@lhcampus.com
Website: http://lhcampus.com/

The Lighthouse Voc-Ed Center, Inc. is an Accredited Private Special Education School for students age 7 to 21.

The Social Learning Center
50 North Plains Highway
Wallingford, CT 06492
Tel: (203) 774 0008 x 310
Contact Name: Lois Silver
Email: lsilver@benhaven.net
Website: http://www.sociallearningcenter.org

Offers social cognitive groups, individual counseling services, individual speech/language therapy, social communication evaluations and professional development.

St. Vincent's Special Needs Autism Services
95 Merritt Boulevard
Trumbull, CT 06611
Tel: (203) 375 6400
Contact Name: Debra A. Rausch
Email: debra.rausch@stvincents.org
Website: http://stvincentsspecialneeds.org

TheraCare's Academy for Young Minds
50 Washington Street, Suite #502
Norwalk, CT 6854
Tel: (888) 355 3255 x 2003
Contact Name: Deborah Mastronardi
Email: deborahmastronardiW@theracare.com
Website: http://www.theracare.com

TheraCare has developed its own curriculum, Developmental Designs for Young Minds.

Vista Vocational and Life Skills Center
1356 Old Clinton Rd.
Westbrook, CT 6498
Tel: (860) 399 8080
Contact Name: Bobbi Guercia

Email: bguercia@vistavocational.org
Website: http://www.vistavocational.org

A community-based post-secondary educational program for young adults with neurological disabilities. Offers vocational training, life skills instruction, counseling and support services.

Legal, Government & Financial Services

Advocacy for Kids, LLC
Fairfield, CT
Tel: (203) 763 4099
Contact Name: Ann McCarthy & Laurie Markus
Email: ann@advocacyforkids.net
Website: http://www.advocacyforkids.net

Founded by education advocates Laurie Markus and Ann McCarthy, Advocacy for Kids is dedicated to securing educational rights for Connecticut children with disabilities.

Advocacy Offices of Faith Filiault
196 Danbury Road
Wilton, CT 06897
Tel: (203) 493 4237
Contact Name: Faith Filiault
Email: faith@advocatewithfaith.com
Website: http://www.advocatewithfaith.com

Special Education, Bullying and Mental Health Advocacy.

Advocacy Solutions
33 Honey Hill Trail
Wilton, CT 6897
Tel: (203) 544 8366
Contact Name: Mary Ann Lombardi / Nancy Byrne
Email: mlombardi@advocacysolutionsct.com
Website: http://www.advocacysolutionsct.com

All About Your Special Child Education Advocacy Services
P.O. Box 323
Middlefield, CT 6455
Tel: (860) 349 1806
Contact Name: Julie Swanson
Email: julieswan@comcast.net
Website: http://www.yourspecialchild.com

Andrew A. Feinstein, Attorney at Law
86 Denison Avenue
Mystic, CT 6355
Tel: (860) 572 8585
Email: feinsteinandrew@sbcglobal.net
Website: http://www.attorneyfeinstein.com

Special education law.

Bureau of Rehabilitation Services
25 Sigourney Street, 11th Floor
Hartford, CT 06106
Tel: (860) 424 4840
Email: brs.dss@ct.gov
Website: http://www.ct.gov/brs/site/default.asp

Vocational Rehabilitation (VR) is a program of the Bureau of Rehabilitation Services which assists persons with significant physical or mental disabilities to prepare for, find or keep a job.

Child Advocacy, LLC
543 Prospect Avenue
Hartford, CT 6105
Tel: (203) 271 3011
Email: childadvocate@cox.net
Website: http://www.childadvocacyllc.com

Department of Housing and Urban Development
20 Church St. 10th Floor
Hartford, CT 06103
Tel: (860) 240 4800
Contact Name: Julie Fagan
Email: CT_Webmanager@hud.gov
Website: http://www.hud.gov/local/index.cfm?state=ct&topic=offices

Education Advocacy, LLC
846 Farmington Ave. Suite 10
West Hartford, CT 06119
Tel: (860) 270 0151
Contact Name: Diane Willcutts
Email: diane.willcutts@gmail.com
Website: http://www.educationadvocacyllc.com

Facing Futures, LLC
70 Bunker Hill Drive
Trumbull, CT 6611
Tel: (203) 261 3211
Contact Name: Maggie Coudriet Siegel
Email: Maggie@FacingFutures.net
Website: http://www.FacingFutures.net

FacingFutures, LLC specializes in advocacy for the special needs community.

Husky Health
55 Farmington Avenue
Hartford, CT 06105-3730
Tel: (1-877-CT-HUSKY (1-(877) 284 8759)
Website: http://www.huskyhealth.com/hh/site/ default.asp

HUSKY Health is the State of Connecticut's public health coverage program for eligible children, parents relative caregivers, senior citizens, individuals with disabilities, adults without children, and pregnant women.

Children up to age 19 may qualify regardless of family income level.

Law Office of Ann E. Rose, LLC
6 Nelson Lane
Newtown, CT 6740
Tel: (203) 304 1332
Email: arose@annroseesq.com
Website: http://www.annroseesq.com

Special education law.

Linda J. Talbert, LLC
161 East Ave. Suite 104
Norwalk, CT 06851
Tel: (203) 899 0745
Contact Name: Linda J. Talbert
Email: LindaTalbert@me.com
Website: http://www.SpecialEducationAdvocateCT.com

Martha L. Gibson
100 Eugene O'Neill Drive
New London, CT 6320
Tel: (860) 227 7492
Email: martha.gibson@ml.com
Website: http://www.fa.ml.com/martha.gibson

Financial planning for families of individuals with special needs.

Office of Protection and Advocacy for Persons with Disabilities
60-B Weston Street
Hartford, CT 6120
Tel: (860) 297 4300
Contact Name: James McGaughey
Email: hn2571@handsnet.org
Website: http://www.ct.gov/opapd

Otto Educational Consulting, LLC
Deep River, CT 06417
Tel: (860) 575 4718 or (860) 767 0755
Contact Name: Carole A. Otto, Director
Email: Ottocarole@gmail.com
Website: http://www.caroleotto.vpweb.com

PLAN of CT
P.O. Box 370312
West Hartford, CT 6137
Tel: (860) 523 4951
Email: director@planofct.org
Website: http://www.planofct.org

Manages trusts, set up by families, for the benefit of their family member with a disability.

Community and Recreation Services

Abilis
50 Glenville St.
Greenwich, CT 06831
Tel: (203) 531 1880
Website: http://www.abilis.us

Support and advocacy for people with developmental disabilities and their families in lower Fairfield County, CT and parts of Westchester County, NY.

Ability Beyond Disability
4 Berkshire Blvd.
Bethel, CT 6801
Tel: (888) 832 8427
Email: info@abilitybeyonddisability.org
Website: http://www.abilitybeyonddisability.org

Community-based support for people with disabilities in the Northeast through community job training and placement, supported living, and recreational and educational opportunities.

Ädelbrook Behavioral & Developmental Services
60 Hicksville Road
Cromwell, CT 06416
Tel: (860) 635 6010
Email: info@adelbrook.org
Website: http://www.adelbrook.org

Ädelbrook is a multi-service agency that provides a range of specialty programs for persons with autism and/or developmental disabilities.

Alternative Services Inc.
84 Linwood Avenue
Colchester, CT 6415
Tel: (860) 823 7155
Contact Name: Dolores Maerkle
Email: d.maerkel@asi-ct.org
Website: http://asi-ct.org

Provides Community Living Arrangements, In-Home support (behavioral services, functional behavioral assessments and Positive Behavior Support Plans) and individualized day service.

ARI of Connecticut: Always Reaching for Independence
174 Richmond Hill Ave.
Stamford, CT 6902
Tel: (203) 324 9258
Website: http://www.arict.org

ASD Fitness Center
307 Racebrook Rd.
Orange, CT 06477
Tel: (203) 553 9508

Email: info@asdfitnesscenter.com
Website: http://www.asdfitnesscenter.com

The ASD Fitness Center is a gym designed specifically to serve individuals who are on the Autism Spectrum.

Autism Family Support Group
Natchaug Hospital
189 Storrs Rd.
Mansfield, CT 06250
Tel: (860) 705 3877
Contact Name: Carleigh Hannah
Email: carleigh.hannah@hhchealth.org

Benhaven
187 Half Mile Road
New Haven, CT 6473
Tel: (203) 239 6425
Contact Name: Larry Wood, Executive Director
Email: lwood@benhaven.org
Website: http://www.benhaven.org

Camp Harkness
301 Great Neck Road
Waterford, CT 6385
Tel: (860) 859 5428
Website: http://www.ct.gov/dds/cwp/view.
asp?a=2653&q=393150

Dedicated for exclusive use by citizens with disabilities, accompanied by their family and friends.

Change a Life Time Companies, Inc.
168 Wainwright Place
Stratford, CT 6614
Tel: (203) 345 8992
Contact Name: Veronica Wilson
Email: changealifetime@yahoo.com

Provides respite care, group home, and day program services for people with ASD.

Chapel Haven, Inc.
1040 Whalley Avenue
New Haven, CT 06515
Tel: (203) 397 1714
Email: admissions@chapelhaven.org
Website: http://www.chapelhaven.org

Provides an array of individualized support services for adults 18+ with ASD and those with developmental and social disabilities.

CLASP Homes
246 Post Road East
Westport, CT 06880
Tel: (203) 226 7895
Website: http://clasphomes.org

Operates group homes and supported apartments throughout Fairfield County, serving adults with autism and related developmental disabilities.

Community Systems, Inc.
295 Alvord Park Road
Torrington, CT 06790
Tel: (860) 482 2887
Contact Name: Catharina Ohm
Email: info@csi-ct.org
Website: http://www.communitysystems.org/
supportsprovided/supportedemployment.html

CSI-Connecticut provides supported employment to persons who may work alone competitively or who may work in supported environments.

Connecticut Autism Spectrum Resource Center
101 N. Planes Road
Wellingford, CT 6492
Tel: (203) 265 7717
Contact Name: Monica Trischitti
Email: monica.asrc@hotmail.com
Website: http://www.ct-asrc.org

Provides information and research to help parents and professionals understand the barriers and challenges people faced with ASD.

Connecticut Parent Advocacy Center (CPAC)
Fair Haven Health Clinic
374 Grand Ave.
New Haven, CT 6513
Tel: (203) 776 3211
Toll Free: (800) 445 2722
Email: cpac@cpacinc.org
Website: http://www.cpacinc.org

Statewide parent training & info center; confidential phone consultations; workshops on various special education topics; resources, groups, and events.

Creative Living Community
60 Church Street
Manchester, CT 6040
Email: creativelivingcommunityofct@gmail.com
Website: http://www.creativelivingcommunityofct.org

Elegant Clinical
448 Spring Street
Windsor Locks, CT 06096
Tel: (860) 413 9509
Contact Name: Karen Lapienski, Ed.D., CEO
Email: KarenL11@aol.com
Website: http://www.elegantclinical.com

Elegant is a day program for those with autism, intellectual disabilities, as well as mental illness.

FAVARH
225 Commerce Drive
P.O. Box 1099
Canton, CT 6019
Tel: (860) 693 6662
Website: http://www.favarh.org

Favarh helps people with intellectual and developmental disabilities live as independently as possible.

FOCUS Center for Autism
126 Dowd Ave
Canton, CT 06019
Tel: (860) 693 8809 or (860) 693 6086
Contact Name: Yvonne Gardner
Email: info@focuscenterforautism.org
Website: http://www.focuscenterforautism.org

FOCUS is a year round licensed, clinical Extended Day Treatment Program specializing in the treatment of children and adolescents (ages 5-18) with ASD.

Friends of Autistic People
974 North Street
Greenwich, CT 6830
Tel: (203) 661 8510
Contact Name: Brita Darany von Regensburg
Email: bridaranyi@aol.com
Website: http://www.autisticadults.com/fap.htm

Advocates services for adults on the entire spectrum of autism.

Hart United
72 Washington Avenue
North Haven, CT 6473
Tel: (203) 234 2200
Email: info@hartinc.org
Website: http://www.hartinc.org

Provides support services, in a variety of settings, to individuals with developmental disabilities throughout Connecticut.

The Kennedy Center
2440 Reservoir Avenue
Trumbull, CT 6611
Tel: (203) 365 8522
Email: hr@kennedyctr.org
Website: http://www.thekennedycenterinc.org

Offers a broad range of programs and services for children, adults, and the elderly with diverse disabilities.

Kids Cooperate
167 Dockerel Rd.
Tolland, CT 06084
Tel: (860) 576 9506

Contact Name: Aaron Weintraub
Email: weintraub.a@gmail.com
Website: http://kidscooperate.com

Child-centered social skills groups with a focus on children and teenagers with ASD, ADHD, and Shyness.

LARC
314 Main Street
Torrington, CT 6790
Tel: (860) 482 9364
Email: larc@litchfieldarc.org
Website: http://www.litchfieldarc.org

LIVECTA Programs (The Light House)
New London County, CT
Tel: (860) 445 7626
Contact Name: Laura Reed
Email: livecta@lvecenter.com
Website: http://www.livectaprograms.com

Community-based residential programs.

MARC of Manchester
376R West Middle Turnpike
Manchester, CT 6040
Tel: (860) 646 5718
Website: http://www.marcct.org

Mosaic
100 Sebethe Drive, Suite A2
Cromwell, CT 6416
Tel: (860) 632 2814
Website: http://www.mosaicinfo.org

Provides service to adults with developmental disabilities in 21 community based residential homes in Bloomfield, Bristol, Coventry, Durham, East Hampton, Farmington, Gales Ferry, Mansfield, Middletown, Oakdale, Portland, West Hartford, and Wethersfield. Supported living apartment programs are also located in Hartford, Avon, Middletown, and Newington.

Ryan Woods Autism Foundation (RWAF)
955 S Main St. Suite B0W
Middletown, CT 06457
Tel: (860) 788 7277
Email: rwaf@comcast.net
Website: http://www.ryanwoodsautismfoundation.org

Helps families with ASD find the resources they need through parent and sibling support groups, as well as, educational after-school and summer therapeutic and recreational opportunities.

Sarah, Inc.
246 Goose Lane, Suite 101
Guilford, CT 6437

Tel: (203) 458 4040
Contact Name: Patricia Bourne, Executive Director
Email: pbourne@sarah-inc.org
Website: http://www.sarah-inc.org

Provides advocacy, services and support for people with intellectual and other disabilities.

Sibling Support Group
2300 Main St.
Glastonbury, CT 06033
Tel: (860) 430 1762
Contact Name: Melissa Albert
Email: MAlbert@autismct.com

Sibling support Groups are available for children ages 7-17 and are facilitated by a licensed psychologist.

St. Vincent's Behavioral Services
1 Lois Street
Norwalk, CT 06851
Tel: (203) 221 8899

St. Vincent's Outpatient Behavioral Health Services in Norwalk offers the following programs: Intensive day and evening programs for adults with mental health and substance abuse disorders. Intensive afterschool treatment program for adolescents with emotional/ behavioral and psychological needs.

Star, Inc.
90 Washington St.
South Norwalk, CT 6854
Tel: (203) 853 6404
Website: http://www.starinc-lightingtheway.org

Provides support, services, and advocacy to help individuals achieve independence, free choice, and personal growth.

STRIDE Adaptive Sports
Ski Sundown
126 Ratlum Road
New Hartford, CT 6057
Tel: (860) 379 7669
Contact Name: Shelly Gambino
Email: shelly_gambino@yahoo.com
Website: http://www.stride.org

Wallingford Parks and Recreation Department
6 Fairfield Boulevard
Wallingford, CT 06492
Tel: (203) 294 2120
Contact Name: Emily Swindelles, Assistant Recreation Program Specialist
Email: emily.swindelles@gmail.com
Website: http://www.town.wallingford.ct.us/Content/ Parks_and_Recreation.asp

Provides inclusion programs but also offers adaptive recreation programs designed specifically for individuals with special needs.

DELAWARE

Doctors, Clinics, Hospitals, and Other Health Services

ADVOSERV of Delaware
4185 Kirkwood St Georges Rd
Bear, DE 19701
Tel: (302) 834 7018
Toll Free: (800) 593 4959
Email: Yamashitam@advoserv.com
Website: http://www.advoserv.com/delaware.html

Bear-Glasgow Dental, LLC
1290 Peoples Plaza
Newark, DE 19702
Tel: (302) 836 3750
Contact Name: Jennifer Buckingham
Email: info@bearglasgowdental.com
Website: http://www.bearglasgowdental.com or http:// www.peninsuladentalmillsboro.com

Child Neurology Clinic
Sanjai C. Rao, DO
3521 Silverside Road
Wilmington, DE 19810
Website: http://www.childneurologyclinic.com

Christine Hoffner Barthold, PhD, BCBA
22 Thistleberry Drive
Newark, DE 19702
Tel: (301) 604 7392
Email: chrisbarthold@bartholdautism.com
Website: http://www.bartholdautism.com

Concord Medical Chiropractic Neurology
6 Sharpley Road
Wilmington, DE 19803
Tel: (302) 668 8082
Contact Name: Marcia Puzzanghera
Email: marcia@concordmedical.org
Website: http://www.concordmedical.org

Meadowwood Hospital
575 South Dupont HIghway
New Castle, DE 19720
Tel: (302) 328 3330
Email: bmason@meadowwoodhospital.com
Website: http://www.meadowwoodhospital.com

Works closely with patients and their families to understand the issues they are facing in order to create an individualized treatment plan.

Peninsula Dental, LLC
26670 Centerview Dr Unit 19
Millsboro, DE 19966
Tel: (302) 297 3750
Contact Name: Sandy Hearn
Email: sandy.peninsuladental@gmail.com
Website: http://www.peninsuladentalmillsboro.com or http://www.bearglasgowdental.com

Offers family and special needs dentistry in a comfortable, affordable office environment.

Practice Without Pressure, Inc.
2470 Sunset Lake Road
Newark, DE 19702
Tel: (302) 832 2800 or (302) 559 0048
Contact Name: Jane Miller
Email: Jane.Miller@pwpde.com
Website: http://www.pwpde.com

Practice Without Pressure is a training and treatment center for people with disabilities who fear or avoid routine care.

Therapy Services

All The Difference (ATD)
Concord Plaza, 3521 Silverside Rd. Quillen Building, Suite 21-2
Wilmington, DE 19810
Tel: (302) 478 0600
Website: http://www.allthedifference.org

Provides pediatric sensory integration, evaluation, and therapy using the DIR/Floortime model.

Autism Delaware Clinical Services
924 Old Harmony Road Suite 201
Newark, DE 19713
Tel: (302) 224 6020
Email: delautism@delautism.org
Website: http://autismdelaware.org/AutismResources/ClinicalServices.aspx

Delaware Early Childhood Center
Mispillion Rd. and West Streets
Harrington, DE 19952
Website: http://www.lf.k12.de.us/decc/earlyintervention.html

DECC's Early Intervention program offers early intervention services assisting children, from birth to three years old, who have developmental delays or disabilities and their families.

Dover Behavioral Health
725 Horsepond Road
Dover, DE 19901
Tel: (302) 741 0140
Contact Name: Mike Gavula
Email: michael.gavula@uhsinc.com
Website: http://www.doverbehavioral.com/

Provides inpatient and outpatient behavioral healthcare services for adolescents and adults.

The Jungle Gym Rehabilitation Center for Children
1695 South State Street Suite 5A
Dover, DE 19901
Tel: (302) 734 1515
Website: http://thejunglegymrehab.com

The Jungle Gym is a Rehabilitation Center providing assessment and treatment, including physical, occupational, speech therapy, and various specialized programs for all infants and children.

Rockford Center
100 Rockford Drive
Newark, DE 19713
Tel: (302) 996 5480
Toll Free: (866) 847 4357
Contact Name: Mike Gavula
Email: Mike.Gavula@uhsinc.com
Website: http://www.rockfordcenter.com/

Southern Delaware Therapeutic & Recreational Horseback Riding, Inc.
P.O. Box 219
Nassau, DE 19969
Tel: (302) 644 1920
Website: http://www.sdtrhr.com

Equine-assisted therapy.

Terry Children's Psychiatric Center
10 Central Avenue
New Castle, DE 19720
Tel: (302) 577 4270
Website: http://dhss.delaware.gov/dhss/main/maps/holloway/terrycpc.htm

Schools and Educational Services

Child's Play By the Bay
1510 Savannah Road
Lewes, DE 19958
Tel: (302) 645 2153

Email: info@childsplaylewes.com
Website: http://www.childsplayde.com

Small progressive preschool and childcare center offering a variety of programs designed to meet the developmental needs of children.

Early CHOICES
New Castle County
New Castle Corporate Commons 2 Reads Way
New Castle, DE 19720
Tel: (302) 323 5370
Website: http://www.lf.k12.de.us/decc/earlychoices.html

Offers special education and related services for three year old children with developmental delays and three and four year old children with speech delays and provides support for their families.

Pilot School
100 Garden Of Eden Rd.
Wilmington, DE 19803
Tel: (302) 478 1740
Email: info@pilotschool.org
Website: http://pilotschool.org

University of Delaware
University of Delaware Newark, DE 19716
Tel: (302) 831 0532
Contact Name: Laura T. Eisenman
Email: eisenman@udel.edu
Website: http://www.udel.edu/cds

Legal, Government & Financial Services

Delaware Disabilities Law Program
Community Legal Aid Society
Community Legal Aid Society, Inc. 144 E. Market Street
Georgetown, DE 19947
Tel: (302) 856 3742
Website: http://www.workworld.org

Delaware Health and Social Services: Division of Developmental Disabilities Services
1056 South Governor's Avenue, Suite 101
Dover, DE 19904
Tel: (302) 744 9600
Website: http://www.dhss.delaware.gov/dhss/ddds/

Community and Recreation Services

Active Day Center
200 White Chapel Drive
Newark, DE 19713

Tel: (302) 533 3543
Contact Name: Michelle Hood
Email: mhood@activeday.com
Website: http://www.activeday.com

Autism Delaware
16394 Samuel Paynter Blvd Suite 201
Milton, DE 19968
Tel: (302) 644 3410
Email: delautism@delautism.org
Website: www.autismdelaware.org

Established by families, advocates for the autism community.

Autism Delaware POW&R
924 Old Harmony Road Suite 201
Newark, DE 19713
Tel: (302) 224 6020
Contact Name: Katina Demetriou
Email: katina.demetriou@delautism.org
Website: http://autismdelaware.org/AdultServices/AboutPOWR.aspx

Productive Opportunities for Work & Recreation or POW&R, assists adults with ASD find and be successful at employment, volunteer activities and recreation.

CHIMES Delaware
254 E. Main Street
Newark, DE 19711
Tel: (302) 731 1504
Website: http://www.chimesdel.org

Provides educational, employment, vocational, residential, habilitative and behavioral health services and supports.

Delaware Division of Vocational Rehabilitation
4425 N. Market Street
Wilmington, DE 19089
Tel: (302) 761 8300
Website: http://dvr.delawareworks.com/

Provides opportunities and resources to eligible individuals with disabilities, to promote employment and independent living.

KenCrest
713 East Basin Rd.
New Castle, DE 19720
Tel: (302) 323 2813
Website: http://www.kencrest.org/

Provides services such as inclusive, preschools, services in the home, community living settings, lifesharing, job coaching, and more.

People's Place
1129 Airport Road
Milford, DE 19963
Tel: (302) 422 8033
Website: http://www.peoplesplace2.com

Identifies the social/mental health needs of Delaware residents and facilitates the provision of services to address those needs.

Transition, Education and Employment Model
461 Wyoming Road
Newark, DE 19716
Tel: (302) 831 8103
Contact Name: Wendy Claiser
Email: wclaiser@udel.edu
Website: http://www.udel.edu/cds/teem.employ.html

The goal of Employment Services is to develop job skills, Assists with job skills training, vocational training and employment opportunities for people with disabilities at the University of Delaware and in the surrounding community.

FLORIDA

Doctors, Clinics, Hospitals, and Other Health Services

Ardalan Pediatric Dentistry
Ardalan Pediatric Dentistry
374 SW Prima Vista Blvd.
Port St. Lucie, FL 34983
Tel: (772) 344 4664
Contact Name: Reza Ardalan, DMD
Email: info@ArdalanDental.com
Website: http://www.ArdalanDental.com

Central Florida Functional Medicine PLLC
Scott Smith, PA
3800 West Eau Gallie Blvd, Suite 105
Melbourne, FL 32766
Tel: (321) 259 7111
Website: www.centralfloridafunctionalmedicine.
com/3.html

Functional medicine practice providing care to individuals (children through adults) with pervasive health conditions, including a focus on children with ASD and other special needs.

Child & Family Institute
3492 Magic Oak Lane
Sarasota, FL 34232
Tel: (941) 379 9110
Contact Name: Michael R Fox, M.D
Website: http://www.thechildandfamily.com

Provides medical and psychological care for children, adolescents, and families.

The Conde Center for Chiropractic Neurology
PAL Clinic Office 2863 Executive Park Drive
Weston, FL 33331
Tel: (954) 603 1632
Email: UPP@thecondecenter.com
Website: http://thecondecenter.com/upp.html

Dentistry for Children & Those with Special Needs
1233 NW 18th Street
Pembroke Pines, FL 33026
Tel: (954) 435 4100

Developmental and Behavioral Pediatrics of South Florida
Judith Aronson-Ramos, MD
5350 West Hillsboro Blvd
Coconut Creek, FL 33073
(954) 531 0847
Contact Name: Dr Ramos
Email: info@draronsonramos.com
Website: http://www.draronsonramos.com

Board-certified developmental & behavioral pediatrician specializing in to the evaluation and treatment of pediatric patients (birth - 25 yrs) with challenges in learning, behavior, development, and social-emotional functioning, including ASD.

FIU Embrace
Modesto Maidique Campus, 885 SW 109th Avenue
PG-5, Suite 131
Miami, FL 33199
Tel: (305) 348 3627
Website: http://health.fiu.edu/resources/programs/fiu-embrace

FIU Embrace is a comprehensive, integrated program of the FIU Herbert Wertheim College of Medicine that provides medical and behavioral health care to adults with ASD.

Frank J. Sierra, DMD, PA Pediatric Dentistry
5420 Webb Rd C2
Tampa, FL 33615
Tel: (813) 889 0780
Email: office@SierraDMD.com
Website: http://www.SierraDMD.com

Dr. Lisa's Family Chiropractic & Natural Health Care
1114 Florida Ave. Suite C
Palm Harbor, FL 34683
Tel: (727) 772 1966
Contact Name: Dr. Lisa Marsh
Website: http://www.mydrlisa.com

Miami Children's Hospital
3200 SW 60th Court Suite 302
Miami, FL 33155
Tel: (305) 662 8300
Website: http://www.mch.com

Nelson Mañé, DC
1602 West Sligh Avenue
Suite 500
Tampa, FL 33604
Tel: (813) 935 4744
Website: www.manecenter.com

Perlmutter Health Center
800 Goodlette Road N Suite 270
Naples, FL 34102
Tel: (239) 649 7400
Contact Name: Dr. David Perlmutter, MD, FACN, ABIHM and Dr. Deborah Post, MSN, ARNP For appointments: Fran Lankford
Email: patientmail@perlhealth.com
Website: http://www.perlhealth.com

Using many traditional and complementary health modalities, provides a comprehensive, fully integrated treatment plan specifically designed for individual patients' needs.

Premier Compounding Pharmacy
2000 PGA Blvd. Suite 5507
Palm Beach Gardens, FL 33408
Tel: (561) 691 4991
Contact Name: Ashley- Marketing Director
Email: info@premiercompounding.com
Website: http://www.premiercompounding.com

A compounding pharmacy that specializes in pediatric customized medications.

Rossignol Medical Center
Dan Rossignol, MD FAAFP, FMAPS
3800 W. Eau Gallie Blvd
Suite 105
Melbourne, FL 32934
Tel: (321) 259 7111
Website: www.rossignolmedicalcenter.com

Provides comprehensive biomedical treatments to children with ASD and other conditions.

Seaside Smiles Pediatric Dentistry
Seaside Smiles Pediatric Dentistry
3725 12th Court Suite B
Vero Beach, FL 32960
Tel: (772) 562 6880
Contact Name: Dr. Mindy
Website: http://www.seasidesmiles.com

Singer Family Chiropractic
9770 S Military Trail B 2-3
Boynton Beach, FL 33436
Tel: (561) 739 9500
Email: docsinger@singerfamilychiropractic.com
Website: http://www.singerfamilychiropractic.com

Smile Builders Pediatric Dentistry
6415 Sheldon Road
Tampa, FL 33615
Tel: (813) 880 0100
Contact Name: Shana Kligerman
Email: smilebuilders@verizon.net
Website: http://www.smilebuilders4kids.com

Vitality Health & Wellness
801 Fourth Street
Miami Beach, FL 33139
Tel: (305) 466 1100
Contact Name: Andrew Levinson, MD
Email: info@vitalitywellness.com
Website: http://www.vitalitywellness.com

Functional, medicine integrative psychiatry, and nutrition.

Wholistic Pediatrics
David Berger, MD
3405 West Fletcher Avenue
Tampa, FL 33618
Tel: (813) 960 3415
Website: www.wholisticfamilycare.com

Pediatric integrative medical practice that seeks to find the cause of health problems, not just treat symptoms.

Therapy Services

ABA Therapy Solutions, LLC
Palm City, FL 34990-2042
Tel: (772) 486 1789 or (772) 486 4870
Contact Name: Linda Peirce, M.Ed., BCBA
Email: linda@abasolutions.org
Website: http://www.abasolutions.org

Amanda Keating and Associates
7320 East Fletcher Ave.
Tampa, FL 33637
Tel: (813) 490 6365
Website: http://www.amandakeating.com

Provides a variety of services including psychological assessments, professional consultation, and therapeutic interventions.

BayCare Behavioral Health
6636 Rowan Rd
New Port Richey, FL 34653
Tel: (866) 762 1743

Website: http://baycare.org/body.cfm?id=944

Provides individual screening and assessment along with individual, family and group psychotherapy with our behavioral therapists. Both outpatient and in-home care is available. Support services include: financial assistance, crisis planning, education plan development and more.

Compass Behavioral & Developmental Consultants, LLC
8638 Reedy Branch Dr.
Jacksonville, FL 32256
Tel: (800) 832 9419
Email: info@compassaid.com
Website: http://www.compassaid.com

Focuses on early intervention for children diagnosed with Autism Spectrum Disorder as well as school aged children and supportive services for adults. Provides Intensive ABA therapies, Discrete Trial Training (DTT), Verbal Behavior Therapy (VBT), and Social Skill Training.

Good Hope Equestrian Training Center
22155 SW 147th Avenue
Miami, FL 33170
Tel: (305) 258 2838
Contact Name: Peggy Bass, Ph.D.
Email: ghetc@bellsouth.net
Website: http://www.goodhopeequestriancenter.com

The Good Hope Equestrian Training Center has an array of services for children, youth & adults diagnosed with Autism Spectrum Disorders: therapeutic horseback riding (ages 4 & up), companion services (ages 5 & up), adult day training (ages 21 & up) & supported employment (ages 18 & up).

Hale Therapy Services, Inc.
12691 Chartwell Drive
Fort Myers, FL 33912
Tel: (239) 691 0765
Contact Name: Jennifer Washburn, MS, OTR
Email: jenwashburn@haletherapy.com
Website: http://www.autismspeaks.org/d

Provides a wide range of therapeutic interventions and support services.

HAPPI Farm
17800 SW 52nd Ct.
Southwest Ranches, FL 33331
(954) 629 8133
Contact Name: Marie Lim, Founder and President
Email: marielim@happifarm.org
Website: http://www.happifarm.org

Provides Animal-Assisted Learning and Equine Therapy. Programs include Therapeutic Horseback Riding, Care of Farm and Exotic Animals and Horticulture.

KIDSology, Inc.
14750 S.W. 26 Street Suite #111
Miami, FL 33185
Tel: (305) 392 0445 or (786) 355 1475
Contact Name: Jesenia "Jessie" Hernandez
Email: jessie@mykidsology.com
Website: http://www.mykidsology.com/

Offers ABA Therapy/ Behavior Modification Therapy, Social Skills Training Groups, and counseling.

Live Well Therapy Group (LWTG)
260 Palermo Ave. Suite 14
Coral Gables, FL 33134
Tel: (305) 455 2782 or (786) 663 6887
Contact Name: Sasha Dimitrjevitch
Email: Sasha@livewelltherapygroup.com
Website: http://www.livewelltherapygroup.com

New Way Day Services, Inc.
8399 NW 66Street
Doral, FL 33166
Tel: (305) 597 3861
Contact Name: Cary Merida

Opportunity, Community, Ability (OCA), Inc.
4917 Eli St.
Orlando, FL 32804
Tel: (407) 808 7837
Contact Name: Silvia Haas
Email: shaas@gooca.org
Website: http://www.gooca.org

Provides programs & services for individuals with Autism or other disabilities ages 4 to adulthood including: Afterschool Program, School Age Summer & School Holiday Camps, Preschool (Pee Wee) Summer Camp, AVT (Adult Vocational Training) Program, AVT Entrepreneurial Program- ShopOCA, Behavior Analysis & Therapy, Social Skills Events, Respite, & Special Olympics Training.

The Ocala Autism Center
1130 SE 18th Place
Ocala, FL 34471
Tel: (352) 390 6656
Contact Name: Delsa Darline
Email: delsadarline@e-Swank.com

Palm Beach Behavioral Health and Wellness, LLC
345 Jupiter Lakes Blvd. Suite 302A
Jupiter, FL 33458
Tel: (561) 429 2397
Contact Name: Dr. Kelly Everson
Email: drkelly@palmbeachbhw.com
Website: http://www.palmbeachbhw.com

Sarkis Family Psychiatry
529 NorthWest 60th St
Gainesville, FL 32607
Tel: (352) 331 5100
Contact Name: Stephanie or Suzy Hoover
Email: info@ehsfamily.com
Website: http://www.ehsfamily.com

School of Thought
15214 80th Drive North
Palm Beach Gardens, FL 33418
Tel: (561) 252 5113
Contact Name: Joyce Albu
Email: Aut2teach@aol.com

Provides assessment and treatment to children, adolescents, and adults with ASD and other neurodevelopmental disorders and develops individualized treatment plans.

TherAbilities Performing Arts Center (TPAC)
225 W. Busch Blvd. Suite #102
Tampa, FL 33612
Tel: (813) 344 0960 or (813) 935 3162
Contact Name: Lourdes Quinones, Founder/Physical Therapist
Email: lourdes@tpackids.com
Website: http://www.tpackids.com

Programs designed and led by Pediatric Physical, Occupational, Speech and Music therapists.

Threshold Center for Autism
3550 N. Goldenrod Road
Winter Park, FL 32792
Tel: (407) 671 7060
Contact Name: Indira Clayton
Email: iclayton@threshold-center.org
Website: http://www.threshold-center.org

Walrus Services, LLC ABA Group
390 S Geronimo Street Suite 104
Miramar Beach, FL 32550
Tel: (850) 650 0053or (321) 689 2072
Contact Name:
Dr. Guy Walden
Email: gwalden@embarqmail.com
Website: http://walrusservices.com

Whispering Manes Therapeutic Riding Center
6255 SW 125th Avenue
Miami, FL 33183
Tel: (305) 909 4343
Contact Name: Robin Bramson
Email: Rbramson@whisperingmanes.org
Website: http://www.whisperingmanes.org

Schools and Educational Services

Abis' Place
10168 West Sample Road
Coral Springs, FL 33065
Tel: (954) 753 4441
Contact Name: Danielle Zimmerman
Email: abisplace@aol.com
Website: http://www.abisplace.com

Atlantis Academy
10193 NW 31st Street
Coral Springs, FL 33065
Tel: (954) 752 7571
Contact Name: Dr. Hershey
Email: ihershey@esa-edcuation.com
Website: http://www.esa-education.com

Special education private school serving students in first through twelfth grades.

Bridge Learning Community
Element Church School 2702 Causeway Center Drive
Tampa, FL 33619
Tel: (813) 317 3227
Contact Name: Bill Beers
Email: billiebeers@gmail.com
Website: http://www.bridgelearningcommunity.org

School and therapy center for children with ASD.

Closing the Gaps Learning Center
24 64 Coral Way
Miami, FL 33145
Tel: (305) 854 3516
Contact Name: Edna Caceres
Email: closingthegaps@bellsouth.net
Website: http://www.closingthegaps.net

Uses the Accelerated Learning Strategies program and offers individualized 9-week educational intervention day programs.

College Internship Program (CIP) Brevard
3692 N. Wickham Rd
Melbourne, FL 32935
Tel: (321) 259 1900, X11
Contact Name: Stephanie Brown, Admissions Coordinator
Email: sbrown@cipbrevard.org
Website: http://www.cipbrevard.org

CIP's full-year postsecondary programs provide young adults with Asperger's, High-Functioning Autism, ADHD, Nonverbal and other Learning Differences with the social, academic, career and life skills necessary for success.

College Living Experience (CLE)
6555 Nova Drive Suite #300
Davie, FL 33317

Tel: (954) 370 5142
Contact Name: Terri Shermett, Program Director
Website: http://www.experiencecle.com

College Living Experience (CLE) is a post-secondary program for students who require additional support with academic, social, independent living skills and career development.

Crossroads School
6249 Atlantic Blvd
Jacksonville, FL 32211
Tel: (904) 652 1282
Contact Name: Larry K Broach
Email: lkbroach@crossroadsschools.com
Website: http://www.crossroadsschools.com

Crossroads is a private Christian school specializing in providing educational services to students with learning disabilities and autism.

Crystal Academy
110 Phoenetia Ave
Coral Gables, FL 33134
Tel: (305) 567 5881 or (786) 261 8160
Contact Name: David Pike
Email: pike_davidr@thecrystalacademy.net
Website: http://www.crystalacademycg.org/ or http://www.caprimaryschool.org/

Crystal Academy and Crystal Academy Primary School are a broad service early intervention center. Primary services are Behavior, Speech and Occupational therapies as well as a full K-5th grade ESE curriculum.

De LaSalle Academy of Fort Myers
8871 De LaSalle Academy Way
Fort Myers, FL 33912
Tel: (239) 245 8212
Contact Name: Lori Moreau
Email: lmoreau@delasallefm.org
Website: http://www.delasallefm.org

De LaSalle Academy is a private, non-profit, non-religious school for children with special needs in grades PreK-12. Offering individualized academic programs and therapies including speech & language, occupational, and counseling. Adopted programs include: Michelle Garcia Winner's Social Thinking Program, DIR/Floortime, Love & Logic, Wilson Language, Fast ForWord.

Emerald Coast Autism Center
200 N. Partin Drive
Niceville, FL 32578
Tel: (850) 279 3000
Contact Name: Staci Berryman
Email: ECAutismCenter@cox.net

Offers both individual ABA tutoring and ABA in a classroom environment. Accepts McKay Scholarship and TriCare. Also provides early intervention services through Florida's Early Steps program.

Florida Children's Academy
116 N. Bumby Ave.
Orlando, FL 32803
Tel: (407) 896 1739
Contact Name: Rachel Rodriguez
Email: Flchacademy@gmail.com
Website: http://www.floridachildrensacademy.com

Early Education for children with Autism and other special needs including occupational, physical and speech therapy for children ages 12 months to 12 years old. Florida McKay scholarships accepted.

Infinite Grace Academy
2108 Lewis Turner Blvd
Fort Walton Beach, FL 32579
Tel: (850) 864 2273
Contact Name: Karen Reid, BCBA
Email: infinitegrace@cox.net
Website: http://www.infinitegraceacademy.com

An ABA based therapeutic school for children with communication difficulties. Focuses on verbal behavior methodology incorporated within the curriculum and individualized plans focusing on behavior reduction, skill acquisition, and educational achievement. Low student to staff ratio from 1:1 - 1:4. Accepts Tricare funding and McKay Scholarship.

The Jericho School
1351 Sprinkle Drive
Jacksonville, FL 32211
Tel: (904) 744 5110
Contact Name: Angelo Martinez, Executive Director
Email: jerichoschool@yahoo.com
Website: http://www.TheJerichoSchool.org

The Jericho School and Clinic is an ABA and VBA based program for children with ASD and other developmental disabilities.

The Learning Academy at USF
13301 Bruce B. Downs Boulevard MHC 2113A
Tampa, FL 33612
Tel: (813) 974 2996
Contact Name: Susan Richmond
Email: srichmond@usf.edu
Website: http://learningacademy.fmhi.usf.edu

The Learning Academy at the University of South Florida is a thirty-week, two-semester transitional program designed to help students with ASD build and enhance skills that will prepare students for the world of work or to further their education.

LYF Inc.
Wesley Chapel, FL 33544
Tel: (813) 469 2455 or (727) 514 2785
Contact Name: Jim Cracchiolo
Email: jc@lyfinc.com
Website: http://www.lyfinc.com
FB: http://www.facebook.com/lyfincpasco

Offers Adult Day Training, Special Standards High School Home School and After-School Care all by certified teachers as well as advocacy services, IEP enforcement, and general information regarding education.

Mailman Segal Center (MSC) for Human Development
Jim & Jan Moran Family Center Village Nova
Southeastern University, 3301 College Ave.
Ft. Lauderdale, FL 33314
Tel: (954) 262 6918
Toll Free: (800) 836 8326
Website: http://www.nova.edu/humandevelopment/index.html

May Institute
1409 Kingsley Avenue, Suite 1A
Orange Park, FL 32073
Tel: (904) 269 0773
Contact Name: William Flood
Email: wflood@mayintitute.org
Website: http://www.mayinstitute.org

Provides educational, rehabilitative, and behavioral healthcare services to individuals with autism spectrum disorder and other developmental disabilities, brain injury, mental illness, and behavioral health needs.

Montessori School of North Miami
695 NE 123rd St.
North Miami, FL 33161
Tel: (305) 893 5994
Contact Name: Evelyn Lopez-Couto
Email: montessorinm@aol.com

Montessori school for children 2–6 years old offering a bilingual inclusion program with ABA therapists available in the school; as well as speech, OT, and PT therapy. Accepts McKay, VPK, also private funding available for ASD children.

Nicky's Place Preschool
7150 W. McNab Road
Tamarac, FL 33321
Tel: (954) 718 9532
Contact Name: Kelly Thompson
Email: kelly@nickysplace.com

Nicky's place is a preschool for special needs and typical children, from ages 2 - 5.

Pinnacle Academy
6215 Lorraine Road
Bradenton, FL 34202
Tel: (941) 755 1400
Contact Name: Dr. Kirstina Ordetx
Email: kordetx@verizon.net
Website: http://www.thepinnacleacademy.com

Pinnacle offers a private education to children, ages 16 months to 18 years of age, who have ASD or a related developmental disorder. The program includes ABA, PRT, IT, PECS, and social skills training.

Project THRIVE
College of Education and Human Services, UNF, 1
UNF Drive Building 57, 3rd Floor, Office 3715
Jacksonville, FL 32224
Tel: (904) 620 1356
Contact Name: Joanna L. Ale, MS
Email: unf.thrive@gmail.com

College transition program for degree-seeking students with ASD at the University of North Florida.

Royal Palm School
6650 Lawrence Rd
Lake Worth, FL 33462
Website: http://www.edline.net/GroupHome.page

South Florida Child Development Center
280 Westward Drive
Miami Springs, FL 33166
Tel: (305) 882 8119
Contact Name: Angela M. Gonzalez, CBA
Email: agonz0170@aol.com
Website: http://www.miamifriendshipschool.com

SFCDC is an educational alternative providing an intensive, educational program for young children with autism & related disorders. ABA, Verbal Behavior, Pivotal Response Training, and Direct Instruction are used.

Sydney's School for Autism
4518 South Manhattan Ave
Tampa, FL 33611
Tel: (813) 835 4591
Contact Name: Jennifer R Wooten/Anita Mauer
Email: info@advancedbehavioralsystems.com
http://www.sydneysschoolhouse.com

Program combines regular education with children having special needs. Sydney's School offers therapy and individualized services.

The Transition Program at Southeastern University
Polk County School Board, ATTN: Transition Services
P.O. Box 391
Bartow, FL 33831
Tel: (863) 534 0930

Contact Name: Karen Toppin
Email: karen.toppin@polk-fl.net
Website: http://www.polk-fl.net/districtinfo/
departments/learning/ese/transition.htm

University of South Florida-St. Petersburg
University of South Florida-St. Petersburg St.
Petersburg, FL 33701
Tel: (727) 873 4662
Contact Name: Jordan T. Knab
Email: jknab@mail.usf.edu
Website: http://www.stpt.usf.edu/disability

The Vanguard School
22000 Highway 27
Lake Wales, FL 33859
Tel: (863) 676 6091
Email: vanadmin@vanguardschool.org
Website: http://www.vanguardschool.org

Westlake Academy
4188 S University Drive
Davie, FL 33328
Tel: (954) 236 2300
Contact Name: Robyn Pepitone
Email: wps4188@yahoo.com
Website: http://www.westlakeschool.com

Provides a year round, individualized, alternative academically based educational program based on ABA and VBA for K–12.

Legal, Government & Financial Services

Center for Autism & Related Disabilities
UF-Jacksonville
6271 St. Augustine Rd. Suite 1
Jacksonville, FL 32217
Tel: (904) 633 0760
Toll Free: (800) 928 8476

Provides free services to individuals with autism and related disabilities, to their families, and to the professionals who work with them.

Children's Medical Services
7000 Lake Ellenor Drive
Orlando, FL 32809
Tel: (407) 858 5555
Contact Name: Adrian Lugo
Email: adrian_lugo@doh.state.fl.us
Website: http://www.cms-kids.com

Florida Division of Vocational Rehabilitation
2002 Old Saint Augustine Road Building A
Tallahassee, FL 32301
Tel: (850) 245 3399

Contact Name: Aleisa McKinlay
Website: http://www.rehabworks.org/

Vocational Rehabilitation (VR) is a federal-state program that works with people who have physical or mental disabilities to prepare for, gain or retain employment.

MetLife Center for Special Needs Planning
New England Financial a MetLife Company 9150 S
Dadeland Blvd, Suite 1600
Miami, FL 33156
Tel: (305) 929 5335
Contact Name: S. Scott Lain
Email: slain@miami.nef.com
Website: http://www.miamiagency.neffirm.com/ecard.
cfm?ID=334418

Community and Recreation Services

Achievers of America
9438 US 19 #141
Port Richey, FL 34668
Tel: (727) 868 5084
Contact Email: steveachievers@yahoo.com
Tel: http://www.achieversofamerica.info

The Achievers of America is a recreational program for individuals with disabilities.

Adolph and Rose Levis Jewish Community Center
Adolph and Rose Levis Jewish Community Center
9801 Donna Klein Boulevard
Boca Raton, FL 33428
Tel: (561) 852 3200
Email: martys@levisjcc.org
Website: http://levisjcc.org

Alliance for Independence, Inc.
1038 Sunshine Dr. E.
Lakeland, FL 33801
Tel: (863) 665 3846
Contact Name: Dan Berman
Email: dberman@afi-fl.org
Website: http://www.afi-fl.org

Angelwood Inc.
PO Box 24925
Jacksonville, FL 32241
Tel: (904) 288 7259
Contact Name: Erin LaVecchia
Email: elavecchia@angelwoodjax.org
Website: http://www.angelwoodjax.org

Summer camp for children with autism and/or DD and a day program for adults with autism and/or DD.

Ann Storck Center
1790 S.W. 43rd Way
Fort Lauderdale, FL 33317
Tel: (954) 584 8000
Website: http://www.annstorckcenter.org

Art & Yoga Works, LLC
1217 NE 16th Ave.
Ft Lauderdale, FL 33304
Tel: (908) 303 5855
Contact Name: Lauren Rosenthal, MPS, ATR
Email: lorirose3@gmail.com

Art Therapy and Yoga Classes for individuals with ASD. Group and individual sessions are available.

Autism Caregivers Connect
1515 Huntington Lane #212
Rockledge, FL 32955
Tel: (321) 433 1437
Contact Name: Kimberly Molina
Email: kmolina73@yahoo.com
Website: http://www.accbrevard.org

Autism Caregivers Connect is a non-profit corporation in North and Central Brevard County for families and caregivers of children, teens, and young adults with ASD. It hosts monthly meetings with guest speakers, caregiver social nights, family get-togethers and teen social events.

Boxing for Life, LLC
Pompano Fitness 1955 N Federal Hwy.
Pompano Beach, FL 33062
Tel: (561) 685 9111
Contact Name: Jay Silverman
Email: Jspunchout@gmail.com

A non-contact boxing program designed for those with special needs.

Creative Clay, Inc.
Cultural Arts Center
1124 Central Avenue
St. Petersburg, FL 33705
Tel: (727) 825 0515
Website: http://creativeclay.org

City of Clearwater Therapeutic Recreation
1501 N. Belcher Rd.
Clearwater, FL 33765
Tel: 727-793 2339 ext. 245 or (727) 793 2320
Website: http://www.myclearwater.com/gov/depts/parksrec/therapeutics.asp

Inclusion and Therapeutic Recreation supervised by a Certified Therapeutic Recreation Specialist.

Dinosaur Playground
4910 Tamiami Trail North
Naples, FL 34103
Tel: (239) 430 7529
Website: http://www.dinoplayground.com

Dolphin Healing Retreats
4421 NE 13th Ave
Oakland Park, FL 33334
Tel: (919) 245 3499
Contact Name: Patricia Schmidt
Email: dolphinhealingretreats@gmail.com
Website: http://www.dolphinhealingretreats.com

Estero Martial Arts & Fitness
10021 Estero Town Commons Place Ste 102B
Estero, FL 33928
Tel: (239) 947 0041
Contact Name: Linda Potter
Email: SenseiLinda@EsteroMartialArts.com
Website: http://EsteroMartialarts.com

Offers a martial arts class for children and adults with special needs.

Ever Care Adult Services
112 18th Street
Belleair Beach, FL 33786
Tel: (727) 581 4101
Contact Name:
Mary Jo Henderson
Email: mhscan@aol.com
Website: http://www.evercareservices.com

Florida Special Arts Center
Florida Special Arts Center
10258 NW 46th Street
Tel: (954) 721 1020
Contact Name: Ellen Kleinert-Cohn, Director
Email: flspecialneedscolorguard@yahoo.com
Website: http://www.flsac.org

Fort Lauderdale Aquatics
501 Seabreeze Boulevard
Fort Lauderdale, FL 33316
Tel: (954) 468 5590
Contact Name: Josee Desmarais
Email: jdesmarais@flaswim.com
Website: http://www.flaswim.com

JARC-FL: Housing and Vocational Training
21160 95th Avenue South
Boca Raton, FL 33428
Tel: (561) 558 2550
Contact Name: Justin Vassi
Email: justinv@jarcfl.org
Website: http://www.jarcfl.org

Noah's Ark of Central Florida, Inc.
2225 East Edgewood Drive Suite 6
Lakeland, FL 33803
Tel: (863) 687 0804
Website: http://noahsarkflorida.org/

Opportunity Services
2740 Oak Ridge Ct. Unit 301
Fort Myers, FL 33901
Tel: (239) 936 2773
Website: http://www.oppserv.org/locations/florida/about-us/

Serves adults seeking job assistance or community immersion and employers.

Palm Beach County Therapeutic Recreation Complex
2728 Lake Worth Road
Lake Worth, FL 33461
Tel: (561) 966 7015
Contact Name: Jackie Lambert
Email: JLambert@pbcgov.org
Website: http://www.pbcgov.com/parks/therapeutic_recreation/

Therapeutic Recreation Services is comprised of three areas of concentration: TR, Special Olympics & VSA.

Parc, Inc.
3190 Tyrone Blvd. North
St. Petersburg, FL 33710
Tel: (727) 345 9111
Email: info@parc-fl.org
Website: http://www.autismpinellas.org

Parc is a non-profit organization whose mission is to provide opportunities for children and adults with developmental disabilities to exercise their independence and experience life to the fullest.

Picasso Einstein, LLC
2114 North Flamingo Rd. #105
Pembroke Pines, FL 33028
Tel: (786) 519 1540 or (954) 655 6597
Contact Name: Nelson & Minerva Santiago, Co-Founders
Email: E4i@picassoeinstein.com
Website: http://www.picassoeinstein.com

Provides services through its E4i program specifically designed to assist families with disabilities to become self-sustainable through self-employment. Also provides inclusion training and consulting for employers and entrepreneurship program development services for schools, colleges, universities and non-profit organizations.

Quest
P.O. Box 531125
Orlando, FL 32853
Tel: (407) 218 4300
Website: http://www.questinc.org

Offers individuals with disabilities choices and opportunities to live more independently.

Saddle Up Riding Club Equine Assisted Activities
6080 94th Avenue
Pinellas Park, FL 33782
Contact Name: Melissa Yarbrough
Email: mkasper@saddleupridingclub.org
Website: http://www.saddleupridingclub.org

Saddle Up Riding Club has Equine Assisted Activities for children and adults ages 3 and up with disabilities.

Special Needs Piano Lessons
Creative Music Ability
310 Taxter Run Ln.
Valrico, FL 33594
Tel: (813) 315 9929 or (863) 773 4480
Contact Name: Linda Lalonde
Email: specialneedspiano@yahoo.com

Spectrum Life Care Services
12260 SW 53rd Street Suite #611
Cooper City, FL 33330
Tel: (954) 499 5794
Toll Free: (866) 628 8476
Contact Name: Concetta
Email: concetta@spectrumlifecare.com
Website: http://www.spectrumlifecare.com

Spectrum Life Care Services offers a variety of in-home personal health and support services.

GEORGIA

Doctors, Clinics, Hospitals, and Other Health Services

Bradstreet Wellness Center
Dr. Jeff Bradstreet, MD, MD(H), FAAFP
4488 Commerce Drive, Suite BBuford, GA 30518Tel: (678) 288 9222Fax: (678) 288 9227
Website: www.drbradstreet.org

Provides medical and nutritional treatment to individuals with ASD and other disorders by, among other things, assessing biomarkers to assist in identifying possible causes of symptoms to treat underlying issues not just the symptoms.

BrightStar Care
Atlanta, GA 30308
Tel: (404) 856 7610
Contact Name: Amber Zanfordino
Email: AtlantaITP@BrightStarCare.com
Website: http://www.BrightStarCare.com

Children's Wellness Center
755 Mt. Vernon Highway NE Suite 150
Atlanta, GA 30328
Tel: (404) 303 1314
Website: http://www.childrenswellnesscenter.com

Coastal Compounding Pharmacy
6709-A Forest Park Dr.Savannah, GA 31406
Tel: (912) 354 5188 or (866) 354 5188
Fax: (912) 354 5445
Email: mail@coastalcompounding.com
Website: www.coastalpharmacyinc.com

Compounding pharmacy.

The Dentistry for the Developmentally Disabled (DDD) Foundation, Inc.
52 Executive Park South, Suite 5203
Atlanta, GA 30329
Tel: (404) 942 0086
Contact Name: Tiffany White, Director of Operations
Email: twhite@dddfoundation.org
Website: http://www.dddfoundation.org

The DDD Foundation, Inc is a non-profit organization offering accessible, comprehensive dental treatment to patients having developmental disabilities in the metropolitan Atlanta area.

Developmental Crossroads, LLC
202 White Street
Marietta, GA 30060
Tel: (770) 428 1128
Contact Name: Dr. Angela Karvounis
Email: drangelajcc@yahoo.com
Website: http://developmentalcrossroads.com

Treating children with ASD using biomedical treatments.

Emory Autism Center (EAC)
The Justin Tyler Truax Building
1551 Shoup Court
Atlanta, GA 30322
Tel: (404) 727 8350
Contact Name: Sheila Wagner, M.Ed., Assistant Director, MONARCH Program Manager
Email: sheila.wagner@emory.edu
Website: http://www.psychiatry.emory.edu/PROGRAMS/autism

The Emory Autism Center is a component of the Department of Psychiatry and Behavioral Sciences at Emory University School of Medicine. Offers diagnosis, family support and treatment, and professional training.

Emory Crawford Long Hospital
550 Peachtree Street NE
Atlanta, GA 30308
Tel: (404) 778 2000
Website: http://www.emoryhealthcare.org/hospitals/euhm

Fresh Start for the Mind, LLC
4080 McGinnis Ferry Rd. Suite 204
Alpharetta, GA 30005
Tel: (404) 808 1161
Email: admin@freshstartmind.com
Website: http://www.freshstartmind.com

Offers comprehensive assessment of cognitive, academic, executive, social emotional, and adaptive functioning to diagnose a variety of conditions including ASD. Also offers behavior management support for families and social skills groups for children.

Genesis Center
104 Colony Park Dr. Suite 800
Cumming, GA 30040
Tel: (678) 947 4454
Contact Name: Mark Sloan
Website: http://www.thegenesiscenter.com

Treats root causes of illness, not just the symptoms. Works to find long-term solutions.

Inner Harbour, LTD
4685 Dorsett Shoals Rd.
Douglasville, GA 30135
Tel: (770) 942 2391
Contact Name: Beverly Watson
Email: beverly.watson@innerharbour.org
Website: http://www.innerharbour.org

Lotus Holistic Health
7002 Hodgson Memorial Dr.
Savannah, GA 31406
Tel: (912) 376 7030 or (919) 426 7787
Contact Name: Alicia Agard
Email: lotusholistichealth@gmail.com
Website: http://www.lotusholistichealth.org

Natural health consultant offering therapies and an individualized treatment plan incorporating a variety of modalities for ASD.

Progressive Medical Center
4646 North Shallowford Road
Atlanta, GA 30338
Tel: (770) 676 6000
Website: http://www.progressivemedicalcenter.com

Uses an integrative medical approach to effectively address the underlying causes of disease.

PSA HealthCare
310 Technology Parkway
Norcross, GA 30092
Tel: (770) 441 1580
Website: http://psahealthcare.com

Provides pediatric home care services for medically fragile children. Offers in-home options for adults with medically fragile conditions.

Dr. Shayne Abelkop, Ph.D., PC
1361 Jennings Mill Rd. Suite 201
Bogart, GA 30622
Tel: (706) 316 1908
Contact Name: Shayne Abelkop
Email: drshayneabelkop@yahoo.com
Website: http://www.drshayneabelkop.com

Spectrum Psychological Services
2551 Roswell Road Suite 525
Marietta, GA 30062
Tel: (404) 987 2531
Contact Name: Dr. Sarah Golsen
Email: sgolsen@spectrum-psychological.com
Website: http://www.spectrum-psychological.com

Provides diagnostic, psychological, and psychoeducational assessment as well as behavior modification and parent training for children with ASD.

Wendi Combes, RN
Jubilee Health
3108 Piedmont Road SuiteSuite 215Atlanta, GA 30305
Tel: (404) 694 0777
Website: www.jubileehealth.org

Therapy Services

Andrea Clifton, LCSW, Ed.S
2320 Heatherton Cir
Dacula, GA 30019
Tel: (770) 338 8721
Contact Name: Andrea Clifton, LCSW, Ed.S
Email: aseadreams@att.net

Individual and therapy services offered for children and adolescents diagnosed with ASD to address issues regarding social skills and communication.

Beyond Limits Therapeutic Riding, Inc.
55 East Greenridge Rd.
Cartersville, GA 30120
Tel: (770) 917 5737
Contact Name: Melissa Adams, Program Assistant
Email: melissa@beyondlimitsriding.org
Website: http://www.beyondlimitsriding.org

Provides therapeutic horseback riding and other services for children and adults.

Calvin Center Therapeutic Riding Program
13550 Woolsey Road
Hampton, GA 30228
Tel: (770) 946 4276
Contact Name: Gretchen Ahrens
Email: gretchen@calvincenter.org
Website: http://www.calvincenter.org

Therapeutic riding for youth and adults with autism.

Chastain Horse Park
4371 Powers Ferry Road
Atlanta, GA 30327
Tel: (404) 252 4244
Website: http://www.chastainhorsepark.org

Therapeutic riding.

Compass Behavioral & Developmental Consultants, LLC
312 North Davis Rd.
Warner Robins, GA 31093
Tel: (800) 832 9419 x 2
Email: info@compassaid.com
Website: http://www.compassaid.com

Early intervention for children diagnosed with ASD and school-aged children and supportive services for adults. Provides Intensive ABA therapies, Discrete Trial Training (DTT), Verbal Behavior Therapy (VBT), and Social Skill Training.

Circus Arts Therapy
206 Rogers Street NE Suite 214
Atlanta, GA 30317
Tel: (404) 549 3000
Contact Name: Carrie Heller
Email: carrie@circusartsinstitute.com
https://circusartsinstitute.com/circus-home

Darling Pediatric Therapies, Inc.
1475 Holcomb Bridge Road Suite 113
Roswell, GA 30076
Tel: (678) 591 3542
Contact Name: Darlene A. Robertson
Email: DARlingot@msn.com
Website: http://www.DarlingPediatricTherapies.com

Occupational Therapy, Speech Language Pathology Physical Therapy and Music Therapy provided in 2 sensory motor gyms and 8 break out rooms.

Debbie Hopkins
Lawrenceville, GA 30043
Tel: (779) 646 7469
Contact Name: Debbie Hopkins
Email: Dhopkins64@hotmail.com

Home-based ABA services provided for children ages 2–6.

Dream Power Therapeutic Equestrian Center
123 Equest Dr.
Canton, GA 30115
Tel: (770) 720 1910 or (770) 654 5430
Contact Name: Gina Little
Email: dreampowertherapy@gmail.com
Website: http://www.dreampowertherapy.org

Therapeutic equestrian program.

Driving Magic, Inc.
P.O. Box 279
Duluth, GA 30096
Tel: (404) 358 4129
Contact Name: Jennifer Lindskoog
Email: drivingmagicinc@aol.com
Website: http://www.drivingmagicinc.org

Therapeutic carriage driving and horsemanship on a 680-acre working farm with individualized lessons and workshops.

GN Integrated Pediatric Therapy
7635 Rock Shadow Ct
Gainesville, GA 30506
Tel: (678) 513 3851
Contact Name: Jill Nurhonen, OTR/L
Email: gillot@comcast.net
Website: http://www.kidsinsync.net

Sensory integration clinic offering OT, ST, and PT for children 0–12 years.

Live Oak Children's Therapy
314-A Stephenson Avenue
Savannah, GA 31405
Tel: (912) 355 3392
Contact Name: Linda Fruin
Email: info@liveoakchildrens.com
Website: http://www.liveoakchildrens.com

May Institute
P.O. Box 870028
Stone Mountain, GA 30087
Tel:770.680.8738
Email: info@mayinstitute.org
Website: http://www.mayinstitute.org

Provides ABA, including to military families of children with ASD.

Milestones ABA
6200 Bradley Park Dr.
Columbus, GA 31904
Tel: (706) 507 4769
Contact Name: Holly Calhoun
Email: hcalhoun@milestonesaba.net

ABA center for children with ASD and other developmental disabilities. Offers tutoring services, center-based services, outreach services, home- or school-based services.

Milton Speech Pathology of Georgia
Alpharetta, GA 30004
Tel: (678) 824 2145 or (404) 719 3991
Contact Name: Amy Squires
Email: amy@miltonspeech.com
Website: http://www.miltonspeechpathology.com

Provides speech therapy in home and in office. Social skills groups are conducted at various locations in the community. Provides functional in-home therapy for children who use augmentative/alternative communication.

Muse For Life
205 Hilderbrand Drive
Sandy Springs, GA 30328
Tel: (404) 943 1063
Contact Name: Craig Martin Canedy
Email: director@museforlife.com
Website: http://www.museforlife.com/index.html

Provides music therapy with individualized treatment plans as well as summer camps and accredited non-traditional academic programming.

Pathways Behavioral Consulting, LLC
Atlanta, GA 30338
Tel: (571) 228 5969 or (404) 465 1818
Contact Name: Becky Lamont, M.Ed., BCBA, President and Founder
Email: becky@pathwaysbehavior.com
Website: http://www.pathwaysbehavior.com

Individualized ABA-based programs.

The Preserve Counseling Center
360 Prospect Place
Alpharetta, GA 30005
Tel: (678) 956 3253
Contact Name: Letitia Barnes, MS, LPC
Email: letitia@preservecounseling.com
Website: http://www.preservecounseling.com

Licensed professional counselor working with individuals and families.

Psychosocial Rehabilitation & Peer Support
207 N. Anderson Drive
Swainsboro, GA 30401
Tel: (478) 289 2619
Website: http://obhs-ga.org

Ray of Hope Counseling Services, Inc.
4255 Wade Green Road, Suite 414
Kennesaw, GA 30144
Tel: (678) 213 2194
Contact Name: Allison O'Hara
Email: a.ohara@rhcounselingservices.com
Website: http://www.rhcounselingservices.com

Soaring Eagles Children's Group
3183 Northbrook Dr
Atlanta, GA 30341
Tel: (770) 314 3201
Contact Name: Otis Farmer
Email: otis@sechildren.com
Website: http://www.sechildren.com

Provides ABA-based programs.

Walker Therapy Center
6625 Highway 53 East, Suite 410
Dawsonville, GA 30534
Tel: (770) 781 4899
Email: info@walkertherapy.com
Website: http://walkertherapy.com

Schools and Educational Services

Alexsander Academy
1090 Powers Place
Alpharetta, GA 30009
Tel: (404) 839 5910
Contact Name: Stefanie Smith
Email: smith@alexsanderacademy.org
Website: http://www.alexsanderacademy.org

Buckhead Prep Inclusion Program
1294 North Druid Hills Road
Atlanta, GA 30319
Tel: (404) 846 2622
Contact Name: Phyllis Patterson
Email: phyllis@buckheadprep.com
Website: http://www.buckheadprep.com

Buckhead Preparatory Preschool at Brookhaven Inclusion Program introduces children with ASD to their toddler, preschool, and prekindergarten classrooms.

Challenged Child and Friends
2360 Murphy Blvd.
Gainesville, GA 30504

Tel: (770) 535 8372
Email: info@challengedchild.org
Website: http://www.challengedchild.org

Inclusion program for children with ASD and other developmental delays.

Creative Academic Solutions
920 Holcomb Bridge Road, Suite 350
Roswell, GA 30076
Tel: (404) 697 0198
Contact Name: Andy Jones
Email: andy-cas@att.net
Website: http://www.creativeacademicsolutions.net

Offers academic and social skills tutoring service for children and teens with special needs. Advocate services for families with children and teens with special needs and improvisational acting classes for children and teens with special needs.

Donna Andrews, Ph.D. Educational Consultant for Individuals with Autism
700 Rocky Ridge Trail
Cornelia, GA 30531
Tel: (706) 878 0887 or (706) 778 8017
Contact Name: Dr. Donna Andrews
Email: drdgandrews@yahoo.com

Provides teacher training, individual work with individuals and their families for issues with education, behavior, social skills instruction, and vocational planning.

The Joseph Sams School
280 Brandywine Boulevard
Fayetteville, GA 30214
Tel: (770) 461 5894
Contact Name: Amy Murray, Principal
Email: info@josephsamsschool.org
Website: http://www.josephsamsschool.org

Kicklighter Academy
7219 Seawright Drive
Savannah, GA 31406
Tel: (912) 355 7633
Contact Name: Ashley Tramontin
Email: AshleyT@krcmail.org
Website: http://www.krcacademy.org

Early care and learning center for all children ages 6 weeks through 6 years.

North Georgia Preparatory
4604 Ball Ground Road Hwy 372
Ball Ground, GA 30107
Tel: (404) 590 9681 or (770) 737 2441
Contact Name: Karen Wylie
Email: northgeorgiaprep@hotmail.com

Porter Academy
200 Cox Road
Roswell, GA 30075
Tel: (770) 594 1313
Email: bramer@porteracademy.org
Website: http://www.porteracademy.org

Summit Autism Center
700 Holcomb Bridge Road St 400
Roswell, GA 30076
Tel: (404) 377 8882
Contact Name: Jennifer Mitchell/ Shauna Courtney
Email: info@summitlearningcenter.org
Website: http://www.summitlearningcenter.org

Offers a variety of educational options year-round for children with ASD.

X'zandria Learning Center
Governor Ridge 1640 Powers Ferry Road
Marietta, GA 30067
Tel: (770) 615 3467
Contact Name: Kay Stevens
Email: xnd04@yahoo.com

Tutoring center specializing in children with learning differences.

Legal, Government & Financial Services

Atlanta Volunteer Lawyers Foundation
235 Peachtree Street N.E. Suite 1750
Atlanta, GA 30303
Tel: (404) 521 0790
Website: http://www.avlf.org

Bass, Bergeron and Smith, PC
420 Creekstone Ridge
Woodstock, GA 30188
Tel: (770) 874 6431
Contact Name: Jim Bass
Email: jim@bbandslaw.com
Website: http://www.bbandslaw.com

Legal representation in areas including Guardianship and Conservatorship, Special Needs Trusts and Wills, IEPs, Social Security and Medicaid Appeals, Divorces involving special needs children, etc.

Calbos Law Firm, LLC
1323 Westchester Ridge
Atlanta, GA 30329
Tel: (404) 667 3794
Contact Name: Christy Calbos

Email: christy@calboslaw.com
Website: http://www.calboslaw.com

Special education law.

Dana H. Carroll, LLC
3330 Cumberland Blvd. Suite 500
Atlanta, GA 30339
Tel: (404) 855 0984
Contact Name: Dana Carroll
Email: danahcarroll@gmail.com
Website: http://www.mariettadisability.com

Legal representation in the areas of Social Security Disability & SSI, Children's SSI, Guardianships, and Student IEPs.

Debbie L Dobbs, MS
Atlanta, GA
Tel: (678) 315 2498
Email: debbie@debbiedobbs.com
Website: http://www.debbiedobbs.com

Help with IEP's, 504 Plans, Medicaid Waivers, Respite & Funding Options.

Department of Behavioral Health & Developmental Disabilities
Atlanta, GA 30303
Tel: (404) 657 2252
Website: http://dbhdd.georgia.gov

Department of Housing and Urban Development
40 Marietta St Five Points Plaza Building
Atlanta, GA 30303
Tel: (404) 331 5136
Contact Name: Ed Jennings, Jr.
Email: GA_Webmanager@hud.gov
Website: http://www.hud.gov/local/index.cfm?state=ga&topic=offices

Heart & Soul Psycho-Educational Advocacy Serv., Inc.
PO Box 681
Union City, GA 30291
Tel: (404) 759 3519
Contact Name: Crystal Calhoun
Email: heartandsouladvocacy@gmail.com
Website: http://www.heartandsouladvocacy.com

Provides educational advocacy & Consulting services including attending school meetings w/parents, analyzing/interpreting IEP's & psychological reports, writing letters, recommending academic/behavior interventions.

Innovative Health Foundation
5050 Research Ct, Suite 800
Suwanee, GA 30024
Tel: (404) 913 9560
Contact Name: Patricia Muesse
Email: patricia@innovativehealthfoundation.org
Website: http://www.innovativehealthfoundation.org

The Innovative Health Foundation (IHF) provides clinical scholarships for children with developmental disabilities including ASD.

The Missing Piece (TMP), LLC
4487 Old Country Way
Snellville, GA 30039
Tel: (678) 939 9070 or (478) 227 8266
Contact Name: Shanna Gairy
Email: sagairytmp@gmail.com
Website: http://www.themissingpiecellc.com

Provides consulting services regarding state Medicaid coverage and access to community resources.

PeachCare for Kids
Tel: (877) GA PEACH or (877) 427 3224
Website: http://www.peachcare.org

Free or low-cost health insurance for Georgia's uninsured children.

The Pollan Law Firm
1801 Peachtree Street Suite 150
Atlanta, GA 30309
Tel: (678) 510 1358
Contact Name: David Pollan
Email: david@pollanlawfirm.com
Website: http://www.pollanlawfirm.com

The Pollan Law Firm is a Special Needs law firm.

Raise Them High
170 Sheringham Dr.
Roswell, GA 30076
Tel: (404) 835 9000
Contact Name: Ann Elliott
Email: ann@raisethemhigh.com
Website: http://www.raisethemhigh.com

Consultants for children with special needs, including assistance with Deeming Waivers, IEP's, and Life Skills.

Vocational Rehabilitation Program
1700 Century Circle Suite 300
Atlanta, GA 30345
Tel: (404) 486 6331
Email: vrpcustomer-service@dol.state.ga.us
Website: http://www.vocrehabga.org/

Worrall Law LLC
109 Anderson Street #100
Marietta, GA 30060

Tel: (770) 425 6060
Contact Name: Steve Worrall
Email: steve@georgiafamilylaw.com
Website: http://georgiaspecialneedslawyer.com

Family estate planning law firm working with families with special needs children.

Community and Recreation Services

Adaptive Aquatics of Georgia (AAG)
Dive Educators 4875 Hog Mountain Rd.
Flowery Branch, GA 30542
Tel: (770) 827 6373
Contact Name: Kristie Snape
Email: ksnape@adaptedswim.com
Website: http://www.adaptedswim.com

Albany Advocacy Resource Center (Albany ARC)
2616 Pointe North Boulevard
Albany, GA 31721
Tel: (229) 888 6852
Contact Name: Laura Calhoun
Email: lcalhoun@albanygaarc.org
Website: http://www.albanyarc.org

Anchor of Hope Foundation, Inc.
41 W Johnston St.
Forsyth, GA 31029
Tel: (478) 994 0438
Website: http://www.anchorofhopefoundation.com

Angel I Am Care
Conyers, GA 30094
Tel: (877) 394 7779
Website: http://www.angeliamcare.com

Provides revolutionary services and resources to families with individuals with special needs, from preschool age to late adulthood.

Annandale Village
3500 Annandale Lane
Sewanee, GA 30024
Tel: (770) 932 4865
Contact Name: Tammy Severino
Email: tammy.severino@annandale.org
Website: http://www.annandale.org

Augusta Paratransit
1535 Fenwick St.
Augusta, GA 30904
Tel: (706) 821 1819
Website: http://www.augustaga.gov/index.aspx?nid=243

Curb to curb van service available to qualifying persons with permanent or temporary disabilities.

Bearfoot Ranch
5150 Oak Grove Circle
Cumming, GA 30028
Tel: (678) 805 RIDE
Contact Name: Edie Ahola
Email: edie@bearfootranch.org
Website: http://www.bearfootranch.org

A comprehensive equestrian center providing riding activities in a safe, effective and compassionate environment, including lessons for those with special needs.

Bobby Dodd Institute
2120 Marietta Blvd. NW
Atlanta, GA 30318
Tel: (678) 365 0071
Contact Name: Lisa Duck
Email: lduck@bobbydodd.org
Website: http://www.bobbydodd.org

Providing assistance to help individuals achieve independence.

Briggs & Associates
2300 Holcomb Bridge Road, Suite 103
Roswell, GA 30076
Tel: (404) 290 6839 or (404) 290 6841
Contact Name: Jennifer Briggs, Owner
Website: http://www.briggsassociates.org

Employment assistance.

Camp Caglewood
P.O. Box 158
Flowery Branch, GA 30542
Tel: (678) 405 9000
Email: info@caglewood.org
Website: http://www.caglewood.org

Offers weekend camping trips and day camps for children and adults with special needs.

Champions for Children
1906 Palmyra Road
Albany, GA 31701
Tel:(229) 439 7061
Contact Name: Teresa Ann Heard
Email: theard@swga-easterseals.org
Website: http://www.championsforchildrenga.org

Clayton County Parks and Recreation
2300 Highway 138 S.E.
Jonesboro, GA 30236
Tel: (770) 477 3766
Website: http://www.claytonparks.com/

The Therapeutic division of Clayton County Parks and Recreation Department offers year round recreational and leisure activities for children and adults with disabilities.

Cobb County Autism Group
Starbucks
1207 Johnson Ferry Road
Marietta, GA 30068
Tel: (770) 861 8800
Contact Name: Nicole Schochet
Email: Lnb0315@gmail.com
Website: http://www.meetup.com/Cobb-County-support-group-Parents-with-ASD-toddlers-kids/

DeKalb Community Service Board
PO Box 1648
Decatur, GA 30031
Tel: (404) 294 3834
Website: http://www.dekcsb.org/

The DeKalb Community Service Board (CSB) is a community-based behavioral health and developmental disabilities services organization located in metropolitan Atlanta, Georgia.

disABILITY LINK
755 Commerce Drive Suite 105
Decatur, GA 30030
Tel: (404) 687 8890
Email: info@disabilitylink.org
Website: http://www.disabilitylink.org

DisABILITY Link is an organization led by and for people with disabilities.

Disabled Friends of America
1208 S. Broad Street
Monroe, GA 30655
Tel: (770) 266 7496
Contact Name: Joseph
Email: csaga@windstream.net

Easter Seals East Georgia
1500 Wrightsboro Rd.
Augusta, GA 30904
Tel: (706) 667 9695
Website: http://www.eastersealseastgeorgia.org

The Elaine Clark Center
5130 Peachtree Blvd.
Chamblee, GA 30043
Tel: (770) 458 3251
Email: information@elaineclarkcenter.org
Website: http://www.elaineclarkcenter.org

Provides a continuum of services for individuals with special needs ages 6 weeks to 22 years old.

Employment First
150 E. Ponce de Leon Ave. Suite 430
Decatur, GA 30030
Tel: (404) 885 1234
Email: info@employmentfirstgeorgia.org

Website: http://www.employmentfirstgeorgia.org/

Employment First Georgia (EFG) is a statewide resource promoting innovative, customized employment practice.

EnAble of Georgia
5101 Buffington Road Building 3453
Atlanta, GA 30349
Tel: (404) 684 5991
Contact Name: Lillian Gibson
Email: administrator@enablega.org
Website: http://www.enablega.org

Providing programs to assist integrating individuals into the community.

Family Home Care
1791 Silver Leaf Ct.
Marietta, GA 30008
Tel: (770) 437 0714
Contact Name: Valentina Lebeau
Email: vlebeau@familyhomecare.us
Website: http://www.familyhomecare.us

Fragile Kids Foundation
3350 Riverwood Pkwy #1400
Atlanta, GA 30339
Tel: (770) 951 6111
Website: http://fragilekids.org

Georgia Advocacy Office
150 E. Ponce De Leon Avenue, Suite 430
Decatur, GA 30030
Tel: (404) 885 1234 or (800) 537 2329
Contact Name: Dr. Joyce R. Ringer
Email: info@thegao.org
Website: http://www.thegao.org

Georgia Community Support and Solutions (GCSS)
1945 Cliff Valley Way, Suite 220
Atlanta, GA 30329
Tel: (404) 634 4222
Contact Name: Kimberly Benjamin
Website: http://www.gacommunity.org

Georgia Options
185 Ben Burton Circle
Bogart, GA 30622
Tel: (706) 546 0009
Website: http://www.georgiaoptions.org

Provides resources and independent living options for people living with developmental disabilities.

GoodLife Care
Marietta, GA 30067
Tel: (770) 783 1415

Contact Name: Paul Wright
Email: paul.wright@goodlifecare.org
Website: http://www.goodlifecare.org

Provides home care nursing services and in-home respite and sitter services for clients with ASD.

Jewish Family & Career Services (JF & CS)
700 14th St. Northwest
Atlanta, GA 30318
Tel: (404) 881 1858
Email: bmdc@jfcs-atlanta.org
Website: http://www.yourtoolsforliving.org

Just People, Inc.
1600 Oakbrook Dr St 530
Norcross, GA 30093
Tel: (770) 441 1188
Contact Name: Nikki Davis
Email: contact@justpeople.org
Website: http://www.justpeople.org

"Just" People, Inc. is a private not for profit agency that provides a wide variety of support services to adults with developmental disabilities, people with Mental Illnesses and Head Injury.

Keeping it Specially Simple (KISS)
755 Vinca Court
Alpharetta, GA 30005
Tel: (404) 932 4140 or (419) 419 9154
Contact Name: Becky Borak
Email: keepingitspeciallysimple@gmail.com
Website: http://www.keepingitspeciallysimple.com/

Assists families and individuals with special needs by supporting, implementing, and advocating for the individual with special needs.

The Kiss Foundation
2858 River Ridge Hill
Decatur, GA 30034
Tel: (678) 698 3986
Contact Name: Donna Johnson
Email: donnajohnson@thekissfoundation.org
Website: http://www.thekissfoundation.org

Support groups for siblings of children with autism and other sensory related disorders.

Maggie's Hope
PO Box 3046
Peachtree City, GA 30269
Tel: (404) 797 6160
Email: recovery@maggieshope.org
Website: http://www.maggieshope.org

Assists with funding for non-traditional treatments, gluten free/casein free foods, school advocates and other therapies not covered by insurance.

Marcus Jewish Community Center of Atlanta
5342 Tilly Mill Road
Dunwoody, GA 30338
Tel: (678) 812 4000
Contact Name: Michael Wise
Email: michael.wise@atlantajcc.org
Website: http://www.atlantajcc.org

Offers the Blonder Family Department for Special Needs.

MARTA Mobility
2424 Piedmont Road, NE
Atlanta, GA 30324
Tel: (404) 848 5000
Website: http://www.itsmarta.com/accessibility-mobility.aspx

MARTA provides ADA Complementary Paratransit Service to eligible persons with disabilities.

Myles-A-Part Foundation
P.O. Box 1345
Roswell, GA 30077
Tel: (678) 575 0014
Website: http://www.mylesapart.org

New Directions
4545 Suwanee Dam Road
Suwanee, GA 30024
Tel: (678) 926 2489 or (678) 640 2489
Contact Name: Mary O'Connell
Email: info@NewDirectionsForAutism.org
Website: http://www.NewDirectionsForAutism.org

New Directions provides an individual focused vocational, behavioral day program.

The Olivia Center for Developmental Disabilities, LLC
Roswell Professional Center 10050 Crabapple Rd, Ste. C-109
Roswell, GA 30075
Tel: (770) 899 5311
Contact Name: Kelly Williams
Email: TheOliviaCenter@yahoo.com

Offers: Community Access, Prevocational Training, Person-Centered Approach, Caregiver Support Workshops, Health & Wellness Workshops, Transition /IEP Support (Tutoring), CPR/First Aid Training Sessions, ISP Goal Support, Volunteer Opportunities, Summer Programs.

Parents Educating Parents and Professionals
8355 Cherokee Blvd. Suite 100
Douglasville, GA 30134
Tel: (770) 577 7771 or (800) 322 7065

Email: united_parent@peppinc.org
Website: http://www.peppinc.org

PEPP, Inc is a non-profit organization that promotes academic achievement, educational rights, and transition for youth with disabilities and disadvantages that may exist based on high-risk indicators such as foster care, juvenile offence, and socio-economics.

Sensations TheraFun™
1704 Chantilly Drive
Atlanta, GA 30324
Tel: (404) 634 3500
Contact Name: Jay Perkins
Email: jayperkins@sensationstherafun.com
Website: http://www.sensationstherafun.com

Sensations TheraFun™ offers a wide range of services to families to satisfy the sensory needs of their children.

Shenanigans Improv
3625 Longfellow Trail
Marietta, GA 30062
Tel: (770) 354 5770
Contact Name: Sandy Bruce
Email: shenanigans.info@gmail.com
Website: http://www.ShenanigansImprov.com

Shenanigans is a fast-paced improv group for tweens, teens, and adults with ASD.

SNAPS - Special Needs and Parent Support
11330 Woodstock Road
Roswell, GA 30075
Contact Name: Robin Mellie
Email: rbmellie@yahoo.com

Social Skills Today
Gwinnett, GA
Tel: (678) 640 2489 or (678) 296 6084
Contact Name: Mary O'Connell
Email: mary@socialskillstoday.com
Website: http://www.socialskillstoday.com

Social skills group activities, community outings, drama club, week-end overnights, day and residential summer camp for children ages 4 to young adult with ASD, sensory integration disorder, and social skills deficits.

Southside Support Incorporated
Fayetteville, GA 30214
Tel: (678) 827 2893
Contact Name: Raissa Chandler
Email: southsideraissa@gmail.com
Website: http://www.southsidesupport.org

Support group for parents of students with ASD and other disabilities.

Spark Your Creativity
4545 Suwanee Dam Rd.
Suwaneee, GA 30024
Tel: (678) 755 7472 or (770) 882 8153
Contact Name: Joy Fofana, M.A., Certified School Counselor, Art Instructor
Email: Sparkyourcreativityclasses@gmail.com
Website: http://www.sparkyourcreativityclasses.com

Provides creative and educational experiences for students of all ages through the Arts.

Special Pops Tennis
3176 Westfield Way
Roswell, GA 30075
Tel: (404) 386 6250
Contact Name: Martha pedrick
Email: mpedrick@mindspring.com
Website: http://www.specialpopstennis.com

Offers an adaptive tennis program for children and adults with intellectual disabilities.

Spectrum Autism Support Group
Suwanee, GA 30024
Tel: (770) 617 8775
Contact Name: Claire Dees
Email: claidee@aol.com
Website: http://www.atl-spectrum.com

Parent-operated group providing support, education, and resources.

Swimmerman Swim School
Jonesboro, Smyrna, Atlanta
Tel: (770) 210 0136
Contact Name: Lynn Hannah
Email: info@swimmerman.com
Website: http://www.swimmerman.com

Wolf Strategic Advice
274 Beverly Rd.
Atlanta, GA 30309
Tel: (312) 371 7740
Contact Name: Kelly Raclin Miller
Email: wolfstrategicadvice@gmail.com
Website: http://www.wolfstrategicadvice.com

Free resource for information regarding services such as schools, doctors, dentists, and therapists.

Working On Work together (WOW) In-Sync, Inc.
2137 Flintstone Dr. Suite E
Tucker, GA 30084
Tel: (770) 939 1100 x 101
Contact Name: Karen Lynn
Email: klynn@wowinsync.org

Job training and mentoring programs and initiatives with support and accommodations for adults with ASD.

HAWAII

Doctors, Clinics, Hospitals, and Other Health Services

Dr. Curtis Takemoto-Gentile
2658 South King Street
Honolulu, HI 96826
Tel: (808) 955 1544
Website: http://www.doctorctg.com/

Family physician providing general care and care to those with ASD.

The Institute For Family Enrichment
91-1841 Fort Weaver Road,
Ewa Beach, Hawaii 96706-1909
Tel: (808) 596 8433
Website: http://www.tiffe.org

Provides a variety of mental health prevention and treatment services to children and families.

Kahi Mohala Behavioral Health Hospital
91-2301 Old Fort Weaver Road
Ewa Beach, HI
Tel: (808) 671 8511
Website: http://www.kahimohala.org/about

Provides inter-disciplinary approach to services, incorporating an integrative perspective in emotional, physical, cognitive and behavioral health care treatment.

Kapi'olani Medical Center for Women & Children
Behavioral Development Clinic
1319 Punahou Street
Honolulu, HI 96826
Tel: (808) 983 6000
Email: info@kapiolani.org
Website: http://www.kapiolani.org
Facebook: https://www.facebook.com/KapiolaniMedicalCenter

Malama Pono Autism Center
100 Kahelu Ave. Suite 112
Mililani, HI 96789
Tel: (808) 450 3080
Contact Name: Taffy Perucci, Clinic Director

Email: TaffyP@mpautismcenter.org

Website: http://www.malamaponoautismcenter.org

Provides individualized treatment programs developed by behavior experts, educators, and health consultants.

Mental Health Kokua
1221 Kapiolani Boulevard, Suite 345
Honolulu, HI 96814
Tel: (808) 737 2523
Website: http://www.mentalhealthkokua.org/

Therapy Services

ABA Positive Support Services
Positive Support Services
94-1221 Ka Uka Blvd,
Unit 108, 3167,
Waipahu, HI 96797
Tel: (808) 292 7968
Contact Name: Catherine Wilson
Email: catherine@positivesupportservices.com
Website: http://positivesupportservices.com

Provides one to one support for children with ASD supervised by a BCBA. Services include ABA, verbal behavior, Floortime, discrete trial training, natural environment training, and respite services.

Aptitude Habilitation Services, Inc.
3-3367 Kuhio Hwy. Unit #204
Lihue, HI 96766
Tel: (800) 991 6070
Website: http://www.aptitudeservices.com/

Provides applied behavioral therapy to children and adults on the autism spectrum.

Autism Behavior Consulting (ABC) Group, LLC
99-950 Iwaena St. Second Floor
Aiea, HI 96701
Tel: (808) 277 7736
Email: info@autismbehaviorconsulting.com
Website: http://www.autismbehaviorconsulting.com
Facebook: https://www.facebook.com/pages/Autism-Behavior-Consulting-Group-Inc/133375266707024

Providing Applied Behavior Analytic Educational and Behavioral Consulting on the island of Oahu, near Honolulu, Hawaii. In clinic, home, or community/school.

Autism Services by Bayada Habilitation
Kapa'a, HI 96746
Tel: (888) 995 0788
Website: http://www.bayada.com/services_autism.asp

Services for children and adults with ASD to assist them with learning, social skills, socialization, and behavior.

Behavior Analysis No Ka Oi, Inc.
560 N Nimitz Hwy. Suite 114B
Honolulu, HI 96817
Tel: (808) 591 1173
Contact Name: Christine Kim Walton, Ph.D., BCBA-D
Email: ckwalton@hawaiibehavioranalysts.com
Website: http://www.hawaiibehavioranalysis.com

Provides assessments and treatment for children with autism and other developmental disabilities, as well as typically developing children with behavior, academic, communication, or social needs.

Dr. William Bolman, MD
Psychiatrist
1600 Kapiolani Boulevard Suite 620
Honolulu, HI 96814
Tel: (808) 944 2597

Hawaii Communication Bridge LLC
1071 Lanui Pl
Honolulu, HI 96817
Tel: (808) 256 1355
Contact Name: Erica Apana, M.S.,CCC-SLP
Email: erica@hawaiicommunicationbridge.com
Website: http://www.hawaiicommunicationbridge.com
Facebook: https://www.facebook.com/hawaiicommunicationbridge

Provides in-home speech/language evaluations and therapy on the island of O'ahu.

Hawaii FI-DO
PO Box 757
Kahuku, HI 96731
Tel: (808) 638 0200
Email: hifido@hawaii.rr.com
Website: http://www.hawaiifido.org

Assistance dogs. The only Certified Training Center on the island of Oahu, Hawaii; also Internationally Accredited under ADI Assistance Dogs International.

Healing Horses, Kauai
PO Box 2082
Kapaa, HI 96746
Tel: (808) 635 4720
Contact Name: Heather Phelps, Director
Email: hhkauai@gmail.com
Website: http://www.HealingHorsesKauai.com
Facebook: https://www.facebook.com/HealingHorsesKauai

Equine-assisted activities and therapies

Maui Center for Child Development
244 Papa Pl, Suite 102
Kahului, HI 96732
Tel: (808) 873 7700

Contact Name: Kiegan Blake
Email: kiegan@otmaui.com
Website: http://mauichilddevelopment.com/
Facebook: https://www.facebook.com/mauichild

Oahu Speech Language Pathology
Medical Arts Building 1010 South King Street B4
Honolulu, HI 96814
Tel: (808) 593 0030
Email: oahuspeech@hawaii.rr.com
Website: http://www.oahuspeech.com

Rehabilitation Hospital of the Pacific
98-1005 Moanalua Road
Aiea, HI 96701
Tel: (808) 486 8000
Website: http://www.rehabhospital.org
Facebook: https://www.facebook.com/
pages/Rehabilitation-Hospital-of-the-
Pacific/171277832893313

Sounding Joy Music Therapy
1314 South King Street Suite 711
Honolulu, HI 96814
Tel: (808) 593 2620
Email: postmaster@soundingjoymt.org
Website: http://soundingjoymt.org

Speech Solutions
725 Kapiolani Blvd. #206
Honolulu, HI 96813
Tel: (808) 596 0099
Contact Name: Debra, Administrative Assistant
Email: admin@speechsolutionshawaii.com
Website: http://www.speechsolutionshawaii.com
Facebook: https://www.facebook.com/
SpeechSolutionsHawaii

Sprouts Therapy, LLC
1210 Wilhelmina Rise Unit B
Honolulu, HI 96816
Tel: (858) 248 7824
Contact Name: Crystal Amelang, OTR/L, SIPT
Email: camelang@sproutstherapy.com
Website: http://www.sproutstherapy4kids.com

Offers intensive occupational therapy services around the island of Oahu, Hawaii.

Teri Holter, LCSW, DCSW, SEP
Makawao, HI 96768
Tel: (808) 205 8055
Contact Name: Teri Holter
Email: RadBalance@aol.com

Therapeutic Horsemanship of Hawaii
P.O. Box 138
Waimanalo, HI 96795
Tel: (808) 342 9036
Email: dana@thhwaimanalo.org
Website: http://www.thhwaimanalo.org

Therapeutic horsemanship sessions may include grooming, saddling, riding, and learning all about horses. Session activities vary depending on rider abilities.

Schools and Educational Services

Autism Comprehensive Educational Services (ACES)
94-849 Lumi'aina St. Suite 201
Waipahu, HI 96797
Tel: (808) 294 7050
Contact Form: https://www.acesaba.com/contact/Oahu
Website: http://www.ACESaba.com

Offers a variety of behavioral and educational services in the home, school, and community.

Cornerstone Educational Preschool
P.O. Box 630275
Lanai City, Hawaii 96763
Tel: (808) 342 3466
Contact Name: Dr. Jennifer Dustow
Email: drdustow@gmail.com
Website: http://www.cornerstoneeducationalpreschool.
com

Loveland Academy Hawaii
1506 Piikoi Street
Honolulu, HI 96822
Tel: (808) 524 4243
Email: receptionist@loveland-academy.com
Website: http://www.lovelandacademyhawaii.com

University of Hawaii
Honolulu, HI 96822
Tel: (808) 956 9199
Contact Name: Robert A. Stodden
Email: stodden@hawaii.edu
Website: http://honolulu.hawaii.edu/disability

Student ACCESS assists in providing equal access to Honolulu Community College facilities, programs, activities, and services to students with disabilities.

Variety School of Hawaii
710 Palekaua Street
Honolulu, HI 96816
Tel: (808) 732 2835
Email: yeevariety@inets.com
Website: http://www.varietyschool.org

Legal, Government & Financial Services

The Advocacy Project
900 Fort Street Mall, 1140
Honolulu, HI 96813
Tel: (808) 384 7325
Contact Name: Keith Peck
Email: Intake@spedlawcenter.com
Website: http://www.spedlawcenter.com

Free and low cost special education legal assistance.

Department of Housing and Urban Development
1132 Bishop St. Suite 1400
Honolulu, HI 96813
Tel: (808) 457 4662
Contact Name: Ryan Okahara
Email: answers@hud.gov
http://www.hud.gov/local/index.
cfm?state=hi&topic=offices

Hawaii Department of Health
801 Dillingham Blvd.
Honolulu, HI 96817
Tel: (808) 587 7564
Website: http://hawaii.gov/health/disability-services/
developmental

Hawaii Disability Rights Center
1132 Bishop Street, Suite 2102
Honolulu, HI 96813
Tel: (808) 949 2922
Email: info@hawaiidisabilityrights.org
Website: http://www.hawaiidisabilityrights.org

Scott C. Suzuki
1013 Poha Lane
Honolulu, Hawaii 96826
Tel: (808) 983 3850
Website: http://www.suzukiaal.com/

Offers legal services regarding special needs planning,
guardianship, and related issues.

Special Needs Hawai'i
737 Bishop St Suite 2910
Honolulu, HI 96813
Tel: (808) 540 3733
Contact Name: Kirk Barth
Email: kbarth@metlife.com
Website: http://www.specialneedshawaii.com

Provides comprehensive financial plans for families
with special needs children or dependents.

State Vocational Rehabilitation
1901 Bachelot Street
Honolulu, HI 96817
Tel: (808) 586 9744
Email: info@hawaiivr.org
Website: http://www.hawaiivr.org

Community and Recreation Services

Abilities Unlimited
414 Kuwili St. Suite 103
Honolulu, HI 96817
Tel: (808) 532 2100
Email: info@winnersatwork.org
Website: http://www.abilitiesunlimitedhi.org

The Arc of Kona
PO Box 127
Kealakekua, HI 96750
Tel: (808) 323 2626
Website: http://www.arcofkona.org

The Arc of Kona is a private nonprofit organization for
persons with disabilities, their advocates and families.

Full Life
120 Keawe Street, Hilo, HI 96720 Suite 202
Hilo, HI 96720
Tel: (808) 935 7699
Contact Name: Stone Wolfsong
Email: stone@fulllifehawaii.org
Website: http://www.fulllifehawaii.org
Facebook: https://www.facebook.com/FullLifeHawaii

Full Life provides services for adults and children on
the Autism Spectrum through the Hawaii State Developmental Disabilities Waiver Contract.

Hawaii Autism Foundation
P.O. BOX 2775
Honolulu, HI 96803
Tel: (808) 233 9144
Email: director@hawaiiautismfoundation.org
Website: http://www.hawaiiautismfoundation.org/
Facebook: https://www.facebook.com/pages/Hawaii-
Autism-Foundation/210379695651774

Helemano Plantation
64-1510 Kam Hwy.
Wahiawa, HI 96786
Tel: (808) 622 3929
Email: helemano808@hawaii.rr.com
Website: http://www.helemano.org

Offers training and employment opportunities for those
with developmental disabilities in its work centers.

Learning Disabilities Association of Hawaii (LDAH)
245 North Kukui Street Suite 205
Honolulu, HI 96817
Tel: (808) 536 9684 X28
Contact Name: Rosie Rowe, Education & Training
Coordinator
Email: BRowe@LDAHawaii.org
Website: http://www.ldahawaii.org
Facebook: https://www.facebook.com/ldahawaii.pti

Provides screening, identification, information, training and mentoring, and public outreach and advocacy.

Hire Abilities Hawaii HI
Tel: (808) 956 9142
Email: millers@hawaii.edu
Website: http://www.hireabilitieshawaii.org

Provides resources to support employment for individuals with disabilities.

Kaua'i Bus
3220 Ho'olako St.
Lihue, HI 96766
Tel: (808) 246 8110
Email: thekauaibus@kauai.gov
Website: http://www.kauai.gov/Government/
Departments/TransportationAgency/ParatransitService/
tabid/574/Default.aspx

Paratransit Service for qualified individuals.

Manawale'a Riding Center
41-170A Waikupanaha St.
Waimanalo, HI 96795
Tel: (808) 352 1523
Email: manawalea2000@yahoo.com
Website: http://www.manawalea.org

Maui Paratransit Program
2145 Kaohu St. #102
Wailuku, HI 96793
Tel: (808) 270 7511
Website: http://www.co.maui.hi.us/index.aspx?NID=607
Facebook: https://www.facebook.com/
countyofmaui?v=wall

ADA paratransit service is an advance reservation, curb to curb service for qualified persons with disabilities.

Responsive Caregivers of Hawaii
98-1247 Kaahumanu Street, #219B
Aiea, Hawaii 96701
Tel: (808) 488 7391
Email: info@rcoh.org
Website: http://www.rcoh.org

Steps, LLC
328 Uluniu St., Ste 201,
Kailua, HI 96734
Tel: (808) 263 5521
Contact Name: Emely Suazo
Email: esuazo@stepshawaii.com
Website: http://www.stepshawaii.com

Provides behavioral consultation and assistance to families navigating healthcare, school, and social systems.

IDAHO

Doctors, Clinics, Hospitals, and Other Health Services

Eagle Canyon Wellness & Sensory Development Center
Monika Buerger, DC
1516 S. Midway
Ammon, ID 83406
Tel: (208) 346 7763
Website: www.eaglecanyonwellness.com

Specializing in natural ways to treat neurodevelopmental disorders, as well as natural health care options for children, adults, and pregnant women.

The Kids' Dentist, pllc
2300 W Everest Ln, #125
Meridian, ID 83646
Tel: (208) 938 6343
Contact Name: Leslie McIntire
Email: mykidsdmd@yahoo.com
Website: http://mykidsdmd.com

Kootenai Medical Center
2003 Kootenai Health Way
Coeur d'Alene, ID 83814
Tel: (208) 765 4800
Website: http://www.kootenaihealth.org/index.
asp?w=pages&r=407&pid=31

Northwest Neurobehavioral Health, LLC
2950 E. Magic View Drive, Suite 140
Meridian, ID 83642
Tel: (208) 955 7333
Contact Name: Jennifer La Jeunesse, LCSW
Email: jlajeunesse@nnhidaho.com
Website: http://www.nnhidaho.com

Spoelstra Family Chiropractic and FOCUS
370 E Kahleen Avenue, Suite 600
Coeur d' Alene, ID 83815
Tel: (208) 667 7434
Contact Name: Dr. Amy Spoelstra
Email: jenniferk@spoelstrachiro.com
Website: http://www.cdahealth.com

Dr. Spoelstra is a pediatric chiropractor that specializes in neurodevelopmental disorders.

St. Luke's Children's Hospital
St. Luke's Children's Hospital
190 E. Bannock St.
Boise, ID 83712
Tel: (208) 381 2222
Website: http://www.stlukesonline.org/boise

Therapy Services

Camp Hippo Pediatric Therapy
7 N. 600 W
Blackfoot, ID 83221
Tel: (208) 782 2267
Contact Name: Kris Jaques
Email: camphippopeds@aol.com
Website: http://www.camphippo.com

Offers pediatric speech, occupational and physical therapy. Services include rock climbing, aquatics, hippotherapy, canine therapy intervention, social communication programs and sensory integration.

The Children's Therapy and Learning Center
449 S Fitness Place
Eagle, ID 83616
Tel: (208) 957 6301
Contact Name: Kari Thompson, OTD, OTR/L
Email: kari@childrenstlc.com
Website: http://www.childrenstlc.com

Consultations, evaluations and screenings for infants through teens, as well as occupational therapy, social skills training, academic acceleration and remediation, nutrition counseling, and developmental room design.

Children's Therapy Place, Inc.
6855 W Fairview Ave Ste 120
Boise, ID 83704
Tel: (208) 323 8888
Contact Name: Hadley Cole
Email: info@childrenstherapyplace.com
Website: http://www.childrenstherapyplace.com

Based in Boise, Idaho, with locations throughout the Treasure Valley. Therapy is offered in both private and group sessions and also conducted at off-clinic sites.

Four Feathers Counseling Center
515 Pine St
Sandpoint, ID 83864
Tel: (208) 627 8988
Contact Name: Rick Verdugo
Email: ttirona@fourfeatherscounseling.com
Website: http://fourfeatherscounseling.com/

Home-Link Trust Inc.
Home-Link Trust Inc.
1110 South Boulevard
Idaho Falls, ID 83402
Tel: (208) 524 6375
Website: http://www.homelinktrust.com

Offers state-of-the-art neurobehavioral intervention services for children and adults with developmental disabilities and traumatic brain injuries.

Idaho Center for Autism
5353 Franklin Road
Boise, ID 83705
Tel: (208) 342 0374
Contact Name: Stephanie Spencer Whipps, M.S., M.Ed. - Executive Director
Email: stephaniewhipps@hotmail.com
Website: http://idahocenterforautism.com

Services include: developmental therapy, habilitative supports and interventions, intensive behavioral intervention (IBI), friends academy, speech therapy, service coordination, educational therapies, counseling, sibling and parent support groups, advocacy, referrals, classes, workshops and continuing education credits and a lending library.

Mental Wellness Centers
1070 Hiline Road
Pocatello, ID 83201
Tel: (208) 478 9081 or (208) 478 4999
Website: http://mwcid.com/

Music Makes Connections
6515 Northview
Boise, ID 83704
Tel: (208) 405 9454
Contact Name: David Brown
Email: davidbrown@musicmakesconnections.com
Website: http://www.musicmakesconnections.com

Provides music therapy in both a one on one and group settings for both adults and children.

Music Therapy of Idaho, LLC
Boise, ID
Tel: (208) 371 9102
Contact Name: Stephanie Leavell, MT-BC
Email: MusicTherapyofIdaho@gmail.com
Website: http://www.MusicTherapyofIdaho.com

Providing board certified music therapists for individual and group sessions in Southwest Idaho.

North Idaho Children's Mental Health
1717 Ontario St.
Sandpoint, ID 83894
Tel: (208) 265 6798
Website: http://www.nicmh.com/

Provides wrap around services to children and their families in North Idaho.

Therapy Express
8024 E. Scardale Court
Boise, ID 83704
Tel: (208) 867 0116
Website: http://therapyexpressidaho.com

Provides pediatric occupational therapy, speech therapy and physical therapy for children from birth to over 21. Specializes in children with sensory integration disorders, autism spectrum disorders, developmental, neurological, musculoskeletal and learning disabilities.

Therapeutic Recreation Services of Idaho
Meridian, ID 83642
Tel: (208) 863 3409
Contact Name: Jodi Deerfield
Email: trsidaho@gmail.com

A recreation therapy program for children and teens with Autism Spectrum Disorders develop social skills using theatre and other expressive activities.

Warm Springs Counseling Center
740 Warm Springs Avenue
Boise, ID 83712
Tel: (208) 343 7797
Contact Name: Stacey Taylor
Email: staylor@childrenshomesociety.com
Website: http://www.childrenshomesociety.com

Warm Springs Counseling Center provides a full array of behavioral health services including diagnostic and treatment services for Autism Spectrum Disorders and Group Therapy for individuals with ASD and their families.

Schools and Educational Services

Boulder Creek Academy
Boulder Creek Academy
378 Emerson Lane

Bonners Ferry, ID 83805
Tel: (877) 348 0848
Contact Name: Shawnale Wilson
Website: http://www.bouldercreekacademy.net

Northwest College Support
211 Coeur d' Alene Ave Suite #102
Coeur d Alene, ID 83814
Tel: (208) 699 6817
Contact Name: Traci
Email: traci@cultivationcounseling.com
Website: http://www.collegesupportnw.com

Legal, Government & Financial Services

C.K. Quade Law, LLC
1501 Tyrell Lane PO Box 1756
Boise, ID 83706
Tel: (208) 367 0723
Contact Name: Char Quade
Email: char@charquadelaw.com

Curtis Webb
Attorney at Law
155 2nd Ave. North P.O. Box 1768
Twin Falls, ID 83301
Tel: (208) 734 1616
Email: curtiswebb@curtiswebb.net
Website: http://www.curtiswebb.net

Idaho Department of Health and Welfare
Boise, ID 83720-0036
Tel: (208) 334 5500
Website: http://www.healthandwelfare.idaho.gov

Idaho Division of Vocational Rehabilitation
650 W. State Street Room 150
Boise, ID 83720
Tel: (208) 334 3390
Contact Email:
department.info@vr.idaho.gov
http://www.vr.idaho.gov/

VR is a state-federal program that assists people with disabilities prepare for, secure, retain or regain employment.

Idaho Medicaid Program
P.O. Box 83720
Boise, ID 83720
Tel: (208) 334 5500
Contact Name: Richard Armstrong
Email: BoydE@dhw.idaho.gov
Website: http://www.healthandwelfare.idaho.gov/Default.aspx?TabId=123

Panhandle Autism Society
P.O. Box 3950
Coeur d'Alene, ID 83816
Tel: (208) 664 4133
Email: panhandleautismsociety@yahoo.com
Website: http://www.panhandleautismsociety.org

The Panhandle Autism Society (PAS) is a non-profit organization serving Idaho's five northern counties. They are a chapter of the Autism Society of America and a United Way Agency of Kootenai County.

Community and Recreation Services

Adventure Island Playground and SplashPad
Meridian & Ustick Roads
Meridian, ID 83646
Tel: (208) 887 3531
Contact Name: Angela Lindig
Email: alindig@juno.com

Community Connections, Inc.
1675 S. Maple Grove
Boise, ID 83709
Tel: (208) 377 9814
Contact Name: Brian Fay
Website: http://www.cciidaho.com/home.html

Assists individuals with disabilities while enhancing their independence.

Community Partnerships of Idaho (CPI), Inc.
3076 N Five Mile Rd.
Boise, ID 83713
Tel: (208) 376 4999
Toll Free: (800) 850 7511
Contact Name: Katherine Hansen, Executive Director
Email: katherine.hansen@mycpid.com
Website: http://www.mycpid.com

Idaho Autism
United States
Email: info@idahoautism.com
Website: http://idahoautism.com

Provides resources to families affected by autism.

Specialized Needs Recreation
P.O. Box 2451 710 East Mullan Ave.
Coeur D'Alene, ID 83814
Tel: (208) 755 6781
Contact Name: Angie Goucher
Email: anggou@aol.com
Website: http://www.snr.bz

Sun Valley Adaptive Sports
Sun Valley Adaptive Sports
PO Box 6791

Ketchum, ID 83340-6791
Tel: (208) 726 9298
Contact Name: Tom Iselin
Email: tom@svasp.org
Website: http://www.svasp.org

SVAS uses sports and recreation as healing for all types of people with all types of disabilities.

Tomorrow's Hope Satellite Services Inc.
1655 W. Fairview Ave. #100
Boise, ID 83702
Tel: (208) 319 0760 or (208) 283 0539
Contact Name: Deb Poole
Email: dpoole@tomorrowshopeinc.org
Website: http://www.tomorrowshopeinc.org
FB: http://www.facebook.com/TommorowsHopeInc

ILLINOIS

Doctors, Clinics, Hospitals, and Other Health Services

Advanced Physicians
2356 N. Elston Ave
Chicago, IL 60614
Tel: (773) 349 1122
Website: http://www.advancedphysiciansgroup.com

Provides an integrated approach to diagnosis and care.

All About Kids Dentistry
1845 E. Rand Rd Suite 203
Arlington Heights, IL 60004
Tel: (847) 870 0475
Contact Name: Victoria Ursitti, DMD

Dental care services for children and adolescents with special needs.

Ann & Robert H. Lurie Childrens Hospital of Chicago
2300 N Children's Plaza Box 16
Chicago, IL 60614
Tel: (312) 227 4000
Toll Free: (800) KIDS DOC
Website: http://www.luriechildrens.org

Associated Dental Specialists
Grove Medical Center, 4160 Route 83 Suite 308
Long Grove, IL 60047
Tel: (847) 634 6166
Email: specialdental@comcast.net
Website: http://www.specialdental.com

Bucktown Dental Associates
2002 North Damen Avenue
Chicago, IL 60647

Tel: (773) 530 3781
Website: http://www.bucktowndentalassociates.com

Chicago Family Health Center
Chicago Family Health Center
9119 S. Exchange Ave
Chicago, IL 60617
Tel: (773) 768 5000
Email:info@chicagofamilyhealth.org
Website: http://www.chicagofamilyhealth.org

Child Diagnostic Clinic
1701 W. Curtis Rd
Champaign, IL 61822
Tel: (217) 365 6200
Website: http://www.carle-clinic.com/Pediatric_
Adolescent/Pages/ChildDiagnostic.aspx

Serves children ages 2-18 years with behavioral, developmental, and learning disorders.

Edward Hospital
Edward Hospital
801 S Washington
Naperville, IL 60540
Tel: (630) 527 3379
Website: http://www.edward.org

Maria Nida V. Barino, M.D
406 West Boughton Road Suite C
Bolingbrook, IL 60440
Tel: (630) 759 1052
Contact Name: Maria Nida V. Barino, M.D

McElroy Pediatric Dentistry, Ltd.
231 S. Gary Avenue Suite 105
Bloomingdale, IL 60108
Tel: (630) 351 4440
Contact Name: Kathy Witowski, Business Mgr.
Email: info@mcelroydds.com
Website: http://www.mcelroydds.com

Provides specialized dentistry for infants, children, adolescents and children with special needs.

Palatine Pediatric Dentistry
600 N. North Ct. Suite 250
Palatine, IL 60067
Tel: (847)-991-4663
Contact Name: Dr. Irwin M. Seidman
Email: iseidmandds@sbcglobal.net
Website: http://www.palatinepediatricdentist.com

Pediatric Developmental Center Advocate Illinois
Masonic Medical Center 3040 N. Wilton St.
Chicago, IL 60657
Tel: (773) 296 7340
Website: http://www.advocatehealth.com/autism

True Health Medical Center
Anju Usman, MD, FAAFP, ABIHM
603 East Diehl Road
Suite 135
Naperville, IL 60563
Tel: (630) 995 4242
Website: www.truehealthmedical.com

Provides integrative and biomedical treatments for individuals with ASD and other conditions.

University of Illinois at Chicago Specialized Care for Children
8609 W Bryn Mawr Avenue, Suite 202
Chicago, IL 60631
Tel: (773)-444-0080
Contact Name: Nivedita Desai
Email: nndesai@uic.edu
Website: http://www.uic.edu/hsc/dscc/

The University of Illinois at Chicago - Division of Specialized Care for Children (DSCC) is the Illinois Title V agency that provides care coordination for families and children with special health care needs.

University of Illinois Medical Center
1740 West Taylor Street
Chicago, IL 60612
Toll Free: (888) 842 1801
Tel: (312) 996 6217
Website: http://uillinoismedcenter.org

The Autism Clinic provides a comprehensive multidisciplinary assessment including a structured diagnostic interview, neuropsychological and psychoeducational assessment, and a neurological examination. Depending on the patient, additional assessments may include genetic and metabolic screening and functional brain imaging.

Yummy Dental
3500 N. Lincoln Ave
Chicago, IL 60657
Tel: (773) 281 8100
Contact Name: Grace Yum, DDS
Email: info@yummydental.com
Website: http://yummydental.com

Dental care services for children and adolescents with special needs.

Will County Medical Associates
2100 Glenwood Avenue
Joliet, IL 60435
Tel: (815) 725 2121
Website: http://www.wcmadoc.com

Therapy Services

Association House of Chicago
1116 North Kedzie Avenue
Chicago, IL 60651
Tel: (773)-772-7170
Website: http://www.associationhouse.org/services/behavioralhealth

Offers a variety of behavioral healthcare services, including prevention, treatment and education. Services are offered in both English and Spanish.

Ben Gordon Center
12 Health Services Drive
DeKalb, IL 60115
(815) 756 4875
Website: http://www.bengordoncenter.org

Offers behavioral health services, therapy and support groups.

Centennial Counseling Center
110 E. Countryside Parkway
Yorkville, IL 60560
Tel: (630) 553 1600
Website: http://www.centennialcounseling.com

Center For Children And Families
Erikson Institute, 451 N LaSalle St. Floor 4
Chicago, IL 60654
Tel: (312) 893 7119
Email: centerforchildrenandfamilies@erikson.edu
Website: http://ccf.erikson.edu

Central DuPage Hospital
Central DuPage Hospital
25 North Winfield Road
Winfield, IL 60190
Tel: (630) 933 1600
Website: http://www.cdh.org

Chicago Comer Children's Hospital
5721 S. Maryland Avenue
Chicago, IL 60637
Toll Free: (888) UCH 0200
Tel: (773) 702 1000
Website: http://www.uchicagokidshospital.org

Illinois Developmental Therapy Association
P.O. Box 1114
Oswego, IL 60543
Contact Name: Lisa Lampman
Email: LisaLampmanDT@aol.com
Website: http://www.illinoisdta.org

Logan-Mason Rehabilitation Center: Mental Health Centers of Central Illinois
760 S. Postville Drive
Lincoln, IL 62656
Tel: (217) 735 1413
https://www.mhcci.org

Provides behavioral health care and rehabilitation services.

Mental Health Centers of Central Illinois- The Childrens Center
5220 S. Sixth Street Road
Springfield, IL 62703
Tel: (217) 757 7700
https://www.mhcci.org

Provides behavioral health care and rehabilitation services.

Mental Health Centers of Central Illinois Memorial Partial Hospitalization Program
901 North First Street
Springfield, IL
Tel: (217) 757 2455
https://www.memorialmedical.com/Services/Behavioral-Health/Default.aspx

Naperville Pediatric Psychology and Development
1220 Hobson Road Suite 216
Naperville, IL 60540
Tel: (630) 548 9235
Contact Name: Dr. Jennifer Manfre
Email: drmanfre@napervilleppd.com
Website: http://www.napervilleppd.com

Provides assessment, consultation, and intervention services (including ABA services, individual, family, and group therapy) to children/adolescents with ASD.

Neurodevelopmental Clinic
Child Psychiatry University of Chicago Medicine, 5841 S Maryland Ave.
Chicago, IL 60637
Tel: (773) 702 3858
Contact Name: Dr. Sharon Hirsch, Director
Email: shirsch@yoda.bsd.uchicago.edu

Specializes in the assessment and diagnosis of children with complex neurogenetic and behavioral needs and collaborates with Development & Behavioral Pediatrics and Pediatric Neurology.

Northern Illinois Academy (NIA)
Sequel Youth and Family Services 998 Corporate Blvd.
Aurora, IL 60502
Tel: (847) 391 8011 or (847) 391 8000
Contact Name: Vanessa Wouk, MSW, LSW, Admission Director

Email: Vanessa.Wouk@sequelyouthservices.com
Website: http://sequelyouthservices.com/html/autism-northernillinois.html

Northern Illinois Academy is a Psychiatric Residential Treatment Facility (PRTF) licensed by DCFS that serves youth ages 6 to 21 and provides an on-site school.

NorthPointe Resources, Inc
3441 Sheridan Rd
Zion, IL 60099
Tel: (847) 872 1700
Website: http://www.northpointeresources.org

Rehabilitation Institute of Chicago
345 E. Superior Street
Chicago, IL 60611
Tel: (312) 238 6812
Contact Name: Julie Zook
Email: jzook@ric.org
Website: http://www.ric.org

Urban Brain and Body, LLC
2551 N Clark St Suite 8
Chicago, IL 60614
Tel: (312) 257 8550 or (217) 246 7688
Contact Name: Seth Franz
Email: seth.franz@urbanbrainandbody.com
Website: http://www.urbanbrainandbody.com

Offers neurofeedback therapy.

Schools and Educational Services

Elmhurst College Adult and Graduate Enrollment
190 Prospect Avenue
Elmhurst, IL 60126
(650) 617 3309
Contact Name: Tim Ahlberg
Email: ahlbergt@elmhurst.edu

Elmhurst Learning and Success Academy
190 S. Prospect Avenue Cureton Hall
Elmhurst, IL 60126
Tel: (630) 617 3752
Email: elsa@elmhurst.edu
Website: http://public.elmhurst.edu/elsa

A four-year program that offers a full-time, post-secondary educational experience to young adults with developmental disabilities.

Options for College Success
820 Davis St Suite 455
Evanston, IL 60201
Tel: (847) 425 4797
Email: info@optionsforcollegesuccess.org
Website: http://optionsforcollegesuccess.org/app/

Prairie State College Disability Services
202 S. Halsted St
Chicago Heights, IL 60411
Tel: (708) 709 3500
Contact Name: Diane Janowiak, Director
Email: djanowiak@prairiestate.edu
Website: http://www.prairie.cc.il.us/ss/ss-disasvcs.html

Think College Illinois
1640 W. Roosevelt Road, Room 405
Chicago, IL 60608
Toll Free: (877)-232-1990
Tel: (312)-413-1407
Website: http://www.thinkcollegeillinois.org

Triton College Center for Students with Disabilities
2000 Fifth Ave
River Grove, IL 60171
(708) 456 0300 X3854
Contact Name: Deborah M Ford
Email: dford@triton.edu
Website: http://www.triton.edu

Turning Pointe Career College
1500 W. Ogden Avenue
Naperville, IL 60540
Tel: (630) 615 6032
Contact Name: Ketra Kuniej
Email: kkuniej@turningpointeaf.org
Website: http://www.turningpointecareercollege.org

Teaches life, social and work readiness skills to assist individuals With ASD.

University of Illinois at Chicago Disability Resource Center
1200 W. Harrison St Room 1190 SSB (MC 321)
Chicago, IL 60607
Tel: (312) 413 2183
Contact Name: Roxana Stupp, Director
Email: drc@uic.edu
Website: http://www.uic.edu/depts/oaa/disability_resources/contact.html

Willowglen Academy Illinois
701 W Lamm Road
Freeport, IL 61032
Tel: (815)-233-6162
Contact Name: Rodger Kinard
Email: rkinard@willowglen-il.com
Website: http://www.willowglen-academy.com

Legal, Government & Financial Services

Abraham Lincoln Centre (ALC)
3858 S Cottage Grove Ave.
Chicago, IL 60653
Tel: (773) 285 1390
Contact Name: Gloria Knight-Hinds, Director of
Behavioral Health Services
Email: gknight@abelink.org
Website: http://www.abelink.org

Cahill & Associates
1155 S. Washington Street Suite 106
Naperville, IL 60540
Tel: (630) 778 6500
Website: http://www.cahillassociateslaw.com

Center for Disability and Elder Law
79 W. Monroe St. Suite 9
Chicago, IL 60603
Tel: (312) 376 1880
Email: info@probonocdel.org
Website: http://www.probonocdel.org

Chicago Lawyers Committee for Civil Rights
100 N LaSalle St.
Chicago, IL 60602
Tel: (312) 630 9744

The public interest law consortium of Chicago's leading
law firms.

DePaul University Special Education Advocacy Clinic
14 East Jackson Boulevard Suite 100
Chicago, IL 60604
Tel: (312) 362 8294
Website: http://www.law.depaul.edu/clinical_programs/
clinical_special_ed.asp

Disabled Workers Program
130 W. Mason St
Springfield, IL 62702
Tel: (217)-524-7514
Website: http://work.illinois.gov/disabpgm.htm

Legal Assistance Foundation of Chicago
111 W. Jackson Blvd. Suite 300
Chicago, IL 60604

Tel: (312) 341 1070
Website: http://www.lafchicago.org

Prairie State Legal Services
102 N. Center, Suite 405
Bloomington, IL 61701
Tel: (309) 827 5021
Toll Free: (800) 874 2536
Website: http://www.pslegal.org

University of Illinois at Chicago Specialized Care for Children
8609 W Bryn Mawr Avenue, Suite 202
Chicago, IL 60631
Tel: (773)-444-0080
Contact Name: Nivedita Desai
Email: nndesai@uic.edu
Website: http://www.uic.edu/hsc/dscc/

The University of Illinois at Chicago - Division of Specialized Care for Children (DSCC) is the Illinois Title V agency that provides care coordination for families and children with special health care needs.

Community and Recreation Services

ALLternative Recreation, Inc
1830 N. Milwaukee Ave Unit A
Chicago, IL 60647
Tel: (773)-278-9230
Contact Name: Sophie Morgan
Email: info@allternativerec.com
Website: http://www.allternativerec.com

Offers various activities through play, social interaction, independent, fine and gross motor skills and music and movement for children ages 18 months to 13 years.

Always Learning While Living
828 Sheridan Road
Highwood, IL 60040
Tel: (847) 454 7219
Contact Name: Barry D, Petersen II
Email: director@alwayslearningwl.org
Website: http://AlwaysLearningWL.org

Always Learning While Living is a day program for adults who have special needs.

American Home Health
1660 B Farnsworth Ave, Suite 3
Aurora, IL 60505
Tel: (630)-236-3501
Contact Name: Edward Lara
Email: Edward.lara@ahhc-1.com
Website: http://www.ahhc-1.com

Provides support services that allow a patient to be at home.

Association of the Developmentally Disabled of Woodford County
200 Moody St
Eureka, IL 61530
Tel: (309) 467 3015
Email: addwc@mtco.com
Website: http://www.addwc.org

Offers community living options, home based support services, employment and training programs, and advocacy.

Association for Individual Development (AID)
309 W New Indian Trail Ct.
Aurora, IL 60506
Tel: (630) 966 4000
Email: info@the-association.org
Website: http://www.the-association.org

Austin Special Chicago
5318 N. Elston Ave.
Chicago, IL 60630
Tel: (773) 282 9992
Contact Name: Marciel Roy Aban
Email: info@austinspecial.org
Website: http://www.austinspecial.org

The Autism Program of Illinois (TAP)
5220 S. 6th St. Rd. Suite 1700
Springfield, IL 62703
Tel: (217) 588 7661
Contact Name: Farah Salim
Email: fsalim@thehopeinstitute.us
Website: http://www.theautismprogram.org/

The Autism Program of Illinois (TAP) is a statewide network of approximately 30 organizations providing diagnosis, treatment, support groups, and resources for those affected by ASD.

Barbara Olson Center of Hope
3206 North Central Avenue
Rockford, IL 61101
Tel: (815) 964 9275
Tel: (815) 964 9388
Website: http://www.b-olsoncenterofhope.org

Provides a variety of vocational, employment, educational, social and habilitative services for teens and adults with developmental disabilities.

Blue Cap
2155 Broadway
Blue Island, IL 60406
(708) 389 8137
Contact Name: Karen Connelly
Website: http://www.blue-cap.org

Serves infants, children and adults with developmental disabilities through community-based educational, therapeutic, vocational and residential opportunities.

Center For Enriched Living
280 Saunders Rd
Riverwoods, IL 60015
Tel: (847) 948 7001
Contact Name: Lauren Berndt
Email: Lauren@CenterForEnrichedLiving.org
Website: http://www.centerforenrichedliving.org

A non-residential, social enrichment and skill-development center.

Challenge Unlimited Incorporated
Challenge Unlimited Incoporated
4 Emmie L Kaus Ln
Alton, IL 62002
Tel: (618) 465 0044
Email: info@cuinc.org
Website: http://www.cuinc.org

Provides work related opportunities to individuals with disabilities.

Charleston 7th Street Day Program
521 7th Street
Charleston, IL 61920
Tel: (217) 348 8798
Website: http://www.ctfillinois.org

Clearbrook
1835 W. Central Road
Arlington Heights, IL 60005
Tel: (847) 870 7711
Contact Name: Bernie Andersen
Email: info@clearbrook.org
Website: http://www.clearbrook.org

Donca, Inc
400 North County Farm Rd
Wheaton, IL 60187
Tel: (630)-665-8169

Donka, Inc. is a non-profit organization providing no-cost computer training and job readiness services to persons with physical and visual disabilities.

Foundation for Autism Services for Today and Tomorrow (FASTT)
500 East Division
Maryville, IL 62062
Tel: (618) 741 6409
Contact Name: Dawn Whalen-Bregenzer, Program Director

Email: program.director@fasttfoundation.org
Website: http://www.fasttfoundation.org

An adult day program providing services to adults with ASD.

Have Dreams
515 Busse Highway Suite 150
Park Ridge, IL 60068
Tel: (847) 685 0250
Website: http://www.havedreams.org

Offers individualized afterschool programs and diagnostic and family support services from early childhood through adulthood.

Homewood Day Program
17341 Palmer Blvd
Homewood, IL 60430
Tel: (708) 922 1532
Website: http://www.ctfillinois.org

Illinois Valley Center for Independent Living
18 Gunia Dr
LaSalle, IL 61301
Tel: (815) 224 3126
Email: ivcil@ivcil.com
Website: http://www.ivcil.com

Invisible Differences
Companies That Care, 954 W Washington Blvd. Suite 430
Chicago, IL 60607
Tel: (312) 661 1010
Contact Name: Marci Koblenz, Founder and President
Email: marcikoblenz@companies-that-care.org
Website: http://www.companies-that-care.org/action/invisible-differences

Supports adolescents and young adults with neurobehavioral and learning disabilities to complete their education and prepare for work.

Knowledge, Creativity, Caring, Development, Dedication (KCCDD) Inc
2015 Windish Drive
Galesburg, IL 61401
Tel: (309) 344 2600
Contact Name: Mary Crittenden, Executive Director
Email: mcrittenden@kccdd.com
Website: http://www.kccdd.com

Lester and Rosalie Anixter Center
2001 N. Clybourn Ave Floor 3
Chicago, IL 60614
Tel: (773) 973 7900 or (773) 973 2180
Email: AskAnixter@anixter.org
Website: http://www.anixter.org

Little City Foundation
1760 W Algonquin Rd.
Palatine, IL 60067
Tel: (847) 358 5510
Website: http://www.littlecity.org

Little Friends Center for Autism
140 N. Wright Street
Naperville, IL 60540
Tel: (630) 355 6533
Contact Name: Kim Bus
Email: kbus@lilfriends.com
Website: http://www.littlefriendsinc.org

Provides services to children and adults with autism and other developmental disabilities.

Open Door Rehabilitation Center
405 South Wells St
Sandwich, IL 60548
Tel: (815) 786 8468
Contact Name: David C. Baker, Executive Director
Website: http://www.odrc.org

Provides vocational, residential, day and community support services to adults with developmental disabilities.

Park Lawn
10833 S. LaPorte
Oak Lawn, IL 60453
Tel: (708) 425 3344
Email: info@parklawn.com
Website: http://www.parklawn.com

Progressive Careers and Housing (PCH)
120 Locust Street
Hoyleton, IL 62803
Tel: (618) 231 1713 or (618) 493 6071
Contact Name: Missy Reed
Email: missyr@phidd.org
Website: http://www.phidd.org

Self Help Enterprises Inc
2300 West LeFevre Road
Sterling, IL 61081
Tel: (815) 626 3115
Email: selfhelpent@yahoo.com
Website: http://selfhelp-sterling.com.

SHORE Community Services
4232 Dempster Street
Skokie, IL 60076
Tel: (847) 982 2030
Contact Name: Debora Braun
Email: dkb.shore@sbcglobal.net
Website: http://www.shoreinc.org

UCP Land of Lincoln
101 N 16th Street
Springfield, IL 62703
Tel: (217) 525 6522
Contact Name: Aimee Gray
Email: ucpll@ucpll.org
Website: http://www.ucpll.org

Tazewell County Resource Centers
21310 State Route 9
Tremont, IL 61568
Tel: (309) 925 2061
Website: http://tcrcorg.com

William M. BeDell Achievement & Resource Center
400 South Main Street
Wood River, IL 62095
Tel: (618) 251 2175
Email: jjohnson@bedellarc.org
Website: http://www.bedellarc.org

INDIANA

Doctors, Clinics, Hospitals, and Other Health Services

Autism Hope and Healing Clinic
616 E. Main Street
Muncie, IN 47305
Tel: (765) 716 8966
Email: info@autismhopeandhealing.com
Website: http://autismhopeandhealing.com

Believes that ASD is caused by a combination of genetic and environmental risk factors and is not a psychiatric disorder, but rather a whole body disease where recovery is possible.

B-Renewed Wellness Solutions LLC
3805 Debbie Ln.
Evansville, IN 47711
Tel: (812) 473 2502
Contact Name: Bonnie Schnautz
Email: bonnie@brenewed.com
Website: http://www.BRenewed.com

Provides wellness education, dietary guidance, and motivational support.

Christian Sarkine Autism Treatment Center
Riley Hospital for Children at IU Health
705 Riley Hospital Dr. Suite 4300
Indianapolis, IN 46202
Tel: (317) 274 8162
Email: kidpsych@iupui.edu

Ernest E. Smith, M.D.
301 East Carmel Drive H400
Carmel, IN 46032
Tel: (317) 582 8290
Contact Name: Leslie Stockton
Email: dbpeds@stvincent.org

Specializes in children with disabilities and developmental and behavioral pediatrics.

Evansville Psychiatric Childrens Center
3300 E. Morgan Ave.
Evansville, IN 47715
Tel: (812) 477 6436
Website: http://www.in.gov/fssa/dmha/6812.htm

Jerry Kartzinel, MDKartzinel Wellness Center
10142 Brooks School Road, Suite 220
Fishers, IN 46037
Tel: (317) 845 8883
Website: www.drjerryk.com

Dr. Kartzinel is a board-certified pediatrician practicing Translational Medicine (translating diverse scientific findings into treatments for patients).

Judy Orthodontics
3920 West 106th Street Suite 150
Carmel, IN 46034
Tel: (317) 471 0100
Contact Name: Jennifer
Email: jenn@davidjudyortho.com
Website: http://www.davidjudyortho.com

Larue D. Carter Memorial Hospital
2601 Cold Spring Road
Indianapolis, IN 46222
Tel: (317) 941 4000
Website: http://www.in.gov/fssa/dmha/6801.htm

Riley Hospital For Children
705 Riley Hospital Drive
Indianapolis, IN 46202
Tel: (317) 944 2060
Website: http://iuhealth.org/riley/child-development/

Using an interdisciplinary team, provides diagnosis, recommendations, and follow-up for children from infancy to adulthood with developmental, behavioral, or learning challenges.

Sanders Weddell Pediatric Dental Specialists
14555 Hazel Dell Pkwy #100
Carmel, IN 46033
Tel: (317) 816 1555
Contact Name: Carrie Dickey
Email: sandersweddell@yahoo.com
Website: http://www.sandersweddell.com

Our office provides specialized dentistry for infants, children, teens, and patients with special health care needs.

St. Mary's Center for Children
3900 Washington Ave. Suite 100
Evansville, IN 47714
Tel: (812) 485 4215
Contact Name: Patient Coordinator
Email: mevers@stmarys.org
Website: http://www.stmarys.org/body.cfm?id=915

Stacie Marcari, DC CNS
75 Executive Drive
Suite G
Carmel, IN 46032
Tel: (317) 846 9355
Website: www.carmelclinic.com

Therapy Services

Acacia Center
819 West Franklin St.
Evansville, IN 47710
Tel: (812) 491 1805
Contact Name: Dr. Gable or Dr. Hines
Website: http://www.acaciacenter.com

Provides psychotherapy, counseling, and psychological assessment.

Autism Hope and Healing Clinic
616 E. Main Street
Muncie, IN 47305
Tel: (765) 716 8966
Email: info@autismhopeandhealing.com
Website: http://autismhopeandhealing.com

Believes that ASD is caused by a combination of genetic and environmental risk factors and is not a psychiatric disorder, but rather a whole body disease where recovery is possible.

Behavior Analysis Center for Autism
11902 Lakeside Dr.
Fishers, IN 46038
Tel: (317) 288 5232
Contact Name: Devon Sundberg
Email: dsundberg@thebaca.com
Website: http://www.thebaca.com

Uses ABA to teach language, social, self-help, academic, daily living and life skills to children with ASD and related disabilities.

Behavior Analysis Center for Autism Preparatory Services
9929 East 126th Street
Fishers, IN 46038

Tel: (317) 436 8961
Contact Name: Leah McKenzie
Email: LMckenzie@thebaca.com
Website: http://www.thebaca.com

Specializes in treating adolescents with ASD, preparing them for either an academic or vocational curricula.

Behavior Specialists of Indiana
2611 A Chicago St.
Valparaiso, IN 46383
Tel: (219) 462 6705
Email: bsinoa@behaviorspecialists.net
Website: http://bsitherapy.com

Behavior Specialists of Indiana, LLC (BSI) specializes in the treatment of individuals diagnosed with ASD and other disorders.

Bierman ABA Autism Center
16414 Southpark Dr.
Westfield, IN 46074
Tel: (317) 815 5501
Email: info@biermanaba.com
Website: http://www.biermanaba.com

Provides services to children with ASD between the ages of 1 and 13, including providing early intervention and personalized and intensive ABA.

Bright Hope Riders of the Wabash Valley, Inc.
6010 E. Devonald Ave.
Terre Haute, IN 47805
Tel: (812) 466 2334
Contact Name: Dianne Mansfield
Email: revmansfield@aol.com
Website: http://terrehaute.com/bright-hope-riders-bhr/

Provides therapeutic horseback riding to persons with developmental disabilities.

Centrality Behavior Support Training
3725 E Southport Rd. Suite F
Indianapolis, IN 46237
Tel: (317) 796 6668
Contact Name: Meagan Dant, MA, BCBA, Clinical Director
Email: meagan@centralitybehavior.com
Website: http://www.centralitybehavior.com

Offers center- and home-based 1:1 ABA, as well as a hybrid program.

Crystal's Behavior Solutions
4221 E. Thompson Road
Indianapolis, IN 46239
Tel: (317) 405 9162
Contact Name: Christy Gray

Email: Christy.Gray@CrystalsBehaviorSolutions.com
Website: http://www.CrystalsABA.com

Uses ABA principles to develop individualized programs.

Disabilities Autism Services of Indiana (D.A.S.I.)
4561 W. Co. Rd. 650 N.
Saint Paul, IN 47272
Tel: (812) 322 4374
Contact Name: Libby Caswell
Email: caswellaba@yahoo.com
Website: http://www.dasikids.com

Provides ABA programs.

Fast Track Autism Services LLC
Tel: (317) 537 0487
Contact Name: Misty Turner-Wade, MA, BCBA
Email: misty@fasttrackautismservices.com
Website: http://www.fasttrackautismservices.com

Provides individualized ABA programs and behavior consultation to children diagnosed with ASD and their families in the Central and East Indiana areas.

Fox Behavior Group
1389 W 86th St. #170
Indianapolis, IN 46260
Tel: (317) 409 6151
Contact Name: Lydia Fox
Email: lydia@foxbehaviorgroup.com
Website: http://www.foxbehaviorgroup.com

Provides personalized at-home ABA therapy treatment plans.

Integrity Behavioral Solutions
Indianapolis, IN 46268
Tel: (317) 914 3176
Contact Name: Alicia Boyll, Director
Email: info@integritybehavioralsolutions.com
Website: http://www.integritybehavioralsolutions.com

Integrity Behavioral Solutions provides ABA-based early intervention and therapy services.

Kidworks, LLC
1120 S. Calumet Rd Suite 3
Chesterton, IN 46304
Tel: (219) 983 9675
Email: reception@kidworksonline.com
Website: http://www.kidworksllc.com

Provides pediatric therapeutic services through Early Intervention Services in Lake, Porter, and LaPorte Counties and at their clinic in Chesterton Indiana.

Life Strategies LLC
5521 W. Lincoln Hwy Ste 105
Schererville, IN 46307
Tel: (219) 359 3272

Contact Name: Autumn Vendramin
Email: contact@life-strategies.net
Website: http://www.life-strategies.net

Provides in-home ABA VB programs are supervised by Board Certified Behavior Analysts.

Little Star Center
Locations in Carmel, Lafayette, Bloomington
Website: http://littlestarcenter.org/

Provides individualized ABA-based programs.

Positive Pathways
13295 Illinois St. Suite 132
Carmel, IN 46032
Tel: (317) 848 4900 or (317) 440 4176
Contact Name: Stephanie Shank
Email: sshankpospath@gmail.com
Website: http://www.positivepathways.net

Provides behavior supports and Music Therapy for individuals with ASD in their main office, at home, and in the community.

Reach High Consulting and Therapy
2101 W. Tapp Road
Bloomington, IN 47403
Tel: (812) 330 4460
Contact Name: Audra Lampkins
Email: alampkins@reachhighconsulting.org
Website: http://www.reachhighconsulting.org

Verbal Behavior Center for Autism
9830 Bauer Drive
Indianapolis, IN 46280
Tel: (317) 848 4774
Contact Name: Sabrina Shannon
Email: sshannon@vbca.org
Website: http://www.vbca.org

Wee Care Therapy
440 Edmond Dr.
Dyer, IN 46311
Tel: (219) 322 1415
Contact Name: Susan Swindeman
Email: weecare@weecaretherapy.com
Website: http://www.weecaretherapy.com

Provides behavioral services, developmental therapy, occupational therapy, physical therapy, and speech/language therapy, and social skills groups.

The Zeilbeck Group LLC
109 Patton St.
LaPorte, IN 46350
Tel: (219) 575 1437
Email: azeilbeck@hotmail.com
Website: http://www.andrewzeilbeckbehaviors.com

Provides Behavior Management Services for psychologically and developmentally disabled individuals in Northwest Indiana.

Schools and Educational Services

College Internship Program (CIP) Bloomington
425 N. College Ave
Bloomington, IN 47404
Tel: (813) 323 0600 x 22
Contact Name: Lori Mangrum, Admissions Coordinator
Email: lmangrum@cipbloomington.org
Website: http://www.cipbloomington.org

The Independence Academy
612 West 42nd Street
Indianapolis, IN 46208
Tel: (317) 926 0043
Contact Name: Susan Le Vay
Email: susanlevay@theindependenceacademy.org
Website: http://www.iaindiana.org/

A private, non-profit school for students in grades 5-12 with high-functioning Autism and Asperger's offering a low student to teacher ratio and a multi-sensory approach.

Indiana Autism Education & Training Center, Inc.
14197 Dove Drive
Carmel, IN 46033
Tel: (317) 573 9610
Contact Name: Sheila Wolfe
Email: sheilawolfe@sbcglobal.net
Website: http://www.aetcinc.org

Interlock
230 South Schroder Road
Muncie, IN 47304
Contact Name: Belinda Hughes
Email: Belinda@InterlockIn.org
Website: http://www.Interlockin.org

Assists and educates families in East Central Indiana and assists special education classrooms in accommodating students with ASD.

Simply Speaking Preschool, LLC and Learning Center
12912 Coldwater Road, Suite A
Fort Wayne, IN 46845
Tel: (260) 417 9443
Contact Name: Janice Anne Cook, Founder
Email: janiceannecook@simplyspeakinglearning
center.com

Services for children ages 2 to 5. Autism services include: Social Skills, Fine and Gross Motor, Sensory Integration, Speech and Language and more.

T.C. Harris School
3700 Rome Drive
Lafayette, IN 47905
Tel: (765) 448 4220
Toll Free: (877) 854 1024
Website: http://www.tcharrisschool.com/

Worthmore Academy
3535 Kessler Boulevard East Drive
Indianapolis, IN 46220
Tel: (877) 700 6516
Contact Name: Brenda Jackson
Email: bjackson@worthmoreacademy.org
Website: http://www.worthmoreacademy.org

Legal, Government & Financial Services

Department of Housing and Urban Development
151 North Delaware St. Suite 1200
Indianapolis, IN 46204
Tel: (317) 226 6303
Contact Name: John Hall
Email: IN_Webmanager@hud.gov
Website: http://www.hud.gov/local/index.
cfm?state=in&topic=offices

Indiana Protection and Advocacy Services
4701 North Keystone Avenue Suite 222
Indianapolis, IN 46205
Tel: (317) 722 5555 or (800) 622 4845
Contact Name: Tom Gallagher
Email: il-ipas@source.isd.state.in.us
Website: http://www.in.gov/ipas

IndyGo Open Door Service
Tel: (317) 917 8747
Website: http://www.indygo.net/pages/open-door-service

Open Door ADA paratransit service is provided for the needs of qualified riders with disabilities.

Vocational Rehabilitation Services
138 E. Lincoln Highway
Schererville, IN 46375
Tel: (219) 864 8163
Website: http://www.in.gov/fssa/ddrs/2636.htm

Community and Recreation Services

About Special Kids (ASK)
7275 Shadeland Avenue
Indianapolis, IN 46250
Tel: (800) 964 4746 or (317) 251 7488
Email: familynetw@aboutspecialkids.org
Website: http://www.aboutspecialkids.org

Active Day Center
Various locations
Tel: (317) 569 0014
Contact Name: Clyde Bolton
Email: cbolton@activeday.com
Website: http://www.activeday.com

Medical adult day care centers.

ADA Complementary ParaTransit Service
100 West 4th Avenue
Gary, IN 46402
Tel: (885) 7555
Website: http://www.gptcbus.com/ada.htm

Paratransit Service is complementary service provided by the Gary Public Transportation Corporation to qualifying residents with disabilities.

ADEC
P.O. Box 398
19670 S.R. 120
Bristol, IN 46507
Tel: (574) 848 7451
Website: http://www.adecinc.com

Provides residential and day services to assist people with disabilities to participate in their community as employees, students, competitors, consumers, advocates, and volunteers.

ARC Opportunities
0235W 300N.
Howe, IN 46746
Tel: (260) 463 2653
Email: info@arcopportunities.org
Website: http://www.arcopportunities.org/aboutus.htm

Asperger Autism Group of Goshen
602 South Eighth Street
Goshen, IN 46526
Contact Name: Christine Guth
Email: cguth@autismgoshen.org
Website: http://www.autismgoshen.org

Autism Advocates of Indiana
P.O. Box 285
Fishers, IN 46038
Tel: (317) 403 4308
Contact Name: Patty Reed
Email: phreed1@aol.com

Seeks to increase and broaden public knowledge and awareness about ASD.

AWS/Benchmark Human Services
Various locations
8515 Bluffton Road
Fort Wayne, IN 46809
Tel: (260) 744 6145
Toll Free: (877) 456 2971
Website: http://awsbenchmark.com/

Bi-County Services
425 E. Harrison Rd.
Bluffton, IN 46714
Tel: (260) 824 1253
Email: info@adifferentlight.com
Website: http://www.bi-countyservices.com

BLAST Youth Group
Speedway United Methodist Church 5065 W. 16th Street
Indianapolis, IN 46224
Tel: (317) 971 2619
Contact Name: Beth DeHoff
Email: bdehoff@iquest.net
Website: http://www.speedway-umc.org/specialneeds.html

A youth group for youth and young adults ages 12 and up with ASD and developmental disabilities.

Bridges of Indiana
Various locations
Tel: (812) 478 0724
Toll Free: (800) 998 0724
Contact Name: Tiffany Smith
Website: http://www.bridgesofindiana.com

Camp Millhouse
25600 Kelly Road
South Bend, IN 46614
Tel: (574) 233 2202
Contact Name: Lea Pitcher
Email: campmillhouse@aol.com
Website: http://www.campmillhouse.org

Camp Millhouse is a residential summer camp for children and adults with mental and physical disabilities.

Camp Red Cedar
3900 Hursh Road
Fort Wayne, IN 46845
Tel: (260) 637 3608
Contact Name: Carrie Perry
Email: redcedar@awsusa.com
Website: http://www.awsredcedar.com

A camp that serves both people with and without disabilities and offers a day camp for children ages 6-18yo with ASD.

Carey Services
2724 South Carey Street
Marion, IN 46953
Tel: (765) 668 8961
Website: http://www.careyservices.com

Cookie Cutters Haircuts for Kids
55 South Raceway
Indianapolis, IN 46231
Tel: (317) 271 3855
Contact Name: Christie
Email: christie@haircutsarefun.com
Website: http://www.haircutsarefun.com

Damar Services, Inc
6067 Decatur Blvd.
Indianapolis, IN 46241
Tel: (317) 856 5201
Contact Name: Carla Bill
Email: carlab@damar.org
Website: http://www.damar.org

Different Like Me Club
Greenwood, IN 46142
Tel: (317) 781 1571
Contact Name: Abbey Parker
Email: abbey@stillpointconsultants.com
Website: http://www.stillpointconsultants.com/news_
and_updates

Easter Seals Crossroads
4740 Kingsway Drive
Indianapolis, IN 46205
Tel: (317) 466 2001
Website: http://www.eastersealscrossroads.org

Evansville Autism Education
1301 Judson Street
Evansville, IN 47713
Tel: (812) 435 8219
Contact Name: Kimberly Sullivan
Email: kim@inautism.org

Four Rivers Resource Services
Linton, IN 47441
Tel: (812) 847 2231
Website: http://www.frrs.org

Gibson County Area Rehabilitation Centers
P.O. Box 5
4207 W. State Rd. 64
Princeton, IN 47670
Tel: (812) 386 6312
Email: gcarc@gcarc.org
Website: http://www.gcarc.org

Hannah & Friends
P.O. Box 1218
Granger, IN 46530
Email: info@hannahandfriends.org
Website: http://www.hannahandfriends.org

Seeks to raise awareness and compassion for those with special needs and offers recreational programs for children and adults with special needs as well as residential services for adults. They also operate a grant program.

Heart of Sailing
1114 N. College Ave.
Bloomington, IN 47404
Tel: (812) 935 7245
Contact Name: George Saidah/ Founder
Email: gsaidah@heartofsailing.org

Introduces sailing to special needs children and adults.

Hopewell Center
5325 S Main St.
Anderson, IN
Tel: (765) 642 0201
Website: http://www.hopewellcenter.org

Indiana Resource Center for Autism
2853 East Tenth St.
Bloomington, IN 47408-2696
Tel: (812) 855 6508
Website: http://www.iidc.indiana.edu/irca

Indiana Resource Center for Families with Special Needs
1703 S. Ironwood Drive
South Bend, IN 46613
Tel: (574) 234 7101
Toll Free: (800) 332 4433
Email: insource@insource.org
Website: http://www.insource.org

IndyGo Open Door Service
Tel: (317) 917 8747
Website: http://www.indygo.net/pages/open-door-service

Open Door ADA paratransit service is provided for the needs of qualified riders with disabilities.

Jacob's Place Inc.
16960 Williamson Lane
Noblesville, In., IN 46062
Tel: (317) 756 7781
Contact Name: Kristine Barnett
Email: kristineshouse@yahoo.com
Website: http://jacobbarnett.com

Operates Youth Sports for Autism, a free program where children with ASD play on teams in an accepting environment, and other programs.

Jubilate Choir for Children with Special Needs
Butler University, 4600 Sunset Ave. Lily Hall, Room 133

Indianapolis, IN 46208
Tel: (317) 940 8065
Contact Name: Lauren Southard
Email: lsouthar@icchoir.org
Website: http://www.icchoir.org/Jubilate

The Indianapolis Children's Choir offers Jubilate, a choir for children with special needs in third through ninth grade.

Lifesong Academy
1900 Stringtown Rd
Evansville, IN 47711
Tel: (812) 490 2826
Contact Name: Brock Quinton
Email: brock@behaviornetworks.com
Website: http://www.lifesongacademy.net

LOGAN Regional Center for Autism
2505 E. Jefferson Blvd.
South Bend, IN 46615
Tel: (574) 289 4831
Contact Name: Leanne D Suarez
Email: leanne@logancenter.org
Website: http://www.logancenter.org

Making Autism Less Scary (MALS) Place
New Haven, IN 46774
Tel: (260) 388 2818
Contact Name: Julie Dennis
Email: MALSPlace2007@gmail.com
Website: http://malsplace2007.webs.com/

An online and live support group to raise awareness.

Meaningful Day Services
640 Patrick Pl.
Brownsburg, IN 46112
Tel: (317) 858 8630
Website: http://www.meaningfuldays.com

Provides therapies, residential and adult day supports.

Noble of Indiana
Various locations
7701 East 21st Street
Indianapolis, IN 46219
Tel: (317) 375 2700
Website: http://www.nobleofindiana.org/

Provides individualized services.

Peak Community Services, Inc.
1416 Woodlawn Avenue
Logansport, IN 46947
Tel: (574) 753 4104
Email: peak@peakcommunity.com
Website: http://www.peakcommunity.com

Provides job training and support.

PIECES Autism Support Group
Terre Haute Regional Hospital
3901 S. 7th Street, Classroom 1
Terre Haute, IN 47802
Tel: (812) 240 0481
Contact Name: Amy Walker
Email: awalker1979@frontier.com

Shults-Lewis Child and Family Services
Po Box 471
Valparaiso, IN 46384
Tel: (219) 464 7669
Contact Name: Raymond Crowder
Email: raycrowder@shultslewis.org
Website: http://www.shultslewis.org

Sycamore Services, Inc.
Various locations
1001 Sycamore Lane
P.O. Box 369
Danville, IN 46122-1474
Tel: (888) 298 6617 or (317) 745 4715
Website: http://www.sycamoreservices.com

Provides individualized training and services to increase independence.

Westside Special Needs Network
5065 W. 16th St.
Indianapolis, IN 46214
Tel: (317) 241 1563
Contact Name: Beth DeHoff
Email: bdehoff@iquest.net
Website: http://www.speedway-umc.org

Young Adult Social Group
ADEC-YMCA PO Box 398
Bristol, IN 46507
Tel: (574) 294 6197 x 105
Contact Name: Viv Blakeslee
Email: blakesleev@adecinc.com
Website: http://www.adecinc.com

A monthly social group for young adults with ASD ages 16-24.

IOWA

Doctors, Clinics, Hospitals, and Other Health Services

Ankeny Children's Dental
800 E. 1st St. Suite E250
Ankeny, IA 50021
Tel: (515) 963 9600
Email: smile@AnkenyChildrensDental.com
Website: http://www.AnkenyChildrensDental.com

Blank Children's Hospital
1200 Pleasant Street
Des Moines, IA 50309
Tel: (515) 241-KIDS
Website: http://www.unitypoint.org/blankchildrens/about-us.aspx

Center for Disabilities and Development
100 Hawkins Drive
Iowa City, IA 52242-1011
Tel: (800) 686 0031
Contact Name: Barbara Thomas
Email: barbara-thomas@uiowa.edu
Website: http://www.uihealthcare.com/cdd

A part of University of Iowa Children's Hospital.

Mental Health Associates
2212 Pierce Street Suite 100
Sioux City, IA 51104
Tel: (712) 255 8323
Contact Name: Scott Cox
Website: http://www.mentalhealthassoc.com

Provides psychological and diagnostic testing, as well as therapy.

Mercy Autism Center
250 Mercy Dr.
Dubuque, IA 52003
Tel: (563) 589 9035
Contact Name: Alyson Beytien
Email: beytiena@mercyhealth.com
Website: http://www.mercy-autism.com

Provides diagnosis, treatment and training for individuals with ASD across the lifespan.

Mills County Public Health
PO Box 209
101 Central
Glenwood, IA 51534
Tel: (712) 527 9699
Contact Name: Julie Lynes
Email: juliel@mcph.us

Patricia McGuire MD FAAP
2215 Westdale Dr. SW
Cedar Rapids, IA 52404
Tel: (319) 365 1006
Contact Name: Maureen Thorpe
Email: office_manager@allchildrenarespecial.com
Website: http://www.allchildrenarespecial.com

Board certified developmental and behavioral pediatrician offering ASD diagnostic evaluations. Also services Springtides, Inc., a nonprofit.

Tanager Place Mental Health Clinic
2309 C Street SW
Cedar Rapids, IA 52404
Tel: (319) 286 4545
Contact Name: Amy March
Email: amarch@tanagerplace.org
Website: http://www.tanagerplace.org/

Offers assessment and measurement for many conditions. Offers ABA in its Autism Spectrum Therapy Program as well as in child psychiatry services, play therapy, music therapy, and counseling.

Therapy Services

Autism Services by Annie
3513 SW Edgewood Ln.
Ankeny, IA 50023
Tel: (515) 865 2928
Contact Name: Annie Novak
Email: anniemnovak@gmail.com

Uses ABLLS assessment, ABA, TEACCH, and VB to address communication, social, and functional academic issues of children with ASD.

Central Rehabilitation Ltd.
950 Office Park Road, Suite 100
West Des Moines, IA 50265
Tel: (515) 224 0979
Toll Free: (800) 357 3422
Contact Name: Brent Cooper, PT
Email: CR84@att.net
Website: http://www.centralrehabilitation.com

Provides physical, occupational and speech therapy, including in-home therapy.

ChildServe
5406 Merle Hay Road
Johnston, IA 50131
Tel: (515) 727 8750
Contact Name: Stacy Carmichael, PhD
Email: stacyca@childserve.org
Website: http://www.childserve.org

Provides diagnostic treatment for ASD, behavior therapy, parent training, cognitive-behavioral therapy, social skills training.

Kids in Harmony, LLC
Des Moines, IA 50310
Tel: (515) 494 4618
Contact Name: Shelly Peterson
Email: mtinharmony@hotmail.com

Provides in-home music therapy services to individuals having special needs as well as adaptive music lessons.

Kristen Henry, Early Autism Behavior Consultant
Sioux City, IA
Contact Name: Kristen Henry
Email: m.k.henry@me.com
Website: http://sites.google.com/site/kristenhenryaba

For children with ASD, addresses behavior and teaches communication, socialization, self-care, and motor schools. Also teaches parents skills to address behaviors.

KMK Consulting, Inc.
5021 Blackhawk Trail
Bettendorf, IA 52722
Tel: (773) 677 4925
Contact Name: Kathryn Kunkel
Email: Akkunkel@hotmail.com

BCBA/SLP providing in-home ABA.

Mercy Riverside Rehab
730 E. 2nd Street
Des Moines, IA 50309
Tel: (515) 643 9800
Website: http://www.mercydesmoines.org

Provides physical, occupational, and speech therapy for infants to adolescents.

Metro West Kids Learning Center
2555 Berkshire Pkwy Suite B
Clive, IA 50325
Tel: (515) 987 8835
Contact Name: Toni Merfeld
Email: toni@metrowestkids.net
Website: http://www.metrowestkids.net

Metro West provides social language groups for high-functioning autism/Asperger's children ages 4-young adult as well as speech and occupational therapy.

Paws & Effect Service Dogs
Box 41442
Des Moines, IA 50311
Tel: (515) 326 4190
Contact Name: Nicole Shumate
Email: nicoleshumate@yahoo.com
Website: http://paws-effect.blogspot.com

Raises, trains, and places service dogs with children and veterans with disabilities.

Speech Rescue
Des Moines, IA 50131
Tel: (515) 276 1474
Contact Name: Melanie Crabb
Email: melanie@speechrescue.com
Website: http://www.speechrescue.com

Provides speech and language therapy as well as ABA and Sensory Integration.

Talk to Me Technologies
323 West 2nd Street
Cedar Falls, IA 50613
Tel: (319) 266 1900
Contact Name: Matthew Dunning
Email: matt@talktometechnologies.com
Website: http://www.talktometechnologies.com

Specializes in augmentative and alternative communication including consultation and evaluation.

West Music - Music Therapy Services
1212 5th Street
Coralville, IA 52241
Tel: (319) 351 2000
Toll Free: (800)-397-9378
Email: musictherapyservices@westmusic.com
Website: http://musictherapy.westmusic.com

Provides 1:1 and group music therapy (both in-office and in-home) as well as recreational music performing groups and adapted lessons.

Schools and Educational Services

Kirkwood Community College Focused Skill Training Program (FST)
6301 Kirkwood Blvd. SW Cedar Hall 2023
Cedar Rapids, IA 52404
Tel: (319) 398 5454
Contact Name: Barbara Mussman, Disabilities Services Director
Email: barb.mussman@kirkwood.edu
Website: http://www.kirkwood.edu/site/index.php?p=31077

Provides educational coaches to enrolled students with HFA or Aspergers Syndrome to work individually to provide academic support and social skills training.

LearningRx
4949 Westown Parkway
West Des Moines, IA 50266
Tel: (515) 964 4142
Contact Name: Maria Stines
Email: maria@learningrx.net
Website: http://www.learningrx.com/west-des-moines/default.htm

St. Ambrose University's Children's Campus
St. Ambrose University
1301 Lombard Street
Davenport, IA 52803
Tel: (563) 333 6000 or (563) 324 2312
Contact Name: Debra Bowson
Email: childrenscampus@sau.edu
Website: http://www.sau.edu/ChildrensCampus.html

Provides an early childhood program for children age 6 weeks to 6 years, with or without disabilities.

University of Iowa REACH Program
The University of Iowa College of Education Lindquist Center
Iowa City, IA 52242
Tel: (319) 384 2127
Contact Name: Dr. Jo Hendrickson
Email: reach@uiowa.edu
Website: http://www.education.uiowa.edu/reach

REACH, a two-year certificate program, offers a living-learning experience integrating into the University of Iowa collegiate experience while gaining a career-focused education.

Legal, Government & Financial Services

Department of Housing and Urban Development
210 Walnut St. Room 239
Des Moines, IA 50309
Tel: (515) 284 4512
Contact Name: Steve Eggleston
Email: IA_Webmanager@hud.gov
Website: http://www.hud.gov/local/index.cfm?state=ia&topic=offices

Mental Health and Disability Services
1305 E. Walnut Street, 5th Floor SE
Des Moines, Iowa 50319-0114
Email: contactdhs@dhs.state.ia.us
Website: http://www.dhs.state.ia.us/mhdd/index.html

MHDS is responsible for planning, coordinating, monitoring, improving and partially funding mental health and disability services.

Vocational Rehabilitation Services
510 E. 12th Street
Des Moines, IA 50319
Tel: (515) 281 4211
Website: http://www.ivrs.iowa.gov/

Community and Recreation Services

Adventures in Social Drama
Des Moines, IA 50310
Tel: (515) 306 0030
Contact Name: Annie Mielke
Email: annie.mielke@asdrama.org
Website: http://www.asdrama.org

Offers a variety of drama classes and programs for individuals with ASD of all ages.

Camp Albrecht Acres
PO Box 50
Sherrill, IA 52073
Tel: (563) 552 1771
Email: info@albrechtacres.org
Website: http://www.albrechtacres.org

Camp Courageous of Iowa
12007 190th Street
PO Box 418
Monticello, IA 52310-0418
Tel: (319) 465 5916
Email: info@campcourageous.org
Website: http://www.campcourageous.org

A year-round respite care and recreational facility for individuals of all ages with disabilities.

Cedar Valley Community Support Services
3121 Brockway Rd.
Waterloo, IA 50701
Tel: (319) 233 1288
Email: info@cvcss.com
Website: http://www.cvcss.com

Champions of Autism & ADHD
2035 Kimball Avenue
Waterloo, IA 50701
Tel: (319) 296 5156 or (319) 233 0380
Contact Name: Dr. Peggy Wainwright
Email: educationalvisions@yahoo.com
Website: http://www.autismchamps.org

Provides resources to families, caregivers, educators, and the community.

Developmental Services of Iowa
535 W Broadway Suite 202
Council Bluffs, IA 51503
Tel: (712) 314 3811 or (866) 511 1386
Email: administrator@dsiowa.com
Website: http://www.dsiowa.com

ECHO PLUS INC
1808 Jackson Avenue PO BOX AF
Spirit Lake, IA 51336
Tel: (712) 336 4052 or (712) 362 2192
Contact Name: Amanda Brewer
Email: abrewer@echoplusinc.com
Website: http://www.echoplusinc.com

ECHO PLUS provides residential services, job training, and job placement to individuals with disabilities in Emmet and Dickinson Counties.

Glenwood Resource Center
711 S. Vine
Glenwood, IA 51534

Tel: (712) 525 1215
Contact Name: Diana Hoogestraat
Email: dhooges@dhs.state.ia.us
https://dhs.iowa.gov/mhds/disability-services/resource-centers/glenwood

GRASP Support Group Southeastern Iowa
Iowa City, IA 52240
Tel: (319) 337 2052
Contact Name: Judy Thayer
Website: http://grasp.org/page/grasp-support-group-southeastern-ia

GRASP is a support group for adults on the Asperger Spectrum.

Hills & Dales
1011 Davis St.
Dubuque, IA 52001
Tel: (563) 556 7878
Contact Name: Casey Leist
Email: cleist@hillsdales.org
Website: http://www.hillsdales.org

The Homestead
8272 NE University Ave
Pleasant Hill, IA 50327
Tel: (515) 957 3371
Contact Name: Evelyn Horton
Email: ehorton@thehomestead.org
Website: http://www.thehomestead.org

Horizons - A Family Service Alliance
819 5th St. SE
Cedar Rapids, IA 52401
Tel: (319) 398 3943
Contact Name: Jennifer Becker, LMHC
Email: jbecker@horizonsfamily.org
Website: http://www.horizonsfamily.org

Horizons Unlimited
3826 460th Ave.
P.O. Box 567
Emmetsburg, IA 50536
Tel: (712) 852 2211
Email: ronaskland@horizons-unlimited.net
Website: http://www.horizons-unlimited.net/

Offers programs including residential, vocational, community employment and day habilitation services.

Iowa Developmental Disability Council Youth Advisory Board
3826 1/2 Douglas Avenue
Des Moines, IA 50310
Tel: (515) 243 4292
Contact Name: Amy Croll
Email: amy@cyconcepts.org

Website: http://www.cyconcepts.org

An opportunity for students with developmental disabilities to engage and to propose ideas to the Iowa Developmental Disabilities Council.

Iowa Family Support Network
Visiting Nurse Services of Iowa
1111 9th St. Suite 320
Des Moines, IA 50314
Tel: (515) 558 9986
Website: http://www.iafamilysupportnetwork.org/

Provides care and resources to families and professionals working with newborns, toddlers, and preschools, and access to community- and group-based services.

Iowa Federation of Families for Children's Mental Health
106 South Booth
Anamosa, IA 52205
Tel: (319) 462 2187
Contact Name: Lori Reynolds
Email: lori@iffcmh.org
Website: http://iffcmh.org

The Larrabee Center
201 E. Bremer Ave. PO Box 155
Waverly, IA 50677
Tel: (319) 352 2234
Email: larrabee@larrabeecenter.org
Website: http://www.larrabeecenter.org

New Choices
2501 18th Street
Bettendorf, IA 52722
Tel: (563) 210 4775
Contact Name: Joe York
Email: jyork@newchoicesinc.com
Website: http://newchoicesinc.com

Optimae Life Services
301 W. Burlington
Fairfield, IA 52556
Tel: (888) 472 1684
Website: http://www.optimaelifeservices.com/optimae-lifeservices/

Optimae provides a variety of employment and educational services.

Regional Autism Assistance Program (RAP)
100 Hawkins Drive #247 CDD
Iowa City, IA 52242
Tel: (866) 219 9119 x 2
Email: Iowa-RAP@uiowa.edu
Website: http://www.chsciowa.org/regional-autism-assistance-program.asp

The Regional Autism Assistance Program (RAP) connects individuals and families suspecting or diagnosed with ASD to ASD resources.

Siouxland Autism Support Group
Sioux City, IA
Email: josh@siouxlandautism.org
Website: http://www.siouxlandautism.org

Serves the Siouxland area in Iowa, Nebraska, and South Dakota.

An all-volunteer organization providing information and support for individuals and families.

Special Kids Special Love
2445 19th St SW po box 1703
Mason City, IA 50401
Tel: (641) 732 5470 or (641) 460 1061
Contact Name: Lacey Carpenter and Vicki Ries
Email: specialkidsspeciallove6@gmail.com
Website: http://www.specialkidsspeciallove.org

Special Kids Special Love is an Autism support group located in Mason City, Iowa, providing families support, tools, and resources.

Spirit Taekwondo
2100 SE 5th Street Pioneer Columbus Community Center
Des Moines, IA 50135
Tel: (515) 202 5289 or (515) 202 5287
Contact Name: Mark Ratekin
Email: info@iowaspirittkd.com
Website: http://www.iowaspirittkd.com

Systems Unlimited
Various Locations
Tel: (319) 337 7326
Email: info@sui.org
Website: http://www.sui.org

KANSAS

Doctors, Clinics, Hospitals, and Other Health Services

Allergy Link, PA Jeremy Baptist, MD PhD
6806 West 83rd Street
Overland Park, KS 66207
Tel: (913) 469 4043
Website: www.allergy-link.com

Treatments for complex medical issues, treating not only symptoms but also causes.

ARH Psychiatric Center
102 Medical Center Drive
Hazard, KS 41701
Tel: (606) 439 1331
Website: http://www.arh.org/our_services/all_services/behavioral_health/inpatient_behavioral_health/hazard.aspx

Children's Mercy
5808 W 110th 5520 College Boulevard
Overland Park, KS 66211
Tel: (913) 696 8000
Website: http://www.childrensmercy.org

Cynthia McMillin, RN, MSN, ARNP
8911 E. Orme, Suite A
Wichita, KS 67207
Tel: (316) 686 7884
Contact Name: Cynthia McMillin, RN, MSN, ARNP
Email: cindy_lee_arnp@yahoo.com

Kansas Center for Autism Research and Training
12600 Quivira Rd. 270 Regnier Hall
Overland Park, KS 66213
Tel: (913) 897 8471
Email: kcart@ku.edu
Website: http://www.kcart.ku.edu

Kansas Neurological Institute
3107 W. 21st Street
Topeka, KS 66604
Tel: (785) 296 5389
Email: rpd@kni.ks.gov
Website: http://srskansas.org/kni

Tish Holub Taylor, Ph.D.
11100 Ash, Suite 202
Leawood, KS 66211
Tel: (913) 738 4177
Email: drtish@tishtaylor.com
Website: http://www.tishtaylor.com

Diagnostic evaluations, behavior management, and individual counseling.

University of Kansas Behavioral Pediatrics
3901 Rainbow Boulevard
Kansas City, KS 66160
Tel: (913) 588 6323
Website: http://www2.kumc.edu/kids/specialty_behavioral.htm

Vision Therapy KC
10875 Grandview Dr., Ste. 2260
Overland Park, KS 66210
Tel: (913) 469 8686
Contact Name: Caroline Metzger

Email: caroline@visiontherapykc.com
Website: http://www.visiontherapykc.com

Therapy Services

Adventure Music Therapy
8227 Renner Rd. #1
Lenexa, KS 66219
Tel: (913) 991 8620
Contact Name: Meredith Ibarra
Email: mibarra1980@gmail.com

Allies in Therapy
8000 Lee Blvd.
Leawood, KS 66206
Tel: (913) 406 3952
Contact Name: Tracy Hadel
Email: thadel@comcast.net
Website: http://www.tracyhadel.com

ASAP Expert Counseling
PO Box 12723
Overland Park, KS 66212
Tel: (913) 952 6696
Contact Name: Teresa Berry
Email: referrals@asapexpertcounseling.com
Website: http://www.asapexpertcounseling.com

Autism Concepts Incorporated (ACI) Learning Centers
6394 College Blvd.
Overland Park, KS 66211
Tel: (913) 663 4100
Toll Free: (800) 345 0448
Contact Name: Nancy Champlin, BCBA
Email: Autism@concepts.com
Website: http://www.acilearningcenters.com

Provides ABA with an emphasis on verbal behavior, for children with ASD and other developmental disabilities.

Autism From the Start
15621 West 87th Street Pkwy Suite 272
Lenexa, KS 66219
Tel: (913).608.7435
Email: care@autismfromthestart.com
Website: http://autismfromthestart.com/

Provides services to toddler through school-aged children in-home, in school, and in the community.

Children's Therapy Group
7620 Metcalf Avenue, Suite M
Overland Park, KS 66204
Tel: (913) 383 9014
Email: ctg@childrenstherapygroup.org
Website: http://www.childrenstherapygroup.org

Programs and services for children from infancy to adolescence.

Empowering Function, LLC
15316 Lowell Avenue
Overland Park, KS 66223
Tel: (913) 961 6819
Contact Name: Christy Hill, MS, OTR/L
Email: christy@empoweringfunction.com
Website: http://www.empoweringfunction.com

Occupational Therapy Practice serving children of all ages.

Exceptional Learners Behavioral Services, LLC
Olathe, KS 66063
Tel: (720) 331 1419
Contact Name: Hillary Ran
Email: ExceptionalLearners@yahoo.com
Website: http://www.ExceptionalLearners.com

Providing in-home assessment, training, consultation and direct implementation of ABA.

Family Consultation Services (FCS) Counseling
560 N. Exposition Street
Wichita, KS 67203
Tel: (316) 352 3267 or (855) 261 2255
Contact Name: Marcy L. Caldwell, LCPC, CAS, Clinical Supervisor
Email: MCaldwell@emberhope.org
Website: http://www.fcscounseling.com

Integrated Behavioral Technologies
304 West
Tonganoxie, KS 66086
Tel: (913) 417 7061
Website: http://www.ibt-inc.org

Kansas City Autism Training Center (KCATC)
4805 W 67th St.
Prairie Village, KS 66208
Tel: (913) 432 5454 or (913) 787 3275
Email: dir.kcatc@yahoo.com
Website: http://www.kcatc.net

KidsTLC
620 South Rogers Road
Olathe, KS 66062
Tel: (913) 324 3628 or (913) 764 2887
Contact Name: Laci Maltbie
Email: lmaltbie@kidstlc.org
Website: http://www.kidstlc.org

A collaborative program for children ages 18 months to 12 years with ASD and other developmental disabilities providing individualized student programming, including ABA.

Little Steps
Edna A. Hill Child Development Center
1000 Sunnyside
University of Kansas
Lawrence, KS 66045
Tel: (785) 864 0502
Email: educare@ku.edu
Website: http://cdc.ku.edu/little-steps

An Early Intervention Program providing individualized learning opportunities to children with developmental disabilities.

Midwest Therapy
PO BOX 4047
Olathe, KS 66063
Tel: (913) 709 9752
Contact Name: Allison Carter
Email: allison@mymidwesttherapy.com
Website: http://www.mymidwesttherapy.com

Pediatric occupational therapy, in-home services provided in Johnson County Kansas and some surrounding areas, specializing in sensory processing, feeding/eating skills, fine motor skills, adaptive/self-help skills.

Noriko Nakamura, MT-BC
Olathe, KS 66051
Tel: (913) 744 1265
Contact Name: Noriko Nakamura, MT-BC
Email: ksmomusictherapy@gmail.com
Website: http://www.ksmomusictherapy.com

Offers individual/group music therapy sessions, adaptive music lessons (piano, guitar, ukulele), and music activities.

No Stone Unturned Therapeutic Learning Center
1133 College Ave. A213
Manhattan, KS 66502
Tel: (785) 587 1825 or (785) 317 0760
Contact Name: Christiana Schadegg
Email: christiana@mathispt.com
Website: http://www.nostoneunturnedtlc.com

Offers occupational therapy, speech therapy, physical therapy, and ABA.

Playabilities for Sensational Kids, LLC
Center for Child and Family Development
4817 W 117th St.
Leawood, KS 64113
Tel: (913) 515 3531
Contact Name: Kelly Reardon, MOTR/L
Email: Kelly@playabilities.org
Website: http://www.playabilities.org

Provides individualized OT services to children within the home, community, or clinic setting, including sensory processing intervention, behavioral intervention and therapeutic play groups including yoga.

Therapeutic Living Solutions
14188 W. 150th Court
Olathe, KS 66062
Tel: (913) 829 7775
Contact Name: Christine Glover
Email: therapists@therapeuticlivingsolutions.com
Website: http://www.therapeuticlivingsolutions.com

Trumpet Behavioral Health
119 Delaware St.
Leavenworth, KS 66048
Tel: (816) 802 6969
Contact Name: Ashley Burkhead
Email: aburkhead@tbh.com
Website: http://www.tbh.com

Provides ABA-based treatment.

Schools and Educational Services

Accelerated Schools of Overland Park
10713 Barkley
Overland Park, KS 66211
Tel: (913) 341 6666
Contact Name: Jane Curran
Email: Jane@acceleratedschoolsop.org
Website: http://www.AcceleratedSchoolsOP.org

Offers full day school with individualized academic programs for students in grades 4 through 12 with ASD and other challenges.

Horizon Academy
4901 Reinhardt Drive
Roeland Park, KS 66205
Tel: (913) 789 9443
Contact Name: Sharyl Kennedy
Email: info@horizon-academy.com
Website: http://www.horizon-academy.org

A private, fully accredited school specializing in serving children with learning disabilities.

Legal, Government & Financial Services

Department for Aging and Disability Services
Behavioral Health Services
915 SW Harrison Docking State Office Building, 9th Floor
Topeka, KS 66612
Tel: (785) 296 3471 or (785) 296 6142
Email: Angela.Hagen@kdads.ks.gov
Website: http://www.kdads.ks.gov/

Disability Rights Center of Kansas
635 SW Harrison, Suite 100
Topeka, KS 66603
Tel: (785) 273 9661
Toll Free: (877) 776 1541
Website: http://www.drckansas.org

A public interest legal advocacy agency advocating for the civil and legal rights of Kansans with disabilities.

Kansas Rehabilitation Services Commission
915 SW Harrison 9th Floor North
Topeka, KS 66612
Tel: (785) 368 8034
Contact Name: Michael Donnelly
Email: rehabilitation.services@srs.ks.gov
Website: http://www.srs.ks.gov/agency/rs/Pages/default.aspx

Scott Wasserman & Associates, LLC
8889 Bourgade
Lenexa, KS 66219
Tel: (913) 438 4636
Contact Name: Scott Wasserman
Email: Scott@yourchild1st.com
Website: http://www.yourchild1st.com

Providing legal services including special education, juvenile law, foster care, custody, and other areas.

Community and Recreation Services

A New Day at Home
Overland Park, KS
Tel: (913) 440 0204
Contact Name: Kimberly Grant
Email: kgrant@anewdayathome.com
Website: http://www.anewdayathome.com

Respite services for families & children with ASD.

Accessible Arts
1100 State Avenue
Kansas City, KS 66102
Tel: (913) 281 1133
Email: accarts@accessiblearts.org
Website: http://www.accessiblearts.org

Asperger Parent Support Group of Topeka
2701 SW Randolph Avenue
Topeka, KS 66611
Tel: (785) 608 2438
Email: aarc_parents@sbcglobal.net

Autism Society of the Heartland
P.O. Box 860984
Shawnee, KS 66286-0984
Tel: (913) 706 0042

Email: Info@ASAHeartland.org
Website: http://www.asaheartland.org

Bethesda Lutheran Communities
14150 113th St
Shawnee Mission, KS 66215
Tel: (913) 906 5000
Contact Name: Mark Trivilino
Email: mark.trivilino@mailblc.org
Website: http://www.bethesdalutherancommunities.org

Community Living Opportunities (CLO)
11627 W. 79th St.
P.O. Box 14395
Lenexa, KS 66285-4395
Tel: (913) 341 9316
Contact Name: Yolanda Hargett
Email: yolandahargett@clokansas.org
Website: http://www.clokansas.org

Provides a full range of services for children and adults with ASD, as well as their families.

Cottonwood, Inc.
2801 W. 31st Street
Lawrence, KS 66047
Tel: (785) 842 0550
Contact Name: Pennie Dubisar-Cross
Email: pdubisarcross@cwood.org
Website: http://www.cwood.org

CLO's Midnight Farm
2084 - B N. 600 Road
Baldwin City, KS 66006
Tel: (785) 979 1889
Contact Name: Yolanda Hargett
Email: yolandahargett@clokansas.org
Website: http://www.midnight-farm.org

Provides rural living, work, therapeutic and recreation opportunities for children and adults with special needs including NARHA therapeutic horseback riding; day service classes, supported employment and special events; day camps; and field trips for special education classes.

Debbie Howard's Gym
655 N Somerset Terr.
Olathe, KS 66062
Tel: (913) 829 3006
Contact Name: Debbie Howard
Email: debbie@debbiehowardsgym.com
Website: http://www.debbiehowardsgym.com

Opportunities for gym time for children with special needs.

The Dream Works
21 N. 12th Street Suite 470
Kansas City, KS 66102
Tel: (913) 281 8695
Email: tdw@thedeamworksinc.com
Website: http://www.thedreamworksinc.com

Social service agency serving Kansas and Missouri and a licensed home health provider.

Easter Seals Capper Foundation
3500 SW 10th Avenue
Topeka, KS 66604-1995
Tel: (785) 272 4060
Contact Name: Linda Burgen
Email: lburgen@capper.easterseals.com
Website: http://www.capper.easterseals.com

Families Together, Inc.
3033 W 2nd St. Suite 106
Wichita, KS 67203
Tel: (316) 945 7747
Toll Free: (888) 815 6364
Email: Wichita@familiestogetherinc.org
Website: http://www.familiestogetherinc.org

Families Together, Inc. is a parent training and information center serving families of children and youth with all disabilities from birth through 21 years old.

Heartspring
8700 E. 29th Street North
Wichita, KS 67226
Tel: (316) 634 8700
Toll Free: (800) 835 1043
Website: http://www.heartspring.org

Heartstrings Community Foundation
7096 W. 105th Street
Overland Park, KS 66212
Tel: (913) 649 5700
Email: info@heartstringscf.org
Website: http://www.heartstringscf.org

Hutchinson Autism Support Group
Hutchinson Public Library
901 North Main
Hutchinson, KS 67501
Tel: (620) 728 0989
Contact Name: Janice Bonham
Email: hutchinsonautism@yahoo.com
Website: http://hutchinsonautismsupportgroup.webs.com

KEYS for Networking
211 West 33rd Street
Topeka, KS 66611
Tel: (785) 233 8732
Toll Free: (800) 499 8732
Website: http://www.keys.org

Provides information, support, and training to families in Kansas whose children who have educational, emotional, and/or behavioral problems.

Lakemary Center
100 Lakemary Drive
Paola, KS 66071
Tel: (913) 557 4000
Contact Name: William Craig
Website: http://www.lakemaryctr.org

Lawrence Autism Society
Lawrence Public Library
Lawrence, KS 66049
Tel: (785) 842 4737
Contact Name: Maria Brockman
Email: lawrenceautismsociety@yahoo.com

The Mission Project
8820 Endsley Ln.
Leawood, KS 66206
Tel: (913) 530 1390
Email: info@themissionproject.org
Website: http://themissionproject.org

Multi Community Diversified Services, Inc.
2107 Industrial Dr.
McPherson, KS 67460
Tel: (620) 241 6693
Email: info@mcds-ks.org
Website: http://www.mcds-ks.org

Parents Sitting for Parents
Kansas City, KS
Contact Name: JasonRadford
Email: JasonRadford2@yahoo.com
Website: http://groups.yahoo.com/group/PS4P-KC

Networking and support group for parents of children with ASD in the Kansas City metro area to support each other with the special needs/struggles they have in finding suitable babysitting.

Rainbows United
340 S. Broadway
Wichita, KS 67202
Tel: (316) 267 KIDS (5437)
Website: http://www.rui.org

Provides community resources and customized services.

Skills to Succeed
413 E Santa Fe St.
Olathe, KS 66061

Tel: (913) 254 0001
Email: info@theskillstosucceed.org
Website: http://www.theskillstosucceed.org

Provides a variety of services to individuals with ASD throughout the lifespan, including teen groups and adult services to support community participation.

Sunflower Supports
3601 SW 29th Street Suite 134
Topeka, KS 66614
Tel: (785) 273 1493 or (785) 273 1195
Email: kathyd@sunflowersupports.kscoxmail.com

Provides residential day services and case management for adults with developmental disabilities.

T Lift
Tel: (785) 312 7054
Email: info@lawrencetransit.org
Website: http://www.lawrencetransit.org/pages/ada-services

T Lift is a door-to-door, shared ride paratransit service for qualified disabled riders.

TARC
2701 SW Randolph Avenue
Topeka, KS 66611-1536
Tel: (785) 232 0597
Contact Name: Mary Ann Keating
Website: http://www.tarcinc.org

Three Rivers
P.O. Box 4152
Topeka, KS 66604
Tel: (785) 273 0249
Toll Free: (800) 555 3994
Website: http://www.threeriversinc.org

Provides education, advocacy, training, and support.

Twin Valley Developmental Services
427 Commerical
Greenleaf, KS 66943
Tel: (800) 748 7416
Website: http://www.twinvalleythriftshop.com

Provides job and life coaching, assisted care, and friendship.

Wichita Paratransit
214 S. Topeka
Wichita, KS 67202
Tel: (316) 337 9476
Website: http://www.wichitatransit.org/Special/Pages/ParatransitGuide.aspx

Wichita Transit's Paratransit Service provides CURB-TO-CURB, SHARED RIDE, accessible van service to qualified disabled riders.

KENTUCKY

Doctors, Clinics, Hospitals, and Other Health Services

Bluegrass Autism Services
PO Box 1673
Danville, KY 40423
Tel: Tel: (859) 516 2360
Email: info@bluegrassautism.com
Website: http://bluegrassautism.com

Provides behavioral analytic services for children and young adults with ASD and other developmental disabilities. Specializes in assessment and consultation for individualized ABA programs, including the Lovaas Method and Verbal Behavior Approach.

Jerry Kartzinel, MD
Kartzinel Wellness Center
13100 Magisterial Drive
Louisville, KY 40223
Tel: (502) 631 1900
Website: www.drjerryk.com

Dr. Kartzinel is a board-certified pediatrician practicing Translational Medicine (translating diverse scientific findings into treatments for patients).

Regional Child Development Clinics
Hart County
1600 Scottsville Road, Suite 100
Bowling Green, KY 42104
Tel: (270) 843 9294
Toll Free: (866) WE-R-RCDC (937-7232)
Email: regionalchilddev@bellsouth.net
Website: http://www.hartcounty.ky.gov/Services/Health/Pages/Regional-Child-Development-Clinics.aspx

Provides diagnostic evaluations and assessments as well as transdisciplinary services, including occupational therapy, speech therapy, physical therapy, behavioral management, and psychological services.

Rockcastle Regional Hospital and Respiratory Care Center
145 Newcomb Avenue
PO Box 1310
Mt. Vernon, Kentucky 40456
Tel: Tel: (606) 256 2195
Website: http://www.rockcastleregional.org

University of Kentucky Pediatric Developmental Disabilities Clinic
Second Floor, Wing D
740 S. Limestone
Lexington, KY 40536
Tel: (859) 323 6211

Contact Name: Phyllis Kirkpatric
Website: http://www.ukhealthcare.uky.edu

Vicco Dental Center, PSC
35 Longfield Circle
Scuddy, KY 41760
Tel: (606) 476 8121
Email: viccodentalcenter@yahoo.com

Therapy Services

Associates in Pediatric Therapy
1900 Midland Trail Suite 1 & 2
Shelbyville, KY 40065
Tel: (502) 633 1007
Contact Name: Jeanne Burnett
Email: kidtherapy@hotmail.com
Website: http://www.kidtherapy.org

A therapeutic clinic practice providing services for children with special needs in Metro Louisville, Lexington and Southern IN.

Bloom Behavior Therapy LLC
333 Broadway Street, Suite 501
Paducah, KY 42001
Tel: (270) 908 0462
Contact Name: Becky Nastally
Email: info@bloombehavior.com
Website: http://www.bloombehavior.com

Specializing in autism intervention (including ABA therapy), school consulting for Western Kentucky.

Bright Start Early Intervention
Henderson, KY 42419
Tel: (270) 860 9594
Contact Name:
Caitlin Conley
Email: brightstartei@gmail.com
Website: http://www.brightstartei.com

Services include consultation, assessment, and development of treatment plans, developmental therapy, and parent/caregiver/teacher workshops and therapy may be provided in-home, school, daycare, or elsewhere.

Cardinal Hill Rehabilitation Hospital
2050 Versailles Road
Lexington, KY 40504
Tel: (859) 254 5701 or (859) 367 7127
Toll Free: (800) 233 3260
Website: http://www.cardinalhill.org

Central Kentucky Riding For Hope
PO Box 13155
Lexington, KY 40583
Tel: (859) 231 7066

Website: http://www.ckrh.org
Equine assisted activities and therapies.

Diocesan Catholic Children's Home
75 Orphanage Road
PO BOX 17007
Fort Mitchell, KY 41017
Tel: (859) 331 2040
Contact Name: Jon Ross
Email: jross@dcchome.org
Website: http://www.dcchome.org

Diocesan Catholic Children's Home is a treatment center for children, ages 6 to 14, who have moderate to severe emotional and/or behavioral problems.

Four Rivers Behavioral Health
425 Broadway
Paducah, KY 42001
Tel: (270) 442 7121 or (270) 442 1452
Website: http://www.4rbh.org

Growing Minds Learning Center
Therapy
1040 Market Street
Henderson, KY 42420
Tel: (270) 827-GMLC(4652)
Email: info@growingmindslearningcenter.com
Website: http://www.growingmindslearningcenter.com

Highlands Center Autism
Therapy – ABA
5080 KY Rt. 321
Prestonburg, KY 41653
Tel: (606) 889 6115
Contact Name: Shelli Deskins
Email: sdeskins@hrmc.org
Website: http://www.highlandsautism.org

Home of the Innocents
1100 East Market Street
Louisville, KY 40206
Tel: (502) 596 1000 or (502) 596 1237
Website: http://www.homeoftheinnocents.org

Provides in-home and in-school support services for children with ASD.

Kaleidoscope, Inc.
10330 Bunsen Way
Louisville, KY 40299
Tel: (502) 495 1662
Contact Name: Tracy Ruth
Email: tracy@kaleidoscopeservices.org
Website: http://www.kaleidoscopeservices.org

Therapeutic structured activities and nursing services.

Kids Can Do Pediatric Therapy Center
440 Whirl-A-Way Drive, Suite 1
Danville, KY 40422
Tel: (859) 239 6670
Website: http://www.emhealth.org/index.php/locations/
kids-can-do-pediatric-therapy-center

Provides speech, occupational, and physical therapy for children from birth-21 years.

Kentuckiana Children's Center
1810 Brownsboro Road
Louisville, KY 40206
Tel: (502) 366 5658 or (502) 366 3090
Website: http://www.kentuckiana.org

The Luci Center
575 Moody Pike
Shelbyville, KY 40065
Tel: (502) 220 4308
Email: info@thelucicenter.org
Website: http://www.thelucicenter.org

PROVIDES therapeutic riding and hippotherapy for individuals with disabilities.

Marshall Pediatric Therapy
105 Windhaven Drive, Suite 1
Nicholasville, KY 40356
Tel: (859) 224 2273
Contact Name: Pam Marshall, OTR/L, Founder/Owner
Website: http://www.mptcares.com

Murray State University Speech and Hearing Clinic
Speech Therapy
125 Alexander Hall
Murray, KY 42071
Tel: (270) 809 2446

Music Therapy Services of Central Kentucky
1 Sperti Drive
Rineyville, KY 40162
Tel: (270) 862 9747
Contact Name: Lorinda Jones
Email: losnotes@infoline.net
Website: http://www.lorindajones.com

New Beginnings Therapy Services, LLC
Therapy
524 MacRander Drive
Berea, Kentucky 40403
Tel: (859) 626 2107
Email: creatingnewbeginnings@gmail.com
Website: http://www.newbeginningstherapyservices.com

New Perceptions
1 Sperti Drive
Edgewood, KY 41017

Tel: (859) 344 9322
Email: contact@newperceptions.org
Website: http://www.newperceptions.org

On the Move Pediatric Therapy
2520 Regency Road, Suite 150
Lexington, KY 40503
Tel: (859) 224 0834
Contact Name: Ashley Godsey
Email: agodsey@onthemovepeds.com
Website: http://www.onthemovepeds.com

Pawsibilities Unleashed
Jeff Town Plaza
1410 Versailles Road
Frankfort, KY 40601
Tel: (888) 759 4920
Contact Name: Tracey Hagan
Email: info@pawsibilitiesunleashed.org

VOLUNTEER dog/handler teams travel throughout Kentucky with therapy dogs. Also provides assistance dogs to people with ASD and other challenges.

Phoenix Preferred Care
PO Box 2
Somerset, KY 42502
Tel: (606) 451 9379
Contact Name: Sandy Coyler
Email: coylerclan@peoplepc.com
Website: http://www.phoenixpreferredcare.com

A private behavioral health agency providing outpatient services to individuals in the Lake Cumberland region.

Regional Child Development Clinics
Hart County
1600 Scottsville Road, Suite 100
Bowling Green, KY 42104
Tel: (270) 843 9294
Toll Free: (866) WE-R-RCDC (937-7232)
Email: regionalchilddev@bellsouth.net
Website: http://www.hartcounty.ky.gov/Services/Health/
Pages/Regional-Child-Development-Clinics.aspx

Provides diagnostic evaluations and assessments as well as transdisciplinary services, including occupational therapy, speech therapy, physical therapy, behavioral management, and psychological services.

Renshaw Early Childhood Center
Western Kentucky University
1906 College Heights Blvd.
Bowling Green, KY 42101

Rider Up Therapeutic Riding Center
1341 West Hwy 1376
East Bernstadt, KY 40729

Tel: (606) 657 0460
Contact Name: Jane Riddle
Email: jane@riderup.org
Website: http://www.riderup.org

A therapeutic horseback riding center.

Square One Specialists in Child & Adolescent Development
6440 Dutchmans Parkway
Louisville, KY 40205
Tel: (502) 896 2606
Contact Name: Melissa Guidry
Email: mguidry@squareonemd.com
Website: http://www.squareonemd.com

University of Louisville Autism Center at Kosair Charities
1405 East Burnett Street
Louisville, KY 40217
Tel: (502) 588-ULAC
Email: ulautism@louisville.edu
Website: http://www.louisville.edu/autism

Verbal Behavior Consulting
1035 Strader Avenue, Suite 125
Lexington, KY 40502
Tel: (859) 899 9201
Website: http://www.verbalbehaviorconsulting.com

Offers client-based behavioral solutions and specializes in treatment for children with ASD and other developmental disabilities based on ABA and VB principles.

Wee Can Autism and Behavioral Consulting, LLC
211 Geri Lane
Richmond, KY 40475
Tel: (606) 416 9220
Website: http://www.weecanabc.com

Wendell Foster's Campus for Developmental Disabilities
815 Triplett Street
PO Box 1668
Owensboro, KY 42303
Tel: (270) 683 4517
Email: info@wfcampus.org
Website: http://www.wfcampus.org

Schools and Educational Services

Carriage House Educational Services and Preschool
13101 Eastpoint Park Blvd.
Louisville, KY 40223
Tel: (502) 253 1293
Contact Name: Mary Horvath, M.Ed.
Website: http://www.carraigehouseps.org

Friends School
901 Breckenridge Lane
Louisville, KY 40207
Tel: (502) 899 1822
Website: http://www.friendsschoollouisville.org

A nonprofit, nonsectarian, family cooperative school for children ages 12 months to 2nd grade.

Kelly Autism Program
Suzanne Vital Clinical Education Complex
Western Kentucky University
WKU 104 Alumni Avenue
Bowling Green, KY 42101
Tel: (270) 745 4527
Email: kellyautismprogram@wku.edu
Website: http://www.wku.edu/kellyautismprogram

Provides services to individuals from the age of seven through adulthood with ASD and includes elementary school, middle school, high school and post-secondary participants including higher education, vocational training, and job support.

Pitt Academy
6010 Preston Highway
Louisville, KY 40219
Tel: (502) 966 6979
Website: http://www.pitt.com

Silver Circles, Inc.
Bardstown, KY
Tel: (502) 348 7551
Contact Name: Catherine Crouse Barnes
Email: silvercirclesinc@gmail.com
Website: http://www.silvercirclesinc.com/

Provides intervention to students from age 2 to adult. with individualized programs including the Irlen Method, Interactive Metronome Therapy, and reading, writing and math programs. They also offer psychological and educational evaluations and sensory profiles.

Summit Academy
11508 Main Street
Louisville, KY 40243
Tel: (502) 244 7090
Tel: (502) 244 8311
Website: http://www.summit-academy.org

Legal, Government & Financial Services

Council on Developmental Disabilities
1151 So. Fourth Street
Louisville, KY 40202
Tel: (502) 584 1239

Email: info@councilondd.com
Website: http://www.councilondd.com

Kentucky Protection and Advocacy
100 Fair Oaks Lane
Frankfort, KY 40601
Tel: (502) 564 2967
Website: http://www.kypa.net

Meinhart Smith & Manning, PLLC
222 E. Witherspoon St. Suite 401
Louisville, KY 40202
Tel: (502) 589 2700
Contact Name: Ethan Manning
Email: ethan@bluegrassjustice.com
Website: http://www.bluegrassjustice.com

Truesdell Law Office
PO Box 1301
Richmond, KY 40475
Tel: (859) 623 6892
Email: truesdelllaw@yahoo.com

Services include Special Needs Trusts, Wills and Estate Planning.

Community and Recreation Services

The Arc of Kentucky
706 E. Main St. Suite A
Frankfort, KY 40601
Tel: (502) 875 5225
Email: arcofky@aol.com
Website: http://www.arcofky.org/

Adanta Group
259 Parkers Mill Rd.
Somerset, KY 42501
Tel: (606) 679 4782
Email: dburdine@adanta.org
Website: http://www.adanta.org

BAWAC
7970 Kentucky Drive
Florence, KY 41042
Tel: (859) 371 4410
Email: info@BAWAC.org
Website: http://www.BAWAC.org

Cedar Lake Lodge
3301 Jericho Road
LaGrange, KY 40031
Tel: (502) 222 7157
Contact Name: Marie Fitzmaurice
Email: mfitzmaurice@cedarlake.org
Website: http://www.cedarlake.org

An adult day health program, provides a person-centered, structured environment for individuals with intellectual and physical disabilities.

Center for Accessible Living
501 S. 2nd Street, Suite 200
Louisville, KY 40202
Tel: (502) 589 6620
Website: http://www.calky.org
More locations in Northern Kentucky and Murray, KY

Dreams With Wings
1579 Bardstown Road
Louisville, KY 40205
Tel: (502) 459 4647
Website: http://dreamswithwings.org

FEAT of Louisville
Families for Effective Autism Treatment
1100 E Market Street
Louisville, KY 40206
Tel: (502) 596 1258

Kamp Kessa
Cedar Fire Farm
758 Beechridge Road
Frankfort, KY 40601
Tel: (502) 747 8041
Website: http://www.cedarfire.net

Lexington Parks and Recreation
545 N. Upper Street
Lexington, KY 40508
Tel: (859) 288 2928
Contact Name: Anessa Snowden
Website: http://www.lexingtonky.gov/index.aspx?page=252

Therapeutic Recreation (TR) programs provide opportunities for persons with disabilities to enjoy activities through recreation, leisure and play.

New Perceptions
1 Sperti Drive
Edgewood, KY 41017
Tel: (859) 344 9322
Email: contact@newperceptions.org
Website: http://www.newperceptions.org

Parents of Adult Autistic Children of Louisville
Louisville, KY 40217
Tel: (502) 214 0592
Contact Name: Elizabeth Stoica
Email: elizabethstoica@ymail.com
Website: http://www.paaclou.com

Parents of Adult Autistic Children of Louisville (PAA-CLou) is a support group for parents and caregivers of autistic adults living in the Louisville and southern Indiana area.

The Point ARC of Northern Kentucky
104 West Pike Street
Covington, KY 41011
Tel: (859) 491 9191
Email: thepoint@thepointarc.org
Website: http://www.thepointarc.org

Special Olympics Kentucky
105 Lakeview Court
Frankfort, KY 40601
Tel: (502) 695 8222
Toll Free: (800) 633 7403
Email: soky@soky.org
Website: http://www.soky.org

Taekwondo for Autistic Children
8140 Dream Street
Florence, KY 41042
Tel: (859) 409 6978 or (859) 781 0995
Contact Name: Dawn Geyer
Email: autism4familiesoutreach@yahoo.com
Website: http://www.tristateata.com

Two Rivers Buddy Ball
3531 Lewis Lane
Owensboro, KY 42301
Tel: (270) 315 9925
Website: http://www.tworiversbuddyball.com

Two Rivers Buddy Ball is a non-profit sports league for individuals ages 5-20 with any disability.

The Hopkins County Family YMCA – Special Needs Swim Instruction
Hopkins County Family YMCA
150 YMCA Drive
Madisonville, Kentucky 42431
Tel: (270) 821 9622
Contact Name: Whitney Johnson
Email: hcymca4@madisonville.com
Website: http://www.hopkinscountyymca.com

YMCA of Central Kentucky – Special Needs Swim Instruction
Beaumont Centre Family YMCA
3251 Beaumont Centre Circle
Lexington, KY 40513
Tel: (859) 219 9622
Contact Name: Kelly Smotherman, Aquatics Director
Email: ksmotherman@ymkacky.org
Website: http://www.ymcacky.org/main/swim

Communicare, Inc.
107 Cranes Roost Court
Elizabethtown, KY 42701
Tel: (270) 765 2605
Website: http://www.communicare.org

Communicare provides a broad spectrum of services aimed to support individuals with developmental disabilities and intellectual disabilities to remain and become a vital part of their communities.

Homeplace Support Service, LLC
1310 Hunstonville Road
Danville, KY 40422
Tel: (859) 936 2010
Contact Name: Ann Skinner
Email: ann.skinner@homeplaceky.com
Website: http://www.homeplacesupportservices.com

Independent Opportunities
400 South Main Street, Suite 200
London, KY 40741
Tel: (606) 877 9209
Contact Name: Wayne Harvey
Email: wharvey@indopp.com
Website: http://www.independentopportunities.com

LOUISIANA

Doctors, Clinics, Hospitals, and Other Health Services

Associates in Pediatric Dentistry (AIPD)
9000 Airline Hwy Suite 100
Baton Rouge, LA 70815
Tel: (225) 924 6622
Website: http://www.aipdbr.com

Children's Center at LSUHSC Shreveport
1450 Claiborne Avenue School of Allied Health Professions
Shreveport, LA 71103
Tel: (318) 813 2960
Contact Name: Nan Massey, MOT, LOTR, Intake Coordinator
Email: nmasse@lsuhsc.edu
Website: http://www.medcom.lsuhscshreveport.edu/alliedhealth

Offers children up to age 21 assistance, assessment, and evaluation services for ASD and other disabilities using a team approach, including speech-language pathology, psychology, marriage and family therapy, occupational therapy, academics, pediatrics, and social work.

Children's Hospital
200 Henry Clay Avenue
New Orleans, LA 70118
Tel: (504) 899 9511
Website: http://www.chnola.org

Dr. Katherine Vo
704 Main Street
Madisonville, LA 70447
Tel: (985) 845 3211
Contact Email: Admin@childrensdentalcottage.com
Website: http://www.childrensdentalcottage.com

Pediatric Dentistry, specializing in treating those with special needs including ASD.

Laurie H. Olson, Ph.D.
3350 Ridgelake Drive Suite 274
Metairie, LA 70002
Tel: (504) 400 9218
Email: lolsonphd@gmail.com
Website: http://www.lolsonphd.com

Louisiana Autism Center
100 Gayven Drive
Ball, LA 71405
Tel: (318) 641 3083 or (318) 641 0444
Contact Name: Shawndrika Anderson
Email: sapsyphd@gmail.com
Website: http://www.louisianaautismcenter.com

Ochsner Child Development Center
Ochsner for Children 1315 Jefferson Hwy.
New Orleans, LA 70118
Tel: (504) 842 3900
Contact Name: Sylvia Williams

Ochsner Child Development Center provides comprehensive medical evaluation and treatment recommendations for children with ASD, including ADOS, developmental testing, genetics, neurology, OT, speech.

Our Lady of the Lake Regional Medical Center
5000 Hennessy Blvd
Baton Rouge, LA 70808
Tel: (225) 765 6565
Website: http://www.ololrmc.com

Smile Stars Pediatric Dentistry
10522 S Glenstone Pl
Baton Rouge, LA 70810
Tel: (225) 769 5377
Email: smilestars@bellsouth.net
Website: http://www.smilestars.com

Tulane Medical Center (TMC)
1415 Tulane Avenue
New Orleans, LA 70112

Tel: (504) 988 5263
Website: http://www.tulanehealthcare.com

Uptown Pediatric Dentistry, Stephen C Holmes, DDS
3715 Prytania St Suite 380
New Orleans, LA 70115
Tel: (504) 896 7435
Contact Name: Stephen Holmes, DDS
Email: schdds@me.com
Website: http://www.uptownpediatricdentistry.com

Therapy Services

Behavioral Intervention Group (BIG)
8180 Siegen Ln.
Baton Rouge, LA 70810
Tel: (225) 757 8002
Email: admin@big-br.com
Website: http://www.big-br.com

Provides applied behavior analysis and verbal behavior services to families and schools with preschool-aged children diagnosed with autism or other developmental disabilities.

Center for Pediatric Therapy (CPT)
220 Civic Center Blvd.
Houma, LA 70360
Tel: (985) 228 0726 or (985) 449 0944
Contact Name: Michele Bower, PT, PCS
Email: michele@therapyforpeds.com
Website: http://www.therapyforpeds.com

The Center for Pediatric Therapy offers individual and group therapy for children from birth to adolescence.

Creating New Connections, LLC
3401 Canal Blvd.
New Orleans, LA 70119
Tel: (504) 231 8981
Contact Name: Christine Tilley, MSEd, BCBA, Owner
Email: Christine@creatingnewconnections.com
Website: http://www.creatingnewconnections.com

Provides ABA and group social skills classes.

Horses of Hope Equine Therapy Program
6860 Bayou Paul Road
St Gabrielle, LA 70776
Contact Name: Rebecca Bombet
Email: rebombet@gmail.com
Website: http://www.rebeccabombet.com

Equine assisted psychotherapy.

Louisiana Autism Center
100 Gayven Drive
Ball, LA 71405
Tel: (318) 641 3083 or (318) 641 0444

Contact Name: Shawndrika Anderson
Email: sapsyphd@gmail.com
Website: http://www.louisianaautismcenter.com

Providing a full range of diagnostic and treatment services including psychological/developmental evaluations, ABA, social skills training, medication management, and parent training/education.

Louisiana State University Health Sciences Center, Communication Disorders Department
1900 Gravier, 9th floor,
New Orleans, LA 70112
Tel: (504) 568 4344 or (504) 568 6520
Contact Name: Meher Banajee
Email: mbanaj@lsuhsc.edu

Speech language therapy services, augmentative and alternative communication services and auditory processing services.

McMains Children's Developmental Center (MCDC)
1805 College Drive
Baton Rouge, LA 70808
Tel: (225) 923 3420
Website: http://www.mcmainscdc.org

Social Services; Psychological Services; Physical Therapy; Occupational Therapy; Speech and Language Therapy; Assistive Technology Assessment; Educational Therapy; and other services.

McNeese Autism Program
Department of Psychology, McNeese State University
4205 Ryan St.
Lake Charles, LA 70605
Tel: (337) 562 4246
Contact Name: Alfred Tuminello, Jr., M.A., B.C.B.A., L.B.A.
Email: MAP@McNeese.edu
Website: http://www.mcneese.edu/autism

The McNeese Autism Program provides comprehensive treatment services for children with ASD and other developmental and behavioral difficulties, including diagnostic testing, intensive early interventions, problematic behavior clinics, social skills groups, language training, pediatric feeding interventions, and family training.

The Missing Piece, Inc.
318 E. Elizabeth St.
Sulphur, LA 70663
Tel: (337) 436 6488
Contact Name: Scott Williamson, BCBA, Director of ABA Services
Email: scott@autismswla.org
Website: http://www.autismswla.org

The Missing Piece is a non-profit ABA clinic.

Sensational Kids Occupational Therapy, LLC
4517 Lorino St.
New Orleans, LA 70006
Tel: (504) 723 2502
Contact Name: Heather Teske
Email: Sensationalkidsot@yahoo.com
Website: http://www.
sensationalkidsoccupationaltherapy.com

Within Reach - Center for Autism
3313 Jurgens St.
Metairie, LA 70002
Tel: (504) 231 6447
Contact Name: Emily Bellaci
Email: Emily@WithinReachNOLA.com
Website: http://www.WithinReachNOLA.com

Within Reach provides Applied Behavior Analysis (ABA) services to individuals with ASD or other developmental disabilities.

Schools and Educational Services

The Chartwell Center
4239 Camp Street
New Orleans, LA 70115
Tel: (504) 899 2478
Email: chartwell@chartwellcenter.org
Website: http://www.thechartwellcenter.org

Serves children with ASD and related disorders age 3 to 21, and offers training and technical support to parents, teachers and other professionals.

The Creative Learning Center of Louisiana
New Orleans, LA 70178-4136
Tel: (504) 975 7961
Contact Name: Sheila Ealey
Email: sheilaealey@yahoo.com

Serving children full day ages 4 to 13.

Greater Baton Rouge Hope Academy
15333 Old Jefferson Hwy.
Baton Rouge, LA 70817
Tel: (225) 293 0141
Website: http://www.hopeacademybr.org

Legal, Government & Financial Services

Louisiana Rehabilitation Services (LRS)
Louisiana Workforce Commission
Baton Rouge, LA 91297
Tel: (225) 219 2225
Toll Free: (800) 737 2958
Contact Name: Mark Martin, Director

Email: mmartin@lwc.la.gov
Website: http://www.laworks.net/WorkforceDev/LRS/LRS_Main.asp

Community and Recreation Services

Ascension Parish Autism Support Group
Ascension Parish Autism Support Group
15297 Stone Hedge Drive
Prairieville, LA 70769
Tel: (225) 622 0323
Contact Name: Sandra Trammell
Email: ascensionparishautism@gmail.com

Autism Answers of Louisiana
1206 JW Davis Drive Suite 105
Hammond, LA 70403
Tel: (985) 549 0836
Contact Name: Jolene Barlow
Email: info@autismanswersofla.org
Website: http://autismanswersla.org/

Autism Services of Southwest Louisiana
3006 Common St.
Lake Charles, LA 70601
Tel: (337) 436 5001
Tel: (866) 603 2273
Email: directcare@bellsouth.net
Website: http://www.autismserviceswla.com/index.html

Autism Society-Louisiana State Chapter, Inc.
P.O. Box 80162
Baton Rouge, LA 70898
Toll Free: (800) 955 3760
Contact Name: Pat Giamanco
Email: autismsociety_lastatechapter@yahoo.com
Website: http://www.lastateautism.org

Camp Tiger
Camp Tiger
LSUHSC Foundation Office of Alumni Affairs
Shreveport, LA 71130
Contact Name: Lindsey Kobetz, Director
Email: lkobet@lsuhsc.edu
Website: http://www.lsumedshv.com/

Evergreen Presbyterian Ministries, Inc.
920 Main St.
Pineville, LA 71360
Tel: (318) 445 4470
Contact Name: Kathy Blackman, Executive Director
Contact Email: kblackman@epmi.org
Website: http://www.epmi.org

Families Helping Families (FHF) of Greater Baton Rouge, Inc.
2356 Drusilla Ln.
Baton Rouge, LA 70809
Tel: (225) 216 7474
Toll Free: (866) 216 7474
Website: http://www.fhfgbr.org

Hand in Hand Autism Services, Inc.
Fort Polk, LA 71459
Tel: (210) 620 6034
Contact Name: Katherine Connor
Email: katherineconnor@handinhandautismservices.com
Website: http://www.handinhandautismservices.com
Facebook: http://www.facebook.com/handinhandautismservices

Louisiana Center for Excellence in Autism
1900 Gravier Room 1035
New Orleans, Louisiana 70112
Tel: (504) 556 7585
Website: http://www.hdc.lsuhsc.edu

Program for Successful Employment
Bossier Parish Community College (BPCC)
6220 E Texas St.
Bossier City, LA 71111
Tel: (318) 678 6192
Contact Name: Rebecca Hanberry, Program Director

Resource Center for Autism Spectrum Disorders (RCASD)
2356 Drusilla Lane
Baton Rouge, LA 70809
Tel: (225) 236 3053
Toll Free: (877) 711 5382
Contact Name: Sandra Trammell
Email: strammell@fhfgbr.org
Website: http://www.rcasd.org

St. Tammany East Autism Network Group
St. Tammany East Autism Network Group Slidell, LA 70461
Contact Name: Anne Galiano
Contact Email: agalianonfhf@bellsouth.net
Website: http://www.fhfnorthshore.org

Strengthening Outcomes with Autism Resources (SOAR)
39041 Old Sawmill Rd
Ponchatoula, LA 70454
Tel: (225) 796 SOAR
Contact Name: Sherri Houin
Email: info@soarwithautism.org
Website: http://www.soarwithautism.org

MAINE

Doctors, Clinics, Hospitals, and Other Health Services

Amy Yasko, PhD NHD AMD FAA
Tel: (207) 824 8501
Website: www.dramyyasko.com

An integrative healthcare practice specializing in chronic inflammation, immunological and neurological disorders, including ASD.

The Barbara Bush Children's Hospital at Maine Medical Center
22 Bramhall Street
Portland, ME 04102
Tel: (207) 662 0111
Website: http://www.bbch.org

Edmund Ervin Pediatric Center
Maine General Medical Center
Edmund Ervin Pediatric Center
Seton Campus 30 Chase Avenue
Waterville, ME 4901
Tel: (207) 872 4390 or (207) 872 4294
Website: http://www.mainegeneral.org/body.cfm?id=75

Franklin Memorial Hospital
111 Franklin Health Commons
Farmington, ME 04938
Tel: (207) 778 6031
Toll Free: (800) 398 6031
Website: http://www.fchn.org

Southern Maine Health Care (SMHC) Developmental-Behavioral Pediatrics
3 Shape Drive
Kennebunk, ME 04043
Tel: (207) 467 8930
Contact Name: Donald R. Burgess, MD
Email: drburgess@smhc.org

Southern Maine Pediatric Dentistry
75 John Robert Rd. Suite 10B
South Portland, ME 4106
Tel: (207) 773 3111
Contact Name: Dr. Whitney Wignall
Website: http://www.mainepedo.com

Spring Harbor Hospital-Developmental Disorders Program
123 Andover Road
Westbrook, ME 04092
Tel: (207) 761 6644
Toll Free: (866) 857 6644

Contact Name: Matthew Siegel
Website: http://www.springharbor.org

Sweetser
50 Moody Street
Saco, ME 04072
Toll Free: (800) 434 3000
Email: info@sweetser.org
Website: http://www.sweetser.org

Therapy Services

Applied Behavior Consultants (ABC), Inc.
110 Marginal Way #289
Portland, ME 04101
Tel: (207) 408 2701
Contact Name: Jill Mullin, MA, M.S.Ed., BCBA
Email: jmullin@appliedbehavior.com
Website: http://www.appliedbehaviorconsultants.com

Christopher Aaron Counseling Center
67 Shaker Road
Gray, ME 04039
Tel: (207) 657 7700
Email: info@christopheraaron.org
Website: http://www.christopheraaron.org

Provides individualized Cognitive Behavioral Therapy and other services for adults and children including in-home support for children and families.

Mainely Kidz PT, Inc.
895 Portland Rd
Saco, ME 04072
Tel: (207) 439 5104
Contact Name: Jen Corbeil, Physical Therapist, Founder
Email: jen@mainelykidzpt.com
Website: http://www.mainelykidzpt.com

Providing physical, occupational and speech therapy services.

Merrymeeting Behavioral Health Associates (MBHA)
76 Pleasant Street
Brunswick, ME 04011
Tel: (207) 721 0214
Website: http://www.merrymeetingbha.com

New England Behavioral Solutions
Meadowbrook Plaza US Route 1
York, ME 3909
Tel: (207) 807 5973
Contact Name: Janet Parent
Email: janet@newenglandbehavior.com
Website: http://www.newenglandbehavior.com

Offers social skills groups, behavioral consultation, and ABA programming.

Pediatric Therapy
York Hospital 57 Portland St.
South Berwick, ME 03908
Tel: (207) 384 7260
Website: http://www.yorkhospital.com/services_
pedirehab.cfm

Occupational, physical and speech therapy.

Tri-County Mental Health Services
143 Pottle Rd.
Oxford, ME 04270
Toll Free: (800) 750 7911
Email: info@tcmhs
Website: http://www.tcmhs.org

Schools and Educational Services

Aucocisco School
126 Spurwink Avenue
Cape Elizabeth, ME 04107
Tel: (207) 773 7323
Website: http://www.aucociscoschool.org

Becket Family of Services
395 Waterville Road P.O Box 9
Norridgewock, ME 4957
Tel: (207) 634 3020 or (207) 831 6460
Contact Name: Steve Tuck
Email: sat72@yahoo.com
Website: http://www.becket.org

KidsPeace New England Autism Spectrum Disorder Residential Program
16 KidsPeace Way
Ellsworth, ME 4605
Tel: (800) 992 9543
Contact Name: Chris Sylvester
Email: chris.sylvester@kidspeace.org
Website: http://www.kidspeace.org/uploadedFiles/
Fact_sheets/fact_sheets_2009/022-0087%20M...

The KidsPeace New England Autism Spectrum Disorder (ASD) Program offers a level of care and treatment specialized for children with moderate ASD.

STRIVE U
28 Foden Road
S. Portland, ME 04106
Tel: (207) 774 6278
Email: eberg@pslservices.org
Website: http://www.pslstrive.org/striveu

STRIVE U provides post-secondary education and training to young adults with developmental disabilities in the realms of residential, employment, and community skills.

Legal, Government & Financial Services

Department of Housing and Urban Development
One Merchants Plaza Suite 601
Bangor, ME 04401
Tel: (207) 945 0467
Contact Name:
William D. Burney
Email: ME_webmanager@hud.gov
Website: http://www.hud.gov/local/index.
cfm?state=me&topic=offices

Division of Vocational Rehabilitation
Bureau of Rehabilitation Services, Maine Department of Labor 185 Lancaster St.
Portland, ME 04101
Toll Free: (877) 594 5627
Website: http://www.maine.gov/rehab

Gibbons Stevens Law Office
7 Wallingford Sq. Suite 206
Kittery, ME 03904
Tel: (207) 703 2950
Contact Name: Mary Gibbons Stevens
Email: Mstevens@gibbonsstevens.com
Website: http://www.gibbonsstevens.com

Provides special education advocacy to students and their families in Maine and Massachusetts.

Murray Plumb Murray
75 Pearl Street
Portland, ME 4104
Tel: (207) 773 5651
Website: http://www.mpmlaw.com

Nelson-Reade Law Office, PC
813 Washington Avenue
Portland, ME 04103
Tel: (207) 828 1597
Contact Name: Patricia A. Nelson-Reade, RN, CELA
Email: pnr@pnrelderlaw.com
Website: http://www.pnrelderlaw.com

Provides special needs planning.

Community and Recreation Services

Bath Area Family YMCA - Special Needs Swim Instruction
303 Centre St
Bath, ME 04530
Tel: (207) 443 4112
Contact Name: Diane Hicks, Aquatics Director
Email: diane@bathymca.org
Website: http://www.bathymca.org/html/swim_
programs.html

Downeast Horizons
77 Union St.
Ellsworth, ME 04605
Tel: (207) 667 2400 X18
Toll Free: (855) 894 3599
Contact Name: Anthony Zambrano, Executive Director
Email: info@dehi.org
Website: http://www.dehi.org

Hope Assocation
85 Lincoln Avenue
Rumford, ME 04276
Tell: (207) 364 4561
Website: http://www.hopeassociation.org/index.html

Provides employment services.

Independence Association
Brunswick, ME 04011
Tel: (207) 725 4371
Toll Free: (877) 653 4760
Website: http://www.independenceassociation.org

John F. Murphy Homes, Inc.
800 Center St.
Auburn, ME 04240
Tel: (207) 782 2726
Website: http://www.jfmhomes.org

Katahdin Friends, Inc.
1024 Central St. Suite A
Millinocket, ME 04462
Tel: (207) 723 9466
Website: http://www.kfimaine.org

Maine Autism Alliance
65 Patterson St
Augusta, ME 04330
Tel: (207) 626 3042
Contact Name: Heidi Bowden
Email: maineautism@aol.com
Website: http://www.maineautism.org

The Progress Center
35 Cottage St.
Norway, ME 04268
Tel: (207) 743 8049
Website: http://www.progresscentermaine.org

Spurwink
899 Riverside Street
Portland, ME 04103
Tel: (207) 871 1200
Toll Free: (888) 889 3903
Email: info@spurwink.org
Website: http://www.spurwink.org

Woodfords Family Services
15 Saunders Way
Westbrook, ME 04092
Tel: (207) 878 9663
Contact Name: Paul A. Nau, PhD, BCBA, Executive Director
Email: pnau@woodfords.org
Website: http://www.woodfords.org

MARYLAND

Doctors, Clinics, Hospitals, and Other Health Services

Children's Choice Pediatric Dentistry
8500 Annapolis Rd. Suite 213
New Carrollton, MD 20784
Tel: (301) 731 8510
Email: info@mychildrenschoicedental.com
Website: http://www.mychildrenschoicedental.com

Cross Keys Dental Associates
2 Hamill Rd. South Quadrangle, Suite 266
Baltimore, MD 21210
Tel: (410) 425 8400
Email: info@crosskeysdentalassociates.com
Website: http://www.crosskeysdentalassociates.com

Dentistry of Bethesda
10401 Old Georgetown Road Suite 204
Bethesda, MD 20814
Tel: (301) 530 2700
Contact Name: Barbara Hornstein
Email: hornsteins@aol.com
Website: http://www.dentistryofbethesda.com

Diane Serex-Dougan, O.D., FCOVD
7954 Harford Road
Baltimore, MD 21234
Tel: (443) 629 5459
Email: dr.diane@verizon.net
Website: http://www.drdiane.net

Provides visual evaluations and vision therapy to individuals with ASD and other disabilities.

Ernesto C. Torres, MD
188 Thomas Johnson Dr Suite 202
Frederick, MD 21702
Tel: (301) 662 2252
Website: http://www.ernestotorresmd.com

General pediatric practice.

Heartlight Healing Arts
9145 Guilford Rd. Suite 100
Columbia, MD 21046

Tel: (410) 880 4215
Contact Name: Pamela Compart, President
Website: http://www.heartlighthealingarts.com

Provides traditional and integrative/functional approaches through a multidisciplinary group of practitioners for children, adults, and families.

Howard County Mental Health Authority
9151 Rumsey Road
Columbia, MD 21045
Tel: (410) 313 7350
Email: hcmha@hcmha.org
Website: http://www.hcmha.org/

Kelly Dorfman MS LND
10828 Tuckahoe Way
Gaithersburg, MD 20878
Tel: (301) 340 2239
Email: office@kellydorfman.com
Website: www.kellydorfman.com

Nutritional consultation in person or by phone for children with ASD and others.

Krause Pediatric & Orthodontic Dental Care
560 Riverside Dr Suite A-205
Salisbury, MD 21801
Tel: (410) 742 1688
Email: info@krausesmiles.com
Website: http://www.krausesmiles.com

Towson University Institute for Well-Being
One Olympic Place Room 200
Towson, MD 21204
Tel: (410) 704 7300
Email: hcaa@towson.edu
Website: http://www.towson.edu/iwb

Trevor Valentine, MD, Developmental and Behavioral Pediatrician
University of Maryland Medical Center
22 S Greene St. 5th Floor
Baltimore, MD 21201
Tel: (410) 706 2300

Washington Adventist Hospital
7600 Carroll Avenue
Takoma Park, MD 20912
Tel: (301) 891 5596
Website: http://www.washingtonadventisthospital.com/WAH/

We Make Kids Smile
3460 Old Washington Rd Suite 200
Waldorf, MD 20602
Tel: (301) 645 6556
Contact Name: Mary Ellen, Office Manager

Email: maryellen@wemakekidssmile.net
Website: http://www.wemakekidssmile.net

Pediatric dental office with an emphasis placed on special needs.

Therapy Services

Autism Consultation & Treatment Center
301 West Main Street
Thurmont, MD 21788
Tel: (301) 271 0400
Contact Name: Dr. Ralph McBee
Email: rmcbee@act-center.net
Website: http://www.act-center.net Home Based Services

Provides intensive behavior therapy for children and teens with ASD based on ABA. Individualized services may include discrete trial teaching, Verbal Behavior, and incidental teaching methods.

The Autism Project
North Beach, MD 20714
Tel: (410) 286 8240
Contact Name: Angel Gaither
Email: theautismproject@cs.com
Website: http://www.theautismproject.info

Programs emphasize social skills, communication, recreation/leisure skills, community skills, daily living skills and the generalization of academic skills.

Equine Therapy Associates
Potomac, MD 20859
Tel: (301) 972 7833
Contact Name: Carol Rae Hansen, Ph.D., Director
Email: Director@equinetherapyassociates.com
Website: http://www.equinetherapyassociates.com

A range of specialized equine instruction and therapies.

Fitness for Health
11140 Rockville Pike Suite 303
Rockville, MD 20852
Tel: (301) 231 7138
Email: info@fitnessforhealth.org
Website: http://www.fitnessforhealth.org

Offers therapeutic exercise, OT, and PT.

Freedom Hills Therapeutic Riding Program
Rolling Hills Ranch 33 Rolling Hills Ranch Ln.
Port Deposit, MD 21904
Tel: (410) 378 3817
Email: fhtrp@freedomhills.org
Website: http://www.freedomhills.org

A therapeutic horseback riding program.

ICAN of Washington, Inc.
5100 Acacia Avenue
Bethesda, MD 20814
Tel: (301) 897 0815
Contact Name: Cynthia Onder, MA., CCC-SLP/BCBA
Email: icanofwashington@hotmail.com
Website: http://www.icanofwashington.com

Dually certified Speech Language Pathologists (SLP) and Board Certified Behavior Analysts (BCBA) provide individual therapy as well implementation of ABA programs, including home programs.

Integrated Therapy Services-Developmental Therapy Services (ITS-DTS), Inc.
10605 Concord St. Suite 100
Kensington, MD 20895
Tel: (301) 933 7880
Contact Name: Kaja Weeks
Email: kaja.weeks@gmail.com
Website: http://www.petitemusique.com

Provides a holistic approach for all ages addressing many issues challenging people with ASD, including: fine and gross motor development, sensory processing disorder, self-regulation, sensory modulation dysfunction, handwriting, speech and language, feeding, augmentative communication, and learning needs.

League for People
1111 E. Coldspring Lane
Baltimore, MD 21239
Tel: (410) 323 0500, X376
Email: tjones@leagueforpeople.org
Website: http://www.leagueforpeople.org

Provides independence through a comprehensive continuum of vocational, rehabilitative, educational, medical, wellness and social services.

Mid-Shore Mental Health Systems, Inc.
28578 Mary's Court, Suite 1
Easton, MD 21601
(410) 770 4801
Contact Name: Holly Ireland
Email: hireland@msmhs.org
Website: http://www.msmhs.org/

Millersville Psychological Services
1110 Benfield Rd. Suite H
Millersville, MD 21108
Tel: (443) 562 1462
Contact Name: Larry Iacarino
Website: http://www.millersvillepsych.com

Services include assessments, counseling/therapy, educational consulting, and tutoring.

Potomac Horse Center (PHC), Inc.—Alternative
14211 Quince Orchard Rd.
North Potomac, MD 20854
Tel: (301) 208 0200
Website: http://www.potomachorse.com

Therapeutic horseback riding lessons.

Reginald S. Lourie Center for Infants and Young Children
12301 Academy Way
Rockville, MD 20850
Tel: (301) 984 4444
Website: http://www.louriecenter.org

Focuses on early identification, treatment and prevention of emotional, behavioral and developmental problems in infants and young children.

Sense-Abilities Pediatric Therapy, LLC
1702 Liberty Rd
Sykesville, MD 21784
Tel: (410) 552 4044
Contact Name: Jamie Hecox
Email: info@senseabilitiestherapy.com
Website: http://www.senseabilitiestherapy.com

Therapeutic and Recreation Riding Center (TRRC), Inc.
3750 Shady Lane
Glenwood, MD 21783
Tel: (410) 489 5100
Website: http://www.trrcmd.org

Provides hippotherapy, participating in competition in the Equestrian Special Olympics, and other therapeutic and education interactions with horses.

Treatment and Learning Centers (TLC)
2092 Gaither Road Suite 100
Rockville, MD 20850
Tel: (301) 424 5200 or (301) 424 5200
Contact Name: Julie Bobrow
Email: JBobrow@ttlc.org
Website: http://www.ttlc.org

Schools and Educational Services

The Auburn School
9545 Georgia Avenue
Silver Spring, MD 20910
Tel: (301) 588 8048
Website: http://www.theauburnschool.org

Baltimore Lab School (BLS)
2220 St. Paul St
Baltimore, MD 21218
Tel: (202) 965 6600 or (410) 261 5500

Contact Name: Katherine Schantz, Head of School
Email: fallon@baltimorelabschool.org
Website: http://www.baltimorelabschool.org

Benedictine Programs and Services
The Benedictine School
Ridgely, MD 21660
Tel: (410) 634 2112
Website: http://www.benschool.org

College Living Experience (CLE)
401 N Washington St. Suite 420
Rockville, MD 20850
Toll Free: (800) 486 5058
Contact Name: Ric Kienzle, Program Director
Website: http://www.experiencecle.com

The Frost School
4915 Aspen Hill Road
Rockville, MD 20853
Tel: (301) 933 3451, X129
Contact Name: Claire Cohen, Director
Email: ccohen@frostschool.org
Website: http://www.frostschool.org

The Frost School is a 12-month special education school, located in Rockville, Maryland, that provides educational services to students ages five to 21 with ASD and other related disorders.

The Harbour School
Annapolis, MD 21409
Tel: (410) 974 4248
Contact Name: Vonnie Callaway, Community Affairs Coordinator
Email: vcallaway@harbourschool.org
Website: http://www.harbourschool.org

Individualized education to students in grade 1 through 12 with learning disabilities, autism, speech language impairments, and other disabilities like ADD/ADHD.

High Road School
7707 German Hill Rd.
Baltimore, MD 21222
Tel: (410) 282 8500
Website: http://www.highroadschool.com

High Road School specializes in serving students facing learning, language, and social challenges.

The Ivymount School, Inc.
11614 Seven Locks Road
Rockville, MD 20854
Tel: (301) 469 0223
Contact Name: Lennie Gladstone
Contact Email: lgladstone@ivymount.org
Website: http://www.ivymount.org

Ivymount School is a non-sectarian, non-public special education day school educating and providing therapeutic services to children and young adults, ages 4-21, with special needs.

Janet and Frank Kelly Autism Center
410 E. Jeffrey St
Brooklyn, MD 21225
Tel: (410) 269 7600 or 4102697600
Contact Name: Sarah Davis
Email: daviss@childrensguild.org
Website: http://www.childrensguild.org

Utilizes the TEACCH approach to educate students grades K-12 and incuding an integrated music and arts program, character education, sensory integration, pre-vocational and vocational training, transition services, as well as included psychiatry, speech therapy, occupational therapy, counseling/social skills training.

The Katherine Thomas School
9975 Medical Center Drive
Rockville, MD 20850
Tel: (301) 738 9691, ext 193
Contact Name: Melanie Roberts, Admissions Coordinator
Email: meroberts@ttlc.org
Website: http://www.ttlc.org

For children preschool through twelfth grade with moderate to severe learning and language disabilities and high-functioning autism.

The One World Center for Autism (OWCA), Inc.
1400 Nalley Ter.
Hyattsville, MD 20785
Tel: (301) 618 8395
Website: http://www.worldforautism.info

Legal, Government & Financial Services

Allegany Core Service Agency
PO Box 1745
Cumberland, MD 21501-1745
Tel: (301) 759 5070
Contact Name: Lesa Diehl
Email: ldiehl@dhmh.state.md.us
Website: http://dhmh.maryland.gov/mha/SitePages/csa.aspx

Baltimore Mental Health Systems, Inc.
201 East Baltimore Street
Baltimore, MD 21202
Tel: (410) 837 2647
Contact Name: Jane Plapinger
Email: jplapinger@bmhsi.org
Website: http://www.bmhsi.org/

Division of Rehabilitation Services (DORS)
Maryland State Department of Education 2301
Argonne Dr.
Baltimore, MD 21218
Tel: (410) 554 9442
Toll Free: (888) 554 0334
Email: dors@dors.state.md.us
Website: http://www.dors.state.md.us

Maryland Core Service Agencies

Core Service agencies are responsible for planning, managing, and monitoring public mental health services at the county level. There is a Core Service Agency in every county and in the city of Baltimore.
Website: www.marylandbehavioralhealth.org

Maryland Department of Health and Mental Hygiene
55 Wade Avenue
Catonsville, MD 21228
Tel: (410) 402 8300
Website: http://www.dhmh.maryland.gov/mha

Maryland Developmental Disabilities Administration
MD
Tel: (410) 767 6500
Website: http://www.dhmh.maryland.gov/dda_md/
serv02.htm

Community and Recreation Services

Abilities Network
8503 LaSalle Road
Towson, MD 21286
Tel: (410) 828 7700
Toll Free: (800) 492 2523
Website: http://www.abilitiesnetwork.org

Active Day Center
1430 Joh Ave. Suite A
Baltimore, MD 21227
Tel: (410) 242 0379
Contact Name: Will Rogers, Director
Email: wrogers@activeday.com
Website: http://www.activeday.com

Medical adult day care centers are a preferred alternative to nursing home or institutional care, providing engaging activities, opportunities for socialization and expert health care dedicated to helping our clients improve daily functioning or delay deterioration.

Anne Arundel County Deparment of Recreation and Parks
Annapolis, MD 21401
Tel: (410) 222 7313
Contact Name: Wendy S Scarborough

Email: rpscar88@aacounty.org
Website: http://www.aacounty.org/RecParks

The Arc Baltimore
7212 York Rd.
Baltimore, MD 21212
Tel: (410) 296 2272
Email: info@thearcbaltimore.org
Website: http://www.baltimorearc.org

ArtStream
620 Pershing Dr.
Silver Spring, MD 20910
Tel: (301) 565 4567
Website: http://www.art-stream.org

Provides both individual and group classes as well as performance opportunities for people with ASD and other disabilities.

Autism Society Montgomery County MD
Olney, MD 20832
Tel: (301) 657 0881
Website: www.autismmontgomerycounty.com

Autism Society of Baltimore-Chesapeake
Baltimore, MD 21234
Tel: (410) 655 7933
Email: info@baltimoreautismsociety.org
Website: www.baltimoreautismsociety.org

B'moreAbilities Special Arts Center
B'moreAbilities Special Arts Center Baltimore, MD
Tel: (443) 769 0507
Contact Name: Zoey Robinson-Budreski
Email: bmoreabilities@gmail.com
Website: http://www.basac.org

Community Services for Autistic Adults and Children (CSAAC)
21515 Zion Rd.
Brookeville, MD 20833
Tel: (240) 912 2220
Contact Name: csaac@cscaac.org
Website: http://www.csaac.org

Community Support Services (CSS), Inc.
Gaithersburg, MD 20877
Tel: (301) 926 2300
Email: css@css-md.org
Website: http://www.css-md.org

Dove Pointe
1219 Mt. Hermon Road
Salisbury, MD 21804
Tel: (410) 341 4472

Email: info@dovepointe.com
Website: http://www.dovepointe.com

Elizabeth Cooney Agency
2 Village Square
Baltimore, MD 21210
Tel: (888) 353 1700
Contact Name: Rhonda Workman
Email: rworkman@elizabethcooneyagency.com
Website: http://www.ElizabethCooneyAgency.com

Provides live-in or hourly staff/nurses for after school care, supply 1:1 staff for day or overnight camp, and additional services.

Eric Lamont Cosby Foundation
1121 Annapolis Road
Odenton, MD 21113
Tel: (301) 356 1680
Contact Name: Yolanda Cosby
Email: elcfoundation@netzero.net
Website: http://elcfoundation.com

Services include: educational advocacy support, autism awareness/early intervention outreach, individualized education program (IEP) development/support, training for parents, community organizations and local businesses, parent resources, and sibling support.

The Greenwell Foundation
Greenwell State Park 25420 Rosedale Manor Lane
Hollywood, MD 20636
Tel: (301) 373 9775
Email: info@greenwellfoundation.org
Website: http://www.greenwellfoundation.org

Haven Universe (HU), Inc.
Rockville, MD 20852
Tel: (301) 841 7412
Contact Name: Lynn Poznanski
Email: lpoznanski@havenuniverse.org
Website: http://www.havenuniverse.org

Howard County Autism Society
10280 Old Columbia Rd. Suite 215
Columbia, MD 21046
Tel: (410) 290 3466
Email: info@howard-autism.org
Website: http://www.howard-autism.org

Innovative Piano, Inc.
Salisbury, MD 21801
Tel: (800) 997 7093
Email: contacts@innovativepiano.com
Website: http://www.innovativepiano.com

ABA-style piano lessons for special needs students.

Itineris Baltimore
2201 Old Court Road
Baltimore, MD 21208
Tel: (443) 275 1100
Email: info@itinerisbaltimore.org.
Website: http://www.itinerisbaltimore.org

Itineris has a Day Program and Supported Employment Program for adults 21 and older.

Jewish Social Services Agency (JSSA)
200 Wood Hill Rd.
Rockville, MD 20852
Tel: (301) 838 4200
Website: http://www.jssa.org

Coordinator and provider of a broad range of clinical and social services for individuals and families residing in the greater Washington metropolitan area.

Linwood Center
3421 Martha Bush Drive
Ellicott City, MD 21043
Tel: (410) 465 1352
Email: admin@linwoodcenter.org
Website: http://www.linwoodcenter.org/

Supported employment in integrated settings, vocational training, recreation, volunteerism and community involvement.

Make Studio
Load of Fun Building 120 W North Ave.
Baltimore, MD 21201
Tel: (443) 627 3502
Email: info@make-studio.org
Website: http://www.make-studio.org

Provides multimodal visual arts programming, including sales & exhibition opportunities, to adults with disabilities.

Maryland Community Connection
6490 Landover Road Suite A9
Landover, MD 20785
Tel: (301) 583 0358
Email: info@marylandcommunityconnection.org
Website: http://www.marylandcommunityconnection.org

Specializes in job finding, training, and retention.

Melwood
5606 Dower House Rd.
Upper Marlboro, MD 20772
Tel: (301) 599 8000
Email: services@melwood.org
Website: http://www.melwood.org

Partnership for Extraordinary Minds
Partnership for Extraordinary Minds
16428 Tomahawk Drive
Gaithersburg, MD 20878
Tel: (301) 444 5225
Contact Name: Staci Daddona
Contact Email: sdaddona@xminds.org

Pathfinders for Autism Resource Center
303 International Cir. Suite 110
Hunt Valley, MD 21030
Tel: (443) 330 5370
Email: info@pathfindersforautism.org
Website: http://www.pathfindersforautism.org

P&J's Life Skills
2909 Churchville Rd.
Churchville, MD 21028
Tel: (410) 322 8659 or (410) 838 0412
Contact Name: Jon Williams
Email: pjslifeskills@gmail.com
Website: http://www.pjslifeskills.com

P&J's Lifeskills provides education, life skills training, and social development to individuals with intellectual, developmental, and emotional disabilities through individual and family respite care, Summer Camps, and weekly group events, targeted at bettering lives and reaching potentials.

Totally Active Kids, LLP
121 E Deer Park Dr
Gaithersburg, MD 20877
Tel: (703) 915 9673
Email: gotakgo@gmail.com
Website: http://www.gotakgo.com

YMCA Bethesda-Chevy Chase - Special Needs Swim Instruction
9401 Old Georgetown Rd
Bethesda, MD 20814
Tel: (301) 530 3725
Contact Name: Blaze Zarev
Email: Blaze.Zarev@ymcadc.org
Website: http://www.ymcadc.org/classes.cfm?category=116

MASSACHUSETTS

Doctors, Clinics, Hospitals, and Other Health Services

Active Healing
Sargent L. Goodchild, Jr.
15 Lexington Avenue
Magnolia, MA 01930

Tel: (978) 525 3608
Email: Sarge@ActiveHealing.org
Website: www.activehealing.org

Treatment based on neurological re-organization using repetitive movements to remap neural pathways.

Judith Mabel, RD PhD CLT
55 Pond Avenue #E103
Brookline, MA 02445
Tel: (617) 232 3073
Website: www.nutritionboston.com

Lurie Center for Autism
MassGeneral Hospital for Children
1 Maguire Road
Lexington, MA 02421
Tel: (781) 860 1700
Email: luriecenter@partners.org
Website: http://www.luriecenter.org

Lydian Center For Integrative Healthcare
777 Concord Avenue
Suite 301
Cambridge, MA 02138
Tel: (617) 876 6777
Website: www.lydiancenter.com

Providing a wide range of alternative healthcare and educational modalities, the center can individualize programs for children and adults to promote total body healing.

Mark Hyman, MD
55 Pittsfield Road
Suite 9, Lenox Commons
Lenox, MA 01240
Website: www.ultrawellnesscenter.com

South Shore Children's Dentistry
223 Route 3A Suite 102
Cohasset, MA 02025
Tel: (781) 383 0003
Contact Name: Julie
Email: julie@drgrazioso.com
Website: http://www.drgrazioso.com

Pediatric dental office specializing in treating children and adults with ASD and other developmental disabilities.

Timothy M. Buie, MD
Pediatric Gastroenterology and Nutrition
55 Fruit StreetBoston, MA 02114-2696
Tel: (617) 726 8705
Fax: (617) 724 2710

And

Lurie Center for Autism1 Maguire Road
Lexington, MA 02421-3114
Tel: (781) 860 1700
Fax: (781) 860 1766
Website: www.massgeneral.org/doctors/doctor.
aspx?id=17260

Specializing in gastrointestinal issues, particularly in children with ASD.

UMass Memorial Medical Center
281 Lincoln St.
Worcester, MA 01605
Tel: (508) 334 1000
Website: http://www.umassmemorial.org

The Weaver Center, LLC
30 Boston Post Road
Wayland, MA 01778
Tel: (508) 358 1112
Email: info@weavercenter.org
Website: http://www.weavercenter.org

Evaluates and treats individuals with learning challenges, attention problems, educational and psychological issues. Individualized treatment plans may include neuropsychological testing, educational testing, projective testing, counseling, school advocacy, tutoring, self-advocacy training.

Therapy Services

Amego, Inc.
33 Perry Avenue
Attleboro, MA 02703
Tel: (508) 455 6200
Contact Name: Sandy Varrieur
Email: SVarrieur@AmegoInc.org
Website: http://www.AmegoInc.org

Psychiatrists, BCBAs, and habilitative therapists providing diagnostic evaluations of children suspected to have ASD and providing individualized behavioral/educational services.

Angelfish Therapy
Tel: (203) 545 0024
Fax: (203) 321 2138
Email: Info@AngelfishTherapy.com
Website: www.angelfishtherapy.com

Aquatic therapy, swim lesson and summer camps with many locations in Connecticut, Massachusetts, New York, and New Jersey.

Berkshire Hills Music Academy
48 Woodbridge Street
South Hadley, MA 01075
(413) 540 9720 X202
Contact Name: Kristen Tillona, Director of Admissions and Marketing
Email: ktillona@berkshirehills.org
Website: http://www.berkshirehills.org

Crystal Springs
38 Narrows Rd.
Assonet, MA 02702
Tel: (508) 644 3101
Email: info@crystalspringsinc.org
Website: http://www.crystalspringsinc.org/

Provides individualized programs including educational and/or residential options, direct therapeutic services and medical, clinical and behavioral services.

Seven Hills Foundation
81 Hope Ave
Worcester, MA 01603
(508) 755 2340
Website: http://www.sevenhills.org

Provides clinical, educational, and community-based supports to children and adults with disabilities.

South Shore Mental Health
500 Victory Rd.
Quincy, MA 02130
Tel: (617) 847 1950
Toll: Free: (800) 852 2844
Website: http://www.ssmh.org

Unique Steps Dance Academy
19 North Washington Street
North Attleboro, MA 02760
Tel: (508) 643 3100
Contact Name: Melissa Medeiros
Email: uniquestepsdance@gmail.com
Website: http://www.uniquestepsdance.com

Therapeutic dance program.

Schools and Educational Services

Cardinal Cushing Centers ACHIEVE Transition Program
405 Washington Street
Hanover, MA 02339
Tel: (781) 826 1559
Contact Name: Michelle Markowitz
Email: mmarkowitz@coletta.org

ACHIEVE is 10 month post-secondary program (1 to 4 years) for students, with mild-moderate intellectual disabilities or ASD who have completed secondary school or a similar program.

The Carroll School
Lincoln, MA 01773
Tel: (781) 259 8342
Email: admissions@carrollschool.org
Website: http://www.carrollschool.org

College and Career Access Project (CCAP)
North Shore Community College (NSCC) 1 Ferncroft Rd.
Danvers, MA 01923
Tel: (781) 593 6722, X6696
Contact Name: Lea Hill, Tutor/Counselor
Email: lhill04@northshore.edu

A noncredit vocational education program for young people with intellectual, developmental or learning disabilities.

College Internship Program (CIP) Berkshire
40 Main St. Suite 3
Lee, MA 01238
Tel: (413) 243 2576, X34
Contact Name: Travis McArthur, Admissions Coordinator
Email: tmcarthur@cipberkshire.org
Website: http://www.cipberkshire.org

Eagleton School
446 Monterey Road
Great Barrington, MA 01230
Tel: (443) 768 3071 Maryland Office of Admissions Coordinator or (413) 528 6377
Contact Name: Al Witmer
Email: awitmer@eagletonschool.com
Website: http://www.eagletonschool.com

Eagleton School is a private year-round residential psycho-educational treatment for boys ages 9-22.

Futures School
100 Cummings Center Suite 157J
Beverly, MA 1915
(978) 993 8096
Contact Name: Erin Dunham
Email: edunham@futuresclinic.com
Website: http://www.futuresbtc.com

ABA-based education and support for academic, social, and behavior needs of children ages 3-22.

May Institute
41 Pacella Park Dr.
Randolph, MA 02368
Tel: (781) 440 0400
Website: http://www.mayinstitute.org

Nashoba Learning Group (NLG)
10 Oak Park Drive
Bedford, MA 01730

Tel: (781) 275 2500
Contact Name: Maureen Vibert
Email: info@nashobalearninggroup.org
Website: http://www.nashobalearninggroup.org

Provides individualized education, training, and intervention services for students aged 3-22 with ASD, and also operates an adult program with ongoing job and community support.

The New England Center for Children (NECC)
Southborough, MA 01772
Tel: (508) 481 1015
Website: http://www.necc.org

Project Forward (PF)
Cape Cod Community College (CCCC) 2240 Iyannough Rd.
West Barnstable, MA 02668
Tel: (508) 362 2131, X4763
Website: http://www.capecod.edu/web/projectforward

A vocational training skills program for students with significant learning difficulties.

Riverview School
551 Route 6A
East Sandwich, MA 02537
Tel: (508) 888 0489
Website: http://www.riverviewschool.org

An independent coeducational boarding school for adolescents and young adults with complex language, learning and cognitive disabilities.

The Threshold Program
Lesley University 29 Everett St.
Cambridge, MA 02138
Tel: (617) 349 8181
Toll Free: (800) 999 1959, X8181
Email: threshold@lesley.edu
Website: http://www.lesley.edu/threshold/

Legal, Government & Financial Services

BenePLAN Services
Toll Free: (877) YES WORK
Website: http://www.beneplan.org

The BenePLAN program provides comprehensive benefits assessment, planning, and assistance to SSI and SSDI beneficiaries, their families and service providers.

The Massachusetts Rehabilitation Commission (MRC)
Massachussets Executive Office of Human Services
Suite 600
Boston, MA 02111

Tel: (617) 204 3600
Toll Free : (800) 245 6543
Contact Name: Charles Carr, Commissioner
Email: Commissioner@mrc.state.ma.us
Website: http://www.mass.gov/eohhs/gov/departments/
mrc

Project IMPACT: Individual Members Planning and Assessing Choices Together

MA
Tel: (617) 204 3854
Website: http://www.communityinclusion.org/project.
php?project_id=23

Provides benefit planning, assistance and outreach for persons with disabilities who receive SSI or SSDI and are interested in working or returning to work.

Community and Recreation Services

3LPlace, Inc.

West Somerville, MA 02144
(914) 980 8423
Contact Name: Andrea Albert, Life College Coordinator
Email: aalbert@3LPlace.org
Website: http://www.3LPlace.org

Adaptive Watersports

Nantucket Community Sailing
Nantucket, MA 02554
Tel: (508) 228 5358
Email: info@nantucketcommunitysailing.org
Website: http://www.nantucketcommunitysailing.org

Asperger's Association of New England (AANE)

Norman-Kent Building, 51 Water St. Suite 206
Watertown, MA 02472
Tel: (617) 393 3824
Email: info@aane.org
Website: http://www.aane.org

Autism Services Association (ASA)

47 Walnut Street
Wellesley Hills, MA 02481
Tel: (781) 237 0272
Contact Name: Sheela M. Smith, Assistant Executive Director, COO
Email: sheelaasa@aol.com
Website: http://www.autismservicesassociation.org

Provides community day supports, day habilitation and supported employment opportunities to young adults and adults with ASD.

Autism Support Center (ASC)

6 Southside Road
Danvers, MA 01923

Tel: (978) 777 9135
Contact Name: Susan Gilroy
Email: asc@ne-arc.org
Website: http://www.ne-arcautismsupportcenter.org

BAMSI

10 Christy's Dr
Brockton, MA 02301
Tel: (508) 580 8700
Contact Email: services@bamsi.org
Website: http://www.bamsi.org

Provides services to adults and children with developmental disabilities, mental illness, behavioral health, and public health needs.

Bridgewell

471 Broadway
Lynnfield, MA 01923
Tel: (781) 593 1088
Email: info@bridgewell.org
Website: http://www.bridgewell.org

Brockton Area Arc, Inc.

1250 West Chestnut Street
Brockton, MA 02301
Tel: (508) 583 8030
Website: http://www.brocktonareaarc.org

CapeAbilities

895 Mary Dunn Rd
Hyannis, MA 02601
(508) 778 5040
Contact Name: Larry Thayer
Website: http://www.capeabilities.org

Center for Human Development (CHD)

332 Birnie Ave.
Springfield, MA 01107
(413) 733 6624
Email: chdinfo@chd.org
Website: http://www.chd.org

The Charles River Center

59 E Militia Heights Rd.
Needham, MA 02492
Tel: (781) 972 1022 or (781) 972 1000
Contact Name: John Grugan, President
Website: http://www.charlesrivercenter.org

Provides employment and job training, residential homes, day habilitation, and recreational programs for children and adults with ASD and other developmental disabilities.

Citizens League for Adult Special Services (CLASS), Inc.

48A N Main St.
North Reading, MA 01864

Tel: (978) 276 0765
Website: http://www.classinc.org

Community Connections, Inc.
127 Whites Path
South Yarmouth, MA 02664
Tel: (508) 362 1140
Toll Free: (800) 308 1321
Website: http://www.communityconnectionsinc.org

Courageous Sailing
Boston, MA 02129
Tel: (617) 242 3821
Website: http://www.courageoussailing.org
At inspire learning, personal growth and leadership.

MGH Aspire
1 Maguire Rd.
Lexington, MA 02421
Tel: (781) 860 1900
Email: mghaspire@partners.org
Website: http://www.massgeneral.org/children/aspire

Minute Man Arc
Carter Center 1269 Main St.
Concord, MA 01742
Tel: (978) 287 7900
Contact Name: Eric Boroush, Director of Operations
Email: eboroush@minutemanarc.org
Website: http://www.minutemanarc.org

The Nemasket Group, Inc.
56 Bridge St.
Fairhaven, MA 02719
Tel: (508) 999 4436
Website: http://www.nemasketgroup.org

New England Village
Pembroke, MA 02359
Tel: (781) 293 5461
Website: http://www.newenglandvillage.org
Offers vocational, educational, and recreational opportunities for residents.

Northeast Arc
64 Holten Street
Danvers, MA 01923
Tel: (978) 762 4878
Website: http://www.ne-arc.org

PRIDE, Inc.
3 Maple St.
Taunton, MA 02780
Tel: (508) 823 7134
Website: http://www.pride-inc.org

Specialized Housing, Inc.
Brookline, MA 02446
Tel: (617) 277 1805, X207
Contact Name: Mary Chris Semrow
Email: mcsemrowshi@gmail.com
Website: http://www.specializedhousing.org
Supportive housing opportunities for adults with disabilities in condominiums and apartments in the greater Boston area and elsewhere.

Toward Independent Learning & Living, Inc. (TILL)
20 Eastbrook Rd. Suite 201
Dedham, MA 02026
Tel: (781) 302 4622 or (781) 302 4600
Contact Name: Dafna Krouk-Gordon, President and Founder
Email: dafna@tillinc.org
Website: http://www.tillinc.org
Offers a range of residential, clinical, family support services and day and vocational programs.

Transitions Centers, Inc.
32 Commercial St.
South Yarmouth, MA 02664
Tel: (508) 398 3333
Contact Name: Chris Spaulding, Executive Director
Email: cspaulding@transitionscenters.org
Website: http://www.transitionscenters.org

Yawkey House of Possibilities (HOPe) at Stonehill College
350 Washington Street
Easton, MA 02356
Tel: (508) 205 0555
Email: houseofpossibilities@comcast.net
Website: http://www.houseofpossibilities.org

MICHIGAN

Doctors, Clinics, Hospitals, and Other Health Services

Autism Collaborative Center (ACC)
EMU 1055 Cornell St.
Ypsilanti, MI 48197
Tel: (734) 487 2890
Contact Name: Dr. Pamela Lemerand, College Supports and Educational Services Director
Email: pamela.lemarand@emich.edu
Website: http://www.accemu.org

Behavioral Resources And Institute for Neuropsychological Services (BRAINS)
3351 Eagle Run Dr. Northeast
Grand Rapids, MI 49525

Tel: (616) 365 8920
Contact Name: Ashley Dodger, Receptionist
Email: staff@brainspotential.com
Website: http://www.brainspotential.com

Budaj Chiropractic
5793 W. Maple Rd. Suite 147
West Bloomfield, MI 48322
Tel: (248) 626 0001
Contact Name: Christy Jackson
Email: budajchiropractic@yahoo.com
Website: http://www.drbudaj.com

Grass Lake Medical Center
12337 E Michigan Ave.
Grass Lake, MI 49240
Tel: (517) 522 8403
Website: http://www.grasslakemedicalcenter.com

Offers a wide range of family medical services, including complementary alternatives.

Hamilton Pediatric Dentistry, PC
3299 Clear Vista Ct. Northeast Suite B
Grand Rapids, MI 49525
Tel: (616) 608 6826
Contact Name: Veronica Hamilton
Email: veronica@veronicahamiltondds.com
Website: http://www.veronicahamiltondds.com

Helen DeVos Children's Hospital
100 Michigan St. Northeast
Grand Rapids, MI 49503
Tel: (616) 39- 9000
Email: contactus@helendevoschildrens.org
Website: http://www.helendevoschildrens.org

Lakes Pediatric Dentistry
3101 Union Lake Rd
Commerce, MI 48382
Tel: (248) 360 2555 or (248) 363 2025
Contact Name: Naila Farooq
Email: lakespediatricdentistry@hotmail.com
Website: http://www.lakespd.com

Oakland Family Wellness
1316 Campbell Rd. Suite 149
Royal Oak, MI 48076
Tel: (248) 397 4664
Contact Name: Elijah Silver, ND
Email: elijahsilvernd@gmail.com
Website: http://www.oaklandfamilywellness.com

Naturopathic health counseling for children and adults with ASD.

Therapy Services

Autism Center of Michigan
428 North Center Street
Northville, MI 48167
Tel: (313) 682 9532
Contact Name:
Michael Wiest MS, LLP, MSW, LMSW
Email: mw6428@hotmail.com
Website: http://autismcenterofmichigan.org

Behavior Therapy services for individuals and families with Autism.

Autism Collaborative Center (ACC)
EMU 1055 Cornell St.
Ypsilanti, MI 48197
Tel: (734) 487 2890
Contact Name: Dr. Pamela Lemerand, College Supports and Educational Services Director
Email: pamela.lemarand@emich.edu
Website: http://www.accemu.org

Offers a full range of on-site therapeutic and diagnostic services and other supports.

Autism Connections
Oakland Judson Center
4410 West 13 Mile Road
Royal Oak, MI 48073
Tel: (248) 837 2047
Contact Name: Emily Besecker
Email: emily_besecker@judsoncenter.org
Website: http://www.judsoncenter.org

Services include in-home ABA programs and behavior consultation for children, teens, and adults with ASD.

Bay-Arenac Behavioral Health
201 Mulholland Rd.
Bay City, MI 48708
Tel: (989) 895 2300
Toll Free: (800) 327 4693
Website: http://www.babha.org

Easter Seals Michigan
2399 E Walton Blvd.
Auburn Hills, MI 48326
Tel: (248) 475 6400
Toll Free: (800) 757 3257
Website: http://mi.easterseals.com

Kids In Motion
2636 South Milford United States
Highland, MI 48357
Tel: (248) 684 9610
Contact Name: Steve Bockmann

Email: marketing@kidsinmotionmi.com
Website: http://www.KidsInMotionMI.com

Specializes in physical, occupational, speech and language, aquatic, sensory integration and music therapy services for ages 0-18 years.

Macomb-Oakland Regional Center (MORC), Inc.
1270 Doris Rd.
Auburn Hills, MI 48326
Tel: (248) 276 8000
Toll Free: (866) 754 3398
Website: http://www.morcinc.org

And

16200 19 Mile Rd.
Clinton Township, MI 48038
Tel: (586) 263- 8700
Toll Free: (866) 807 6940

Offers ABA, social skills training, and other services.

Michigan Abilities Center
7286 West Ellsworth Road
Ann Arbor, MI 48103
Tel: (734) 622 9500
Email: MACinfo@MichiganAbillitiesCenter.org
Website: http://www.MichiganAbilitiesCenter.org

Equine-assisted therapies including hippotherapy, therapeutic riding, equine-assisted psychotherapy, equine-assisted learning and other recreational activities.

SunShine Therapy, LLC
214 South Main Street Suites 208 & 209
Ann Arbor, MI 48104
Tel: (734) 646 3149
Email: SunShineTherapy@hotmail.com

Totally Social
South Lyon, MI 48178
Tel: (248) 200 6003
Contact Name: Sabra Evans
Email: totallysocialasd@gmail.com
Website: http://www.totallysocialasd.com

Services include social skills groups, recreational opportunities, 1:1 social tutoring/educational tutoring, legal advocacy and family consultation.

Schools and Educational Services

Ann Arbor Academy
111 E Mosley St.
Ann Arbor, MI 48104
Tel: (734) 747 6641
Email: office@annarboracademy.org
Website: http://www.annarboracademy.org

College preparatory curriculum for children with learning differences.

The Gray Center
100 Pine Street Suite 121
Zeeland, MI 49464
Tel: (616) 748 6030
Email: info@thegraycenter.org
Website: http://www.thegraycenter.org

Services for Students with Disabilities (SSD)
University of Michigan, 505 S State St. Haven Hall, G-664
Ann Arbor, MI 48109
Tel: (734) 763 3000
Contact Email: ssdoffice@umich.edu
Website: http://ssd.umich.edu

Legal, Government & Financial Services

Children's Educational Services and Support (ACCESS)
Jackson, MI 49202
Toll Free: (888) 834 4340
Email: info@accesseducationmi.com
Website: http://www.accesseducationmi.com

Offers special education advocacy services.

Amy R. Tripp, Esq.
2127 Spring Arbor Road
Jackson, MI 49203
Tel: (517) 787 7600
Email: tripp@mielderlaw.com

Michigan Protection and Advocacy Services (MPAS)
129 W Baraga Ave. Suite A
Marquette, MI 49855
Tel: (906) 228 5910
Toll Free: (866) 928 5910
http://www.mpas.org

Community and Recreation Services

4th Wall Theatre Company
MI
Tel: (313) 212 8864
Contact Name: Katie Mann
Email: 4thwallkids@gmail.com
Website: http://www.4thwallkids.com
FB: http://www.facebook.com/4thwallkids

4th Wall Theatre Company is a mobile theatre.

A-Ride
Tel: (734) 973 6500
Email: aatainfo@theride.org
Website: http://www.theride.org/aride.asp

A-Ride is a shared-ride transportation service for qualified disabled individuals.

The Arc of Livingston
1044 Durant Dr. Suite 1
Howell, MI 48843
(517) 546 1228
Contact Name: Patti Nowak, Executive Director
Email: pnowak@arclivingston.org
Website: http://www.arclivingston.org

Autism Spectrum Partners Providing Instruction Recreation and Enrichment (ASPPIRE), Inc.
Holt, MI 48842
Tel: (989) 272 2977
Contact Name: Bob Steinkamp
Email: bsteinkamp@asppireofmidmichigan.com
Website: http://www.asppireofmidmichigan.com

Autism Support Group of Genesee County (ASGGC)
4476 S Dort Hwy.
Burton, MI 48439
Tel: (810) 742 5404
Email: ASGGC@yahoo.com
Website: http://www.geneseeautism.org

Belightful Yoga
Royal Oak, MI 48073
Tel: (248) 761 6815
Contact Name: Lisa Ballo
Email: info@belightfulyoga.com
Website: http://www.belightfulyoga.com
Belightful Yoga is mobile yoga company.

Building Bridges
Oak Park, MI 48237
Tel: (248) 736 0404
Contact Name: Cheryl Wells
Email: buildingbridges4autism@yahoo.com
Provides in-home training to both the clients and their parents/caregivers and educates community service providers.

Damon's H.O.U.S.E. Inc.
Hands of Understanding Socialization Encounters
Damon's H.O.U.S.E. Inc.
11900 E. McNichols
Detroit, MI 48205
Tel: (313) 245 2731
Contact Name: Mrs. Clara Newman
Email: damonhouse@aol.com
Website: http://damonshouse.org

The Guidance Center
13101 Allen Rd.
Southgate, MI 48195
Tel: (734) 785 7700
Website: http://www.guidance-center.org

Homes for Autism
Birmingham, MI 48012
Tel: (586) 477 0493
Email: info@homesforautism.org
Website: http://www.homesforautism.org

Michigan Alliance for Families (MAF)
1325 S. Washington Ave
Lansing, MI 48910
(800) 552 4821
Email: info@michiganallianceforfamilies.org
Website: http://www.michiganallianceforfamilies.org
Provides information, support and education to families of students with disabilities (birth to age 26) who receive special education services.

Michigan APSE
801 Hazen St. PO Box 249
Paw Paw, MI 49079
Tel: (269) 427 6650
Contact Name: Richard Bowser
Email: rbowser@vbcmh.com
Website: http://www.apsemi.org/
An organization dedicated to the growth and expansion of supported employment.

Moka
3391 Merriam St.
Muskegon, MI 49444
Tel: (800) 644 2434
Email: contact@moka.org
Website: http://www.moka.org

Residential Opportunities, Inc.
1100 South Rose Street
Kalamazoo, MI 49001
Tel: (269) 343 3731
Contact Name: Beverly Reed
Email: breed@resopp.org
Website: http://www.residentialopportunities.org

Totally Social
South Lyon, MI 48178
Tel: (248) 200 6003
Contact Name: Sabra Evans
Email: totallysocialasd@gmail.com
Website: http://www.totallysocialasd.com
Totally Social offers supports/services for individuals on the autism spectrum, their families and their community within western Oakland, Livingston and northern Washtenaw counties. Supports offered include tailored seminars focusing on common ASD challenge areas, ASD education & training within home/community.

Direct services include social skills groups, recreational opportunities, 1:1 social tutoring/educational tutoring, legal advocacy and family consultation.

MINNESOTA

Doctors, Clinics, Hospitals, and Other Health Services

Children's Hospitals and Clinics of Minnesota
345 N Smith Ave.
St. Paul, MN 55102
Tel: (651) 220 6000
Website: http://www.childrensmn.org

Counseling Services of Southern Minnesota
1306 Marshall St.
Saint Peter, MN 56082
Tel: (507) 931 8040
Website: http://www.counseling-services.org

Provides psychological testing and evaluations with recommendations for treatment.

The Dental Specialists
12180 Business Park Blvd. North
Champlin, MN 55316
Tel: (952) 926 1065
Contact Name: Tieg Selberg
Email: tselberg@thedentalspecialists.com
Website: http://www.thedentalspecialists.com

Dentistry for Children & Adolescents
Centennial Lakes Medical Center 7373 France Ave. South
Edina, MN 55435
Tel: (952) 831 4400
Email: edina@childrensdent.com
Website: http://www.childrensdent.com

Eagan Child and Family Care
2530 Horizon Dr.
Burnsville, MN 55337
(651) 209 8640
Email: office@eaganchildandfamily.com
Website: http://www.eaganchildandfamily.com

Fraser
2400 W 64th St.
Minneapolis, MN 55423
(612) 861 1688
Email: fraser@fraser.org
Website: http://www.fraser.org

Provides a range of services including early childhood services, autism evaluations and services, mental health services, neuropsychology, and rehabilitation.

Holland Center
10273 Yellow Circle Dr.
Minnetonka, MN 55343
Tel: (952) 401 9359
Fax: (952) 401 9805
Email: info@hollandcenter.com
Website: www.hollandcenter.com

A pediatric habilitation and rehabilitation treatment center for children with ASD offering, among other things: 1:1 ABA/VB programs; OT, ST, biomedical treatments, nutritional treatments, assessments and consultations, and hyperbaric oxygen therapy.

Mayo Eugenio Litta Children's Hospital
1216 2nd St. Southwest
Rochester, MN 55902
Tel: (507) 255 5123
Website: http://www.mayoclinic.org/childrenshospital

Neurodevelopmental Pediatrics
Gillette Children's Specialty Healthcare
200 University Ave. East
St. Paul, MN 55101
Tel: (651) 290 8701
Website: http://www.gillettechildrens.org

Newbridge Clinic
2720 West 43rd Street
Suite 206
Minneapolis, MN 55410
Tel: (612) 730 2237
Website: www.newbridgeclinic.com

Treatment for chronic conditions for all family members, holistic pediatric practice and other care.

Park Nicollet Alexander Center
8455 Flying Cloud Dr.
Eden Prairie, MN 55344
Tel: (952) 993 2498
Website: http://www.parknicollet.com/alexandercenter

RiverView Health
323 S. Minnesota St
Crookston, MN 56716
Tel: (218) 281 9747
Contact Name: Andrea Reynolds
Email: areynolds@riverviewhealth.org
Website: http://riverviewhealth.org

Provides outpatient OT, PT, and Speech-Language therapy to children with ASD. The practice also has family practice physicians and pediatricians.

Rosenberg Center: Assessment and Treatment for Children and Families
1935 County Road B2 West Suite 100
Roseville, MN 55113
Tel: (651) 636 4155
Contact Name: Amy Lesher
Email: Amy.Lesher@rosenbergcenter.com
Website: http://www.rosenbergcenter.com

University of Minnesota Amplatz Children's Hospital
2450 Riverside Ave.
Minneapolis, MN 55455
(612) 365 1000
Website: http://www.uofmchildrenshospital.org

Therapy Services

Center for Speech, Language & Learning
6230 10th St. Suite 220
Oakdale, MN 55128
Tel: (651) 739 2300
Website: http://www.csllinc.com

Primarily a pediatric facility, but also works with adolescents and some adults.

Courage Center
3915 Golden Valley Road
Minneapolis, MN 55422
Tel: (763) 588 0811
Website:http://www.couragecenter.org

Holland Center
10273 Yellow Circle Dr.
Minnetonka, MN 55343
Tel: (952) 401 9359
Website: http://www.hollandcenter.com

Holland is a Pediatric Habilitation & Rehabilitation Treatment Center for children with ASD.

St. David's Center for Child & Family Development
3395 Plymouth Rd.
Minnetonka, MN 55305
(952) 939 0396
Website: http://www.stdavidscenter.org

Provides services in: early intervention; speech, occupational, physical, music, feeding therapy; counseling; social skills training; and in-home and community-based support for children and adults.

West Metro Learning Connections (WMLC), Inc.
5215 Edina Industrial Blvd. Suite 400
Edina, MN 55439
Tel: (952) 322 7922
Website: http://www.wmlc.biz

Schools and Educational Services

Central Lakes College
Central Lakes College Brainerd, MN 56401
Tel: (218) 855 8058
Contact Name: Suresh Tiwari
Email: stiwari@clcmn.edu
http://www.clcmn.edu/disabilityservices

LearningRx Center
7270 Forestview Ln. North Suite 100
Maple Grove, MN 55369
Tel: (763) 746 5850
Website: http://www.learningrx.com

Minnesota Life College (MLC)
7501 Logan Ave. South Suite 2A
Richfield, MN 55423
Tel: (612) 869 4008
Website: http://www.mnlifecollege.org

Saint Paul College: A Technical & Community College
235 Marshall Avenue Office of Enrollment Services, room 1302
Saint Paul, MN 55102
Tel: (651) 846 1547
Contact Name: Caidin Riley
Email: caidin.riley@saintpaul.edu
Website: http://www.saintpaul.edu/CurrentStudents/Pages/DisabilityServices.aspx?Title=U2V...

Legal, Government & Financial Services

Metropolitan Center for Independent Living
1600 University Ave. W. Suite 16
St. Paul, MN 55104
Tel: (651) 646 8342
Website: http://www.mcil-mn.org

Minnesota Department of Human Services: Children's Mental Health Division
PO Box 64985
St. Paul, MN 55164-0985
Tel: (651) 431 2321 or (651) 431 2321
Email: DHS.info@state.mn.us
Website: http://www.dhs.state.mn.us/

Vocational Rehabilitation Services
Department of Employment and Economic Development
St. Paul, MN 55101
Toll Free: (800) 328 9095
Website: http://www.positivelyminnesota.com/JobSeekers/People_with_Disabilities

Community and Recreation Services

Aspergers Network Support (ANSwer)
12930 30th Ave. North
Plymouth, MN 55441
Tel: (763) 227 5059
Email: info@aspergersmn.org
Website: www.aspergersmn.org

The Association of People Supporting Employment First
1940 Garfield St.
Minneapolis, MN 55418
Tel: (612) 789 2063
Contact Name: Steve Piekarski
Email: pike002@msn.com
Website: www.mnapse.org/

Autism Society of Minnesota
2380 Wycliff Street #102
St. Paul, MN 55114
Tel: (651) 647 1083
Email: info@ausm.org
Website: www.ausm.org

Boost! Learning Enrichment Programs, Inc.
1601 E Highway 13 Suite 209
Burnsville, MN 55337
Tel: (952) 807 1081
Email: info@boostlearningenrichment.com
Website: http://www.boostlearningenrichment.com

Dodge Nature Center
365 Marie Ave. West
West St. Paul, MN 55118
Tel: (651) 455 4531
Website: http://www.dodgenaturecenter.org

Erik's Ranch and Retreats
Edina, MN
Tel: (612) 396 7829
Contact Name: Kathryn Nordberg, CEO
Email: Kathryn@eriksranch.org
Website: http://www.eriksranch.org

Foss Swim School®
9455 Garland Lane
Maple Grove, MN 55311
Tel: (763) 416 8993
Website: http://www.fossswimschool.com

Heartstrings Unlimited, Inc.
4742 W 129th St.
Savage, MN 55378
(651) 260 0936
Contact Name: Sara M. Hartgraves, Co-Founder/
Executive Director
Email: sara@heartstringsunlimited.org
Website: http://www.heartstringsunlimited.org

Hope Adult Day Center
4016 Bloomington Ave
Minneapolis, MN 55407
Tel: (612) 822 1720 or (612) 328 4819
Contact Name: Christiana Greene
Email: olufumi@aol.com

In The Company of Kids Creative Arts Center
Colonial Shopping Center 13710 Nicollet Ave.
Burnsville, MN 55337
Tel: (952) 736 3644
Contact Name: Bonnie Kaye, Artistic Director, Teacher,
Autism Education Professional, Consultant
Email: bonnie.companyofkids@yahoo.com
Website: http://www.cokartscenter.com

JK Martial Arts
Groves Academy 3200 Highway 100 South
Minneapolis, MN 55416
United States
See map: Google Maps
Tel: (763) 253 9016 or (612) 703 3348
Contact Name: Joyce Brekke/Katherine Engstrom
Email: sensei@jk-martial-arts.com
Website: http://www.jk-martial-arts.com

Teaches karate customized to learning needs using structured, methodical, and repetitious teaching methods that incorporate auditory, visual, and tactile senses.

Kaposia, Inc.
8100 Wayzata Blvd.
Golden Valley, MN 55426
Tel: (763) 231 3570
Email: hennepinservices@kaposia.com
Website: www.kaposia.com

Offering employment supports.

Lifetrack Resources
2218 Central Ave. Northeast
Minneapolis, MN 55418
Tel: (651) 788 8855
Website: www.lifetrackresources.org

Lifeworks Services, Inc.
2965 Lone Oak Dr. #160
Eagan, MN 55121
Tel: (651) 454 2732
Website: www.lifeworks.org

Merrick, Inc.
3210 Labore Rd.
Vadnais Heights, MN 55110
Tel: (651) 789 6200

Email: info@merrickinc.org
Website: www.merrickinc.org

Provides adult day & memory care, day training & habilitation, and supported employment. Also an approved Ticket to Work Employer Network.

Midwest Special Services, Inc.
900 Ocean St.
St. Paul, MN 55106
Tel: (651) 778 1000
Website: www.mwsservices.org

Provides individualized programs and supports to adults with intellectual and physical disabilities. Offers a range of program components designed to meet employment aspirations and educational, social, and recreational needs as well.

Opportunity Partners
5500 Opportunity Court
Minnetonka, MN 55343
Tel: (952) 938 5511
Email: info@opportunities.org
Website: www.opportunitypartners.org

PAI
4453 White Bear Parkway
White Bear Lake, MN 55110
Tel: (651) 426 2484
Contact Name: Lynn Bradshaw, Director
Email: lbradshaw@paimn.org
Website: www.paimn.org

A day training and habilitation program to serve adults with intellectual/developmental disabilities.

PossAbilities
1803 3rd Ave. Southeast
Rochester, MN 55904
(507) 281 6116
Email: posm@possabilities.org
Website: http://www.possabilities.org

Customized support, employment, life enrichment, retirement, school to work transition, and youth recreation.

Reach for Resources
Eisenhower Community Center,
1001 Highway 7 #235
Hopkins, MN 55305
(952) 988 4177
Website: http://www.reachforresources.org

Provides support and training to individuals and families with cognitive disabilities to maximize their independence, teach them how to use existing resources, and integrate into the community.

St. Croix Trail Blazers
Majestic Pines Farm
Afton, MN 55001
Tel: (651) 353 5125 or (651)-230-2581
Email: stcroixtrailblazers@yahoo.com
Website: http://www.stcroixtrailblazers.org

A Minnesota Special Olympics and Adapted Equestrian Team.

True Friends
10509 108th St. Northwest
Annandale, MN 55302
Tel: (952) 852 0101
Toll Free: (800) 450 8376
Email: info@truefriends.org
Website: http://www.truefriends.org

Offers resident camps, day camps, respite services, therapeutic riding, and much more at five sites.

Upstream Arts, Inc.
3501 Chicago Ave South
Minneapolis, MN 55407
Tel: (612) 331 4584
Contact Name: Julie Guidry, Executive Director
Email: julie@upstreamarts.org
Website: http://www.upstreamarts.org

Fosters creative communication and social independence through the power of arts education.

West Central Industries (WCI)
900 Highway 15 South
Hutchinson, MN 55340
Tel: (320) 234 7515
Website: http://www.westcentralindustries.com

Provides employment training and placement assistance in West Central Minnesota.

MISSISSIPPI

Doctors, Clinics, Hospitals, and Other Health Services

Autism Clinic at Mississippi State University
299 Morrill Road Box Building, 2nd Floor
Mississippi State, MS 39762
Tel: (662) 325 2568
Contact Name: Daniel Gadke, Ph.D.
Email: schoolpsychservices@colled.msstate.edu

Konnections Autism Resources and Services Center
305 Joyce Avenue
Long Beach, MS 39560
Tel: (228) 324 8301

Contact Name: Tonya Turbville, Ed.S.
Email: tecautism@yahoo.com

Diagnostic and evaluation resources for individuals and families with ASD and related challenges.

North Mississippi Medical Center (NMMC)
830 South Gloster Street
Tupelo, MS 38801
Tel: (662) 377 3000
Toll Free: (800) 843 3375
Website: http://www.nmhs.net

School Psychology Service Center
USM, 118 College Dr. #5025
Hattiesburg, MS 39401
Tel: (601) 266 5255
Website: http://www.usm.edu/school-psychology/school-psychology-service-center

The University of Mississippi Speech and Hearing Clinic
George Hall, 352 Rebel Dr. Room 100
University, MS 38677
Tel: (662) 915 7271
Email: umcdshc@olemiss.edu

Therapy Services

Beyond Therapy Pediatric Group, PLLC
115 W. Jackson Street Suite F
Ridgeland, MS 39157
Tel: (601) 853 9747
Contact Name: Judy Lindsay
Email: judy@bptherapygroup.com
Website: http://www.bptherapygroup.com

Offers a team approach to services for children with ASD, providing individualized programs in clinical and home/community settings.

Laskin Therapy Group, PA
207 West Jackson Street Suite 2
Ridgeland, MS 39157
Tel: (601) 362 0859 or (601) 212 0870
Contact Name: Rebecca Laskin
Email: rebecca@laskintherapygroup.com
Website: http://www.laskintherapygroup.com

Provides integrated, teach approach for OT, PT, speech therapy.

Simple Strokes Therapy
83 Airways Place
Southaven, MS 38671
Tel: (662) 349 8787
Website: http://www.simplestrokestherapy.com

Warren-Yazoo Mental Health Service
3444 Wisconsin Avenue
Vicksburg, MS 39180
Tel: (601) 638 0031
Website: http://www.warren-yazoo.org

Schools and Educational Services

Autism Center of North Mississippi (ACNM)
Spanish Village Complex, 146 S Thomas St. Suite E
Tupelo, MS 38801
Tel: (662) 840 0974
Email: info@autismcenternms.com
Website: http://www.autismcenternms.com

Provides comprehensive educational and behavioral services to families and schools to support students with ASD and related challenges.

Jackson Autism Center (JAC)
6712 Old Canton Rd. Suite 5
Ridgeland, MS 39157
Tel: (769) 218 9596
Contact Name: Dr. Rebecca Mullican
Email: dr.rmullican@gmail.com
Website: http://www.jacksonautismcenter.com

Provides individualized supports for educational, social, communication and language, behavioral, and self-help goals.

Helping Hands Learning Academy
Helping Hands Learning Academy
P.O. Box 1428
Southaven, MS 38671
Tel: (901) 216 1486
Contact Name: Vargas Clark
Email: vclark@helpinghandsacademy.net
Website: http://www.helpinghandsacademy.net

Serves children ages 1-5 using ABA-based methods including Discrete trials, Incidental teachings, and Pivotal Response Training.

Magnolia Speech School
733 Flag Chapel Road
Jackson, MS 39209
Tel: (601) 922 5530
Contact Name: Dr. Tina Atkins, Executive Director
Email: tina.atkins@magnoliaspeechschool.org
Website: http://www.magnoliaspeechschool.org

A private pre-k to 8th grade school for children with a variety of speech and/or hearing challenges.

Services for Students with Disabilities
01 Montgomery Hall
Mississippi State, MS 39762
Tel: (662) 325 3335

Website: http://www.sss.msstate.edu/disabilities

The University of Southern Mississippi-Gulf Coast Autism Project
730 E Beach Blvd.
Long Beach, MS 39560
Tel: (228) 863 1755
Email: timothy.morse@usm.edu

Operates an Autism Demonstration School for students with autism, ages Preschool-Second grade.

Legal, Government & Financial Services

Mississippi Department of Mental Health (DMH)
239 N Lamar St. Robert E. Lee Building, 1101
Jackson, MS 39201
Tel: (601) 359 1288
Website: http://www.dmh.ms.gov

Mississippi Department of Rehabilitation Services (MDRS)
1281 Highway 51
Madison, MS 39110
Toll free: (800) 443 1000
Website: http://www.mdrs.state.ms.us

Community and Recreation Services

The Baddour Center
3297 Highway 51 South
Senatobia, MS 38668
Toll Free: (888) 4BADDOUR
Website: http://baddour.org

Central Mississippi Autism Support Group
149 Dry Creek Road
Magee, MS 39111
Tel: (601) 594 9314
Contact Name: Pam Dollar
Email: pkdollar@bellsouth.net

Gulf Coast Autism Support Nework
3109 Bienville Boulevard
Ocean Springs, MS 39564
(228) 588 3016
Contact Name: Patty Gautier
Email: pattygautier@yahoo.com

Jigsaw MSU
Mississippi State, MS 39762
Tel: (662) 341 3322
Contact Name: Sandy Devlin
Email: sandy3033@gmail.com

Provides advocacy and consultation services as well as

summer camp experience for adolescent males with high functioning autism on Mississippi State University campus.

Living Independence For Everyone (LIFE) of Mississippi
1051 Cliff Gookin Blvd.
Tupelo, MS 38801
Tel: (662) 844 6633
Contact Name: Emily Word, Regional Coordinator
Website: http://www.lifeofms.com

T.K. Martin Center for Technology and Disability
326 Corner Rd.
Mississippi State University, MS 39762
Tel: (662) 325 1028
Website: http://www.tkmartin.msstate.edu

Together Enhancing Autism Awareness in Mississippi (TEAAM)
Mize, MS 39116
Tel: (601) 782 9005
Toll Free: (866) 993 2437
Email: takeaction@TEAAM.org
Website: http://www.TEAAM.org

MISSOURI

Doctors, Clinics, Hospitals, and Other Health Services

Aarons, Kurt, D.D.S.
4411 Belleview Avenue
Kansas city, MO 64111
Tel: (816) 531 2070
Email: info@aaronsdds.com
Website: http://www.kurtaaronsdds.com/

Burrell Behavioral Health
3401 Berrywood Dr.
Columbia, MO 65201
Tel: (573) 777 8401
Contact Name: Bradley Morgan
Email: bradley.morgan@burrellcenter.com
Website: http://www.burrellcenter.com/

Offers comprehensive psychological assessments for adults suspected of having ASD.

Children's Mercy Hospital
2401 Gillham Road
Kansas City, MO 64108
Tel: (816) 234 3000
Website: http://www.childrens-mercy.org

Crossing Back to Health
16216 Baxter Road, Suite 110

Chesterfield, MO 63017
Tel: (636) 778 9158
Contact Name: Anne Dresch
Email: Anned@CrossingBacktoHealth.com
Website: http://www.CrossingBacktoHealth.com

Dr. Jay Kessinger
411 E. Hwy 72
Rolla, MO 65401
Tel: (573) 341 8292
Contact Name: Lucy Nash
Email: Lucy@drkessinger.com
Website: http://www.drkessinger.com
Provides natural healthcare treatments.

Kartzinel Wellness Center
Jerry Kartzinel, MD
4101 Mexico Road, Ste H,
St. Peters, MO 63376
Tel: (636) 922 4472
Website: www.drjerryk.com
Dr. Kartzinel is a board-certified pediatrician practicing Translational Medicine (translating diverse scientific findings into treatments for patients).

Midwest Institute for Neurological Development (MIND)
144 Chesterfield Commons East Rd.
Chesterfield, MO 63005
Tel: (636) 537 9800
Contact Name: Sarah Porzelt, Program Director
Email: info@mi4nd.com
Website: http://www.mi4nd.com
Provides evaluation and management of neurobehavioral and neurodevelopmental disorders.

Pediatric Education Dietitian Services
254 Clarkson Rd
Ellisville, MO 63011
Tel: (636) 227 7337
Contact Name: Barb Linneman, MS, RD, LD
Email: barb@pedsinc.com
Website: http://www.pedsinc.com
Provides services addressing both nutrition and feeding issues for children with ASD.

St. Louis Children's Hospital
Baxter at Clarkson
St. Louis, MO 63017
Tel: (314) 454 5420
Website: http://www.stlouischildrens.org

Thompson Center for Autism and Neurodevelopmental Disorders
University of Missouri
205 Portland Street

Columbia, MO 65211
Tel: (573) 882 6081
Toll Free: (888) 720 0015
Contact Name: Abby Tuttle
Email: thompsoncenter@missouri.edu
Website: http://thompsoncenter.missouri.edu

Therapy Services

Advocate 4 U Behavior Therapy, LLC
9409 E. 65th Street
Kansas City, MO 64133
Tel: (816) 812 4898
Contact Name: Lisa M. Booth, BS, ABA
Email: advocate4ubt@aol.com
Provides ABA therapy as well as advocacy services.

Applied Behavior Services, LLC
1601 McQuade Dr.
St. Peters, MO 63376
Tel: (314) 369 4235
Contact Name: Lisa Gilbertsen
Email: Lisa@HelpWithBehavior.com
Website: http://www.HelpWithBehavior.com

Behavior Solutions, Inc.
44 Portwest Ct
O'Fallon, MO 63303
Tel: (636)2650407
Contact Name: Angie Peeler
Email: apeeler@behsolutions.com
Website: http://www.behsolutions.com

Services include: early intervention, behavioral assessments/supports, parent and professional training, social skills, communication and language skills, school based consultation, schoolwide PBIS supports and training, adult services, and managing severe behavior problems.

Behavior Therapy Services
242 Pennington Lane
Chesterfield, MO 63005
Tel: (636) 675 4032
Contact Name: Melissa Vendt
Email: vendt.behaviortherapyservices@gmail.com

Behavioral Learning Center, LLC
230 N. Belcrest Ave. Suite A
Springfield, MO 65802
Tel: (417) 616 3180
Contact Name: Ginger Crabtree
Email: GCrabtree@ABA2Learn.com
Website: http://www.ABA2Learn.com
Provides ABA assessment and treatment services.

Best Abilities, LLC
9510 Page Ave.
Saint Louis, MO 63114, 63303
Tel: (314) 322 3027 or (314) 435 4063
Contact Name: Margaret Dannevik
Email: mdannevik@bestabilities.com
Website: http://www.bestabilities.com

ABA-based services include functional behavior assessment, verbal behavior, discrete trial training, augmentative communication, autism spectrum disorders, developmental delays, and parent education for children birth to 5 years.

Bill & Virginia Leffen Center for Autism
formerly Ozark Center for Autism
3230 Wisconsin Ave.
Joplin, MO 64804
Tel: (417) 347 7850
Website: http://www.freemanhealth.com/
leffencenterforautism

Provides ABA-based services for birth–21 years.

Collaborative Family Associates
777 S. New Ballas Rd. Suite 328W
Saint Louis, MO 63141
Tel: (314) 993 2474
Website: http://www.wellness.com/dir/2489724/
counselor/mo/saint-louis/collaborative-family-
associates#referrer

Exceptional Equestrians of the Meramec Valley
P.O. Box 1384
Washington, MO 63090
Tel: (636) 390 2141
Email: eemv@sbcglobal.net
Website: http://www.eemv.org

Gateway Education & Therapy
1281 N. Hwy 47
Union, MO 63084
Tel: (636) 583 0788
Contact Name: Kimberly Helm
Email: gatewaycenter@me.com
Website: http://www.gatewayeducationandtherapy.org

Offers speech and language therapy, behavioral therapy, social skills classes, classes focused on sensory integration, tutoring, assessments and consultations, school support, a summer camp, and a parent support group.

Great Strides Behavioral Consulting (GSBC)
2560 Metro Blvd.
Maryland Heights, MO 63043
Tel: (314) 715 3855
Contact Name: Amy Streff, Executive Director
Email: amy@greatstrides.cc
Website: http://www.greatstrides.cc

Green, Maxville and Associates
2743 Russell Blvd
Saint Louis, MO
Tel: (573) 864 9743 or (573) 424 2948
Contact Name: Dale Maxville
Email: greenmaxville@hotmail.com

Provides ABA therapy to children with ASD and behavior therapy to adults with developmental disabilities, as well as providing support and advocacy.

Leaps and Bounds, Inc.
324 Jungermann Road
St. Peters, MO 63376
Tel: (636) 928 5327
Email: info@LeapsAndBoundsKids.com
Website: http://www.LeapsAndBoundsKids.com

A pediatric therapy center.

Ozanam
421 E. 137th St
Kansas City, MO 64145
Tel: (816) 508 3687
Contact Name: Bart Ewing MSE -Autism. LCSW, LSCSW
Email: be3687@ozanam.org
Website: http://ozanam.org

Provides programs/interventions to help adolescents on the higher end of the autism spectrum with severe behavior issues remain in their home and return to their home schools.

Thorson Therapy, LLC
301 Sovereign Court, Suite 211
Ballwin, MO 63011
Tel: (314) 952 2426
Contact Name: Bryan Thorson
Email: bryanthorson@me.com

Schools and Educational Services

ABLE Program
Longview Community College
Lee's Summit, MO 64081
Tel: (816) 672 2366
Contact Name: Dr. Joan Bergstrom, Director
Email: Joan.Bergstrom@mcckc.edu
Website: http://www.mcckc.edu/?qlinks=ABLE Program

Provides support and skills to help disabled students progress into a college program.

Adult Continuing Education for Persons with Developmental Disabilities
Institute for Human Development Health Sciences
Bldg, Third Floor
2220 Holmes St., Room 340

Kansas City, MO 64108
Tel: (816) 672 2207
Website: http://www.ihd.umkc.edu/ACED

Designed to teach independent living skills and provide life-enhancing experiences.

Center for Autism Education
105 Sheriff Dierker Ct.
O'Fallon, MO 63366
Tel: (636) 978 7785
Contact Name: Tony Bryan
Email: tbryan@teachautism.org
Website: http://www.teachautism.org

Good Shepherd School for Children
1170 Timber Run
St. Louis, MO 63146
Tel: (314) 469 0606
Email: goodshepherd@goodss.org
Website: http://www.goodss.org

An early childhood education and therapy center serving children with and without special needs, ages six weeks to six years, and up to age 18 years for therapy services.

Howard Park Center
15834 Clayton Rd.
Ellisville, MO 63011
Tel: (636) 227 2339
Website: http://www.howardparkcenter.org

Missing Piece Learning Company
PO Box 901863
Kansas City, MO 64190-1863
Tel: (913) 522 4775
Contact Name: Lisa Miller
Email: missingpiecekc@gmail.com

Partners in Behavioral Milestones
10330 Hickman Mills Dr. Building II
Kansas City, MO 64137
Tel: (816) 501 5138
Contact Name: Tara Bernbeck
Email: info@behavioralmilestones.com
Website: http://www.behavioralmilestones.com

Offers in-home ABA consultations and training, a private school (Milestones Academy), residential group homes (Community Support Partners), ABA therapy, IEP consultation, behavior management training, and workshops.

Rainbow Center
900 NW Woods Chapel Road
Blue Springs, MO 64015-2622
Tel: (816) 229 3869
Email: peggy.britton@rainbow-center.org
Website: http://www.rainbow-center.org

Provides an intensive therapy program within an academic environment.

T.H.R.I.V.E. Program at the University of Central Missouri
University of Central Missouri
Warrensburg, MO 64093
Email: thrive@ucmo.edu
Website: http://www.ucmo.edu

A 2-year residential college experience to help intellectually challenged young adults to build skills for transitioning from home to independence.

Legal, Government & Financial Services

Bellatrix, PC
165 N Meramec Ave. 2nd Floor
Clayton, MO 63105
Tel: (314) 526 0040
Toll Free: (800) 449 8992
Email: e.intake@bellatrixlaw.com
Website: http://bellatrixlaw.com

Department of Housing and Urban Development
1222 Spruce St. Suite 3.203
St. Louis, MO 63103
Tel: (314) 418 5400
Contact Name: James Heard
Email: MO_Webmanager@hud.gov
Website: http://www.hud.gov/local/index.
cfm?state=mo&topic=offices

Developmental Disabilities Resource Board of Clay County
920 South Kent Street - Suite B
Liberty, MO 64068
Tel: (816) 792 5255
Email: ddrbcc@sbcglobal.net
Website: http://www.macdds.org/Counties/clay.html

Dickerson Oxton Law Firm
435 Nichols Rd. Suite 200
Kansas City, MO 64112
Tel: (816) 977 2080
Website: http://www.dickersonoxton.com

Division of Vocational Rehabilitation
3024 Dupont Circle
Jefferson, MO 65109
Tel: (877) 222 8963
Email: info@vr.dese.mo.gov
Website: http://dese.mo.gov/vr/

Educational Advocacy of Southeast Missouri
918 West Cape Rock Drive
Cape Girardeau, MO 63701

Tel: (573) 253 6884
Contact Name: Shannon Nevill -Registered Nurse
Email: shannon.nevill@gmail.com

Providing educational advocacy to parents in Southeastern Missouri.

Hal Cox, Educational Coach
2334 Olive Street
St Louis, MO 63103
Tel: (314) 421 0090
Email: hcox@stldd.org
Website: http://www.stldd.org

Special education advocates in St. Louis.

Jim Heuer
3827 McClay Road
Saint Peters, MO 63376
Tel: (636) 925 3000
Toll Free: (800) 536 9993
Contact Name: Jim Heuer
Email: jheuer@moneyconcepts.com

Financial planning for those with special needs dependents.

Law Offices of Thomas E. Kennedy, III, L.C.
230 S. Bemiston Ave. Suite 800
St. Louis, MO 63105
Tel: (314).872.9041 or 618.474.5326
Contact Name: Heather Navarro
Email: Hnavarro@tkennedylaw.com
Website: http://www.tkennedylaw.com

Private public interest law firm representing clients in special education law, disability discrimination and other civil rights matters in Missouri and Illinois.

Martha C. Brown & Associates, LLC
220 W Lockwood Ave. Suite 203
Saint Louis, MO 63119
Tel: (314) 962 0186
Contact Name: Colleen Brown, Legal Assistant
Email: cbrown@elderlawstlouis.com
Website: http://www.elderlawstlouis.com

Special needs legal planning.

Missouri Parents Act (MPAct)
8301 State Line Road, Suite 204
Kansas City, MO 64114
Tel: (800) 743 7634
Email: info@ptimpact.org
Website: http://www.ptimpact.org

Missouri Protection and Advocacy Services
P.O. Box 6187
Fulton, MO 65251
Tel: (573) 592 2738
Email: mopasjc@earthlink.net

Website: http://www.moadvocacy.org

Community and Recreation Services

Accessible Recreation
Springfield-Greene County Park Board
Springfield, MO 65803
Tel: (417) 837 5808
Contact Name: Cyrus Taylor
Email: ctaylor@springfieldmo.gov
Website: http://www.springfieldmo.gov/1196/Accessible-Recreation

Achievements Unlimited
9510 Page Ave
St. Louis, MO 63132
Tel: (314) 733 0056
Contact Name: Angela Craven, MS, BCBA, LBA
Email: acraven@bestabilities.com

Day program with behavior support, speech therapy, and OT that focuses on community involvement and vocational training for adults with autism and other developmental disabilities who display challenging behavior.

Action For Autism St. Louis
16052 Swingley Ridge Rd. Suite 205
Chesterfield, MO 63017
Tel: (636) 449 0352
Email: info@afastl.org
Website: http://www.afastl.org

Adam Morgan Scholarship Fund
PO Box 532
St. Peters, MO 63376
Contact Name: Rachel Morgan
Email: Rachel@amfunrun.org
Website: http://adammorganfoundation.org

Autism Works
915 East H Highway
Liberty, MO 64106
Tel: (816) 721 7196
Contact Name: Glenna Love
Email: Autismworkskc@gmail.com
Website: http://autism-works.org/

The Betty and Bobby Allison Miracle League Ball Field
Springfield-Greene County Park
Board 301 E. Talmage St.
Springfield, MO 65803
Tel: (417) 837 5808
Website: http://www.springfieldmo.gov/823/Miracle-League-Ball-Field

The Betty and Bobby Allison Miracle League Ball Field allows individuals ages 5 and up with disabilites to hit, run, catch and play ball.

Boone County Family Resources
1209 East Walnut Street
Columbia, MO 65201
Tel: (573) 874 1995
Email: agency@bcfr.org
Website: http://www.bcfr.org

Bridges Community Support Services
309 N. Jefferson, Suite 370
Springfield, MO 65806
Tel: (417) 865 7929
Toll Free: (800) 427 2699
Contact Name: Regional Director, Eric H. Cantu
Email: ecantu@bridgesofmissouri.com

Residential services include both part-time in-home supports and supported living homes with 24 hour assistance.

Community Support Services of Missouri
2312 Annie Baxter
Joplin, MO 64804
Tel: (417) 624 4515
Website: http://www.cssmo.org

Developing Potential, Inc.
120 W. Walnut Street
Independence, MO 64050
Tel: (816) 252 0086
Email: dpotentialinc@aol.com
Website: http://www.developingpotential.org

Developmental Center of the Ozarks
1545 E. Pythian
Springfield, MO 65802
Tel: (417) 831 1545
Contact Name: Executive Director - Allan McKelvy
Email: amckelvy@dcoonline.com
Website: http://www.dcoonline.com

Family Advocacy and Community Training
800 Friedens Road, Suite 200
St. Charles, MO 63303
Tel: (636) 949 2425
Email: dgould@factmo.org
Website: http://www.factmo.org

Friends of Marvell House
1534 Reale Avenue
St. Louis, MO 63138
Tel: (314) 249 5339
Contact Name: Herice Vereen
Email: hbcarter@charter.net
A 24 hour daycare facility for children and young adults with ASD.

Handi Wheels Paratransit Service
820 E. Miller St.
Jefferson City, MO 65101
Tel: (573) 634 6477
Website: http://www.jeffcitymo.org/publicworks/transit/handiwheels.html

High Hope Employment Services, Inc.
611 W. Third St. Suite 1
Milan, MO 63556
Tel: (660) 265 4614
Email: info@hhesinc.com
Website: http://hhesinc.com/services_supported.shtml
Supported employment.

Judevine Center for Autism
22 Gravois Station Rd.
House Springs, MO 63051
Tel: (800) 780 6545
Contact Name: Karen Draeger
Email: Contactus@judevine.org
Website: http://www.judevine.org

KEEN St. Louis
PO Box 69010
Saint Louis, MO 63169
Tel: (314) 259 5980
Contact Name: Kelle Franklin
Email: kfranklin@keenstlouis.org
Website: http://www.keenstlouis.org

One-to-one recreational opportunities for children and young adults with developmental disabilities at no cost to their families and caregivers.

Learning Disabilities Association of St. Louis
13537 Barrett Parkway Drive, Suite 110
Ballwin, MO 63021
Tel: (314) 966 3088
Email: info@ldastl.org
Website: http://www.ldastl.org

MERS/Goodwill
2545 South Hanley Road
St. Louis, MO 63144
Tel: (314) 647 7453 or (314) 646 2278
Contact Name: Jennifer Glassmeyer
Email: jglassmeyer@mersgoodwill.org
Website: http://mersgoodwill.org

Vocational planning and placement services, along with job coaching. Also offers a variety of activities and resources.

Midwest Adult Autism Project
11786 Westline Industrial Drive
St. Louis, MO 63146

Tel: (314) 983 9230
Contact Name: Rick Goolsby
Email: rgoolsby@headinjuryctr-stl.org
Website: http://headinjuryctr-stl.org/chismain/

A full day, Monday through Friday service for adults with severe autism.

Missouri Advocates for Families Affected by Autism (MOAFAA)
1200 SE London Way
Lees Summit, MO 64081
Tel: (816) 554 3017
Contact Name: Sherri Tucker
Email: autism@kc.rr.com
Website: http://moafaa.blogspot.com

Missouri Family to Family
UMKC Institute for Human Development
215 W. Pershing Rd., 4th Floor
Kansas City, MO 64108
Tel: (800) 444 0821
Website: http://www.mofamilytofamily.org

NextStep for Life
3875 Plass Rd.
Mapaville, MO 63065
Tel: (636) 282 4400 or (636) 933 0244
Email: info@nextstepforlife.org
Website: http://www.nextstepforlife.org

Nova Center of the Ozarks
524 S. Union Ave
Springfield, MO 65802
Tel: (417) 889 3121
Email: ccline@novacenter-sgf.com
Website: http://www.novacenteroftheozarks.org

Our Special Grandkids
St. Louis, MO
Contact Name: Nan Goldberg
Email: nansgrls2@aol.com

Our Special Grandkids is a support group formed by and for grandparents (and other grands) who have grandchildren with ASD.

Paraquad, Inc.
5240 Oakland Avenue
St. Louis, MO 63110
Tel: (314) 289 4200 or (314) 289 4252
Email: contactus@paraquad.org
Website: http://www.paraquad.org

Pathways To Independence
200 South Hanley Road, Suite 507
Clayton, MO 63105

Tel: (314) 863 0202
Contact Name: Craig Strohbeck
Email: craig@pathways2independence.com
Website: http://www.pathways2independence.com

People First of Missouri
PO Box 30142
Kansas City, Missouri 64112
Tel: (800) 558 8652
Email: missouripeoplefirst@gmail.com
Website: http://www.missouripeoplefirst.org/

Rising Abilities
P.O. Box 3515
Camdenton MO. 65020
Tel: (417) 650 8352
Email: amarks@risingabilities.org
Website: http://www.risingabilities.org/risingabilities/

Provides a safe, educational and fun environment for campers with special needs utilizing the resources at the Bennett Spring State Park.

ShowMe Aquatics & Fitness
2085 Bluestone Dr.
St. Charles, MO 63303
Tel: (636) 896 0999
Email: showmeaquatics@showmeaquatics.org
Website: http://showmeaquatics.org

SOAR: Social Opportunities and Respite
Developmental Disabilities Resource Board
1025 Country Club Road
St. Charles, MO 63303
Tel: (636) 949 2546
Website: http://www.ddrb.org

Special Needs Scouts
Unit #2250 St Joseph, MO 64439
Tel: (913) 396 2716
Contact Name: Teresa Julian
Email: jtjulian2003@yahoo.com
Website: http://jtjulian2003.tripod.com

SPENSA
4659 Tauneybrook Drive
St. Louis, MO 63128
Tel: (314) 487 5111
Contact Name: Susan Quante, Soccer Coordinator
Email: Suziek@aol.com
Website: http://www.spensa.org

A St. Louis based soccer program for young people with disabilities, ages 5-21.

St. Louis Life
929 Rolling Thunder Dr.
O'Fallon, MO 63368
Tel: (636) 561 1900
Contact Name: Andy Conover
Email: aconover@stlouislife.org
Website: http://www.stlouislife.org

St. Louis Life is a community-based, residential program for young adults with developmental disabilities.

Sunnyhill, Inc.
11140 So. Towne Square Ste. 101
St. Louis, MO 63123
Tel: (314) 845 3900
Website: http://www.sunnyhillinc.org

Sunnyhill, Inc. provides tailored residential, recreational and educational opportunities for children and adults with developmental disabilities.

Support Innovations
13422 Clayton Rd #214
Saint Louis, MO 63131
Tel: (314) 205 0588
Contact Name: Joann Becker
Email: Info@supportinnovations.com
Website: http://www.supportinnovations.com

Day services for adults with developmental disabilities.

Tailor Institute
611 North Fountain Street
1 University Plaza, MS 9450
Cape Girardeau, MO 63701
Tel: (573) 339 9552
Website: http://www.thetailorinstitute.org/

Transitional Life Solutions, LLC
Ladue, MO 63124
Tel: (314).983.2727 or 314.560.6159
Contact Name: Renau Bozarth
Email: rboza@sbcglobal
Website: http://www.transitionallifesolutions.com

Transitional Life Solutions serves young adults, aged 16-26 with a diagnosis of Asperger's Syndrome, or higher level ASD.

West-Central Independent Living Solutions
710 N. College Ste. D
Warrensburg, MO 64093
Tel: (660) 422 7883
Toll Free: (800) 236 5175
Email: wils@iland.net
Website: http://www.w-ils.org

MONTANA

Doctors, Clinics, Hospitals, and Other Health Services

Children's Clinic of Billings
1232 North 30th Street Suite 200
Billings, MT 59101
Tel: (406) 238 6600 or (406) 238 6624
Contact Name: Marian Elizabeth Kummer, MD FAAP and Laura R Nicholson. MD FAAP
Website: http://www.childrensclinicofbillings.com

Julia Turner Nutrition
PO Box 62
McLeod, MT 59052
Tel: (406) 930 2772
Contact Name: Julia Turner, MMSc, RD, LN
Email: julia@juliaturnernutrition.com
Website: http://www.juliaturnernutrition.com

Develops a customized nutrition action plan to help individuals meet their health and wellness goals. Her areas of expertise include autism, ADHD and related disorders.

Therapy Services

Big Sky Therapeutic Services, PLLC
Big Sky Therapeutic Services, PLLC Great Falls, MT 59405
Tel: (406) 240 2045
Contact Name: Brett E. Gilleo, MSC, LCPC
Email: begilleo@gmail.com
Website: http://www.bigskytherapy.com

The Child Development Center
T214 Ft. Missoula
Missoula, MT 59804
Tel: (406) 549 6413 (Missoula)
Tel: (406) 755 2425 (Kalispell)
Contact Name: Karlyn Gibbs
Email: kgibbs@childdevcenter.org
Website: http://www.childdevcenter.org

Center and home-based services for children and young adults including ASD screening, evaluation and diagnosis, Part C Infant & Toddler Early Intervention, Child Autism Waiver Services, and Insurance Services.

Daly Communication: Speech-Language Therapy
Highway 78 PO Box 1163
Columbus, MT 59019
Tel: (406) 579 0819
Contact Name: Christine Daly
Email: Dalycommunicationslp@gmail.com
Website: http://www.dalyspeechlanguagetherapy.com

A private speech and language practice and treatment plans may include hippotherapy as part of individualized treatment plans.

Full Circle Autism & Developmental Services
1903 S Russell St
Missoula, MT 59801
Tel: (406)-532-1615
Contact Name: Beth Brewer
Email: bethb@fullcirclemhc.com
Website: http://www.fullcirclemhc.com

Pediatric Occupational Therapy Services
P.O. Box 1752
Bozeman, MT 59771
Tel: (406) 600 8366
Contact Name: Kara Cannon, OTR/L
Email: kara@functional-fundamentals.com

Pediatric Therapy Clinic (PTC), Inc.
1610 Poly Dr.
Billings, MT 59102
Tel: (406) 259 1680
Contact Name: Traci Sell, M.S./CCC-SLP, BCBA
Website: http://www.ptcbillings.com

Provides speech, occupational, physical and ABA therapy to children from birth - 21 years of age.

P.L.A.Y. Project
2825 Stockyard Rd., Ste. A23
Missoula, MT 59808
Tel: (406) 850 2977
Contact Name: Audrey Pierce-Seeley
Email: audreys@esgw.org
Website: http://www.esgw-nrm.easterseals.com or http://www.playproject.org

A play-based, developmental, parent training intervention based on DIR/Floortime.

RiteCare Speech, Language & Hearing Clinic
Curry Health Center, Lower Level University of Montana, 634 Eddy Ave.
Missoula, MT 59812
Tel: (406) 243 2405
Contact Name: Jennifer Closson, MS, CCC-SLP, Director of Pediatric Services
Email: jennifer.closson@mso.umt.edu
Website: http://coehs.umt.edu/departments/csd/

STEP, Inc.
644 Grand Avenue Suite 1
Billings, MT 59101
Tel: (406) 248 2055
Contact Name: Amy Olsen
Email: amyo@step-inc.org
Website: http://step-inc.org

STEP, Inc. supports individuals with disabilities in central Montana, providing home and community based education, developmental screenings & evaluations and resource coordination.

Schools and Educational Services

Chief Charlo Elementary School
Missoula Co. Public Schools
5600 Longview
Missoula, MT 59803
Tel: (406) 542 4005, x 4959
Contact Name: Keely Hammontree
Email: kahammontree@mcps.k12.mt.us
Website: www.mcpsmt.org/chiefcharlo

Cold Springs School
Missoula Co. Public Schools
2625 Briggs
Missoula, MT 59803
Tel: (406) 542 4010
Contact Name: Tracy Hardy
Email: thardy@mcps.k12.mt.us
Website: http://www.mcps.k12.mt.us/portal/coldsprings/Home/tabid/360/Default.aspx

Developmental Educational Assistance Program
DEAP 2200 Box Elder
Miles City, MT 59301
Tel: (406) 234 6034
Toll Free: (800) 224 6034
Contact Name: Sandy Peaslee
Email: speaslee@deapmt.org
Website: http://www.deapmt.org

Lame Deer Public Schools
Elementary, Junior High and High School
PO Box 96
Lame Deer, MT 59403
Tel: (406) 477 6305 or (406) 477 8900
Contact Name: Sid Richardson
Email: sidrichardson@lamedeer.k12.mt.us
Website: http://lamedeer.k12.mt.us/

Lincoln-McKinley Primary School
Havre Public School System
801 4th Street
Havre, MT 59501
Tel: (406) 265 9619 x 322
Contact Name: ĐruAnne Earll
Email: earlld@lm.havre.k12.mt.us
Website: http://www.havre.k12.mt.us/193410512175415540/site/default.asp

SPECIAL LEARNING 1-ON-1 LLC
1122 East Main Suite 4
Bozeman, MT 59715
Tel: (406) 580 2640
Contact Name: Shawna Heiser MS BCBA
Email: speciallearning1on1@gmail.com
Website: http://www.speciallearning1on1.com

Serves children with a variety of cognitive and behavioral disorders, particularly those with needs in language production, cognitive delays, and behavioral disorders.

Legal, Government & Financial Services

Andree Larose, Attorney, Morrison, Motl & Sherwood, PLLP
401 N. Last Chance Gulch
Helena, MT 59601
Tel: (406) 442 3261
Contact Name: Administrative Assistant
Email: info@mmslawgroup.com
Website: http://www.mmslawgroup.com

Department of Housing and Urban Development
901 Front St. Suite 1300
Helena, MT 59626
Tel: (406) 449 5050
Contact Name: Erik Amundson
Email: MT_Webmanager@hud.gov
Website: http://www.hud.gov/local/index.
cfm?state=mt&topic=offices

Montana Vocational Rehabilitation
111 North Last Chance Gulch Suite 4C
Helena, MT 59604
Toll Free: (877) 296 1197
Website: http://www.dphhs.mt.gov/vocrehab/
index.shtml

Procedural Safeguards in Special Education
Montana Office of Public Instruction
Tel: (406) 444 4429
Website: http://www.opi.mt.gov/PDF/SpecED/guides/
ProcSafegrdsSpEdbooklet.pdf

Community and Recreation Services

AWARE Inc.
205 E. Park Ave
Anaconda, MT 59711
Tel: (406) 563 8117
Email: info@aware-inc.org
Website: http://www.aware-inc.org

Christikon Camp
1108 24th Street West
Billlings, MT 59102

Tel: (406) 656 1969
Email: christikon@aol.com
Website: http://www.christikon.org

Eagle Mount Bozeman
6901 Goldenstein Lane
Bozeman, MT 59715
Tel: (406) 586 1781
Contact Name: Mary Peterson
Email: maryp@eaglemount.org
Website: http://www.eaglemount.org

Provides therapeutic recreation for persons with physical and mental disabilities and children with cancer. Activities include horseback riding, swimming, skiing, cycling, ice skating, fishing, rafting, and more.

Erik's Ranch and Retreats
Bozeman, MT
Tel: (406) 451 2722
Contact Name: Kathryn Nordberg, CEO
Email: Kathryn@eriksranch.org
Website: http://www.eriksranch.org

Erik's Ranch & Retreats provides safe and unequaled living, working, social and recreational environments for young adults with ASD.

Exceptional Family Connections
502 S 19th Ave Suite 200
Bozeman, MT 59718
Tel: (406) 577 6485
Contact Name: Heather Boyes
Email: haboyes@gmail.com
Website: http://exceptionalfamilyconnections.com

Provides a variety of services to children with special needs and their families including respite care, behavioral support, family support, advocacy, and consultation.

Farm in the Dell International, Inc.
Helena, MT
Tel: (406) 449 9394
Email: farminthedell@qwest.net
Website: http://farminthedell.org

Provides residential and vocational opportunities.

Job Connection, Inc.
1501 14th St. W Suite 220
Billings, MT 59102
Tel: (406) 245 6323
Email: rita@jobconnection.org
Website: http://www.jobconnection.org/

Missoula YMCA - Special Needs Swim Instruction
3000 S Russell St
Missoula, MT 59801
Tel: (406) 721 9622

Contact Name: Rose Kahane, Director of Aquatics
Email: rkahane@ymcamissoula.org
Website: http://www.ymcamissoula.org/index.
php?page=adaptive

Montana Autism Society of America
North Central Chapter
Montana Autism Society of America Great Falls, MT
59403
Tel: (406) 868 8083
Website: http://www.montanaasa.org/

Montana Community Autism & Asperger's Network
MT-CAAN
Montana Community Autism & Asperger's Network
Missoula, MT
Contact Name: Denise Dahlberg
Email: mtcaan@gmail.com
Website: http://www.manta.com/

Parents, Let's Unite for Kids (PLUK)
516 North 32nd Street
Billings, MT 59101
Tel: (406) 255 0540
Toll Free: (800) 222 7585
Email: info@pluk.org
Website: http://www.pluk.org

R.A.V.E
PO Box 80185
Billings, MT 59108
Tel: (406) 237 0025
Toll Free: (888) 882 1927
Website: http://www.rsdinc.org/recadv.html
Vacation and recreational opportunities.

NEBRASKA

Doctors, Clinics, Hospitals, and Other Health Services

Beatrice State Developmental Center
Care Facilities
3000 Lincoln Blvd.
Beatrice, NE 68310
Tel: (402) 223 6600
Email: elton.edmond@dhhs.ne.gov
Website: http://www.hhs.state.ne.us/dip/ded/bsdcindex.
htm

Boys Town Pediatrics
Pediatrics
14080 Boys Town Hospital Road
Omaha, NE 68010
Tel: (402) 778 6920 or (402) 778 6900

Website: http://www.boystownpediatrics.org
https://www.facebook.com/BoysTownPediatrics

Children's Hospital
8200 Dodge Street
Omaha, NE 68114-4113
Tel: (402) 955 3900
Website: http://www.chsomaha.org

Healthy Start Chiropractic & Wellness, PC
5445 Red Rock Lane, Suite 300
Lincoln, NE 68516
Tel: (402) 423 4325
Email: info@healthystartchiro.com
Website: http://www.healthystartchiro.com
A certified pediatric chiropractor that specializes in neurosensory disorders. Along with chiropractic adjustments, address nutritional issues, immune deficits, and provides neurosensory integration therapy for autistic children.

Midlands Pediatrics, PC
401 E. Gold Coast Road, Suite 325
Papillion, NE 68046
Tel: (402) 592 1700
Contact: Dr. Ai Lan Kobayashi
Email: akobayashi@pol.net
Website: http://www.kobayashi.yourmd.com/

Munroe-Meyer Institute (MMI) for Genetics and Rehabilitation
Services and Support
985450 Nebraska Medical Center
Omaha, NE 68198
Tel: (402) 559 6430
Toll Free: (800) 656 3937 X96430
Email: munroemeyer@unmc.edu
Website: http://www.unmc.edu/mmi/
https://www.facebook.com/MunroeMeyerInstitute

Towner County Memorial Hospital
25 S. College Drive Suite 14
Devils Lake, NE 58301
Tel: (701) 968 4411
Toll Free: (800) 943 3337
Contact: Russell Warren Petty, MD FAAP
Website: http://www.tcmedcenter.com

Therapy Services

Behavioral Health Solutions, PC
917 Wildwood Ln. Suite 153
Nebraska City, NE 68410
Tel: (402) 216 0561
Email: shelly@bhsne.com
Website: http://www.bhsne.com

Behavioral Health Specialists, Inc.
900 W Norfolk Ave
Norfolk, NE 68701
Tel: (402) 370 3140
Website: http://www.4bhs.org

Children's Respite Care Center
2010 N. 88th Street
Omaha, NE 68137
Tel: (402) 496 1000
Email: info@crccomaha.org
Website: http://www.crccomaha.org/
https://www.facebook.com/CRCComaha

Offers occupational, physical, speech, and feeding therapy for children with physical, sensory, cognitive, orthopedic, feeding, and communication needs.

Columbus Speech Therapy
2656 33rd Avenue
Columbus, NE 68601
Tel: (402) 564 1212
Email: dnormanolson@gmail.com

Communication Works Speech & Language Services
1540 South 70th St. Suite 101
Lincoln, NE 68506
Tel: (402) 480 3152
Email: toni@comworkslincoln.com
Website: http://www.comworkslincoln.com

Handprints and Footsteps Pediatric Therapy Clinic
5930 Vandervoort Drive Suite A
Lincoln, NE 68516
Tel: (402) 420 2099
Email: handprints@windstream.net
Website: http://www.handprintsandfootsteps.com

Heartland Speech and Language Services
8055 O St. Suite S110
Lincoln, NE 68510
Tel: (402) 327 2500
Email: laurasteffensen@hotmail.com
Website: http://heartlandspeech.com

Provides pediatric speech, language and feeding therapy services.

Kelli Krause
Speech and Language Therapy
410 Augusta Avenue
Bellevue, NE 68005
Tel: (402) 201 4635

Kristin R. Purington, MS, LBA-MO, BCBA
Plattsmouth, NE 68048
Contact: Kristin R. Purington, MS, LBA-MO, BCBA
Tel: (402) 312 9272

Email: krpurington@icloud.com
Provides ABA to all ages with a wide range of areas addressed.

Lovaas Institute for Early Intervention
P.O. Box 21845
Lincoln, NE 68542
Tel: (402) 328 0283
Email: Clarissa Kroll: ckroll@lovaas.com
Website: http://www.lovaas.com

STE Consultants
Omaha, NE 68183
Tel: (510) 665 9700
Email: penelope@steconsultants.com
Website: http://www.steconsultants.com
https://www.facebook.com/pages/STE-Consultants-LLC/157995444230973

Provides ABA services.

Success 4 Kids Therapy
Mental Health Therapist
Family Strategies
11414 W Center
Omaha, NE 68028
Contact: Tina Gunn
Tel: (402) 658 5181
Email: gunn2@cox.net
Website: http://www.tinamgunn.com
https://www.facebook.com/Success4KidsTherapy

Schools and Educational Services

Aurora Preschool
409 J Street
Aurora, NE 68818
Tel: (402) 694 6707

Public school providing individualized programs that may include early childhood special education and speech-language therapy, physical therapy, occupational therapy, hearing services, and vision services.

Autistic Kids are Amazing
Omaha, NE 68132
Email: autistickidsareamazing@gmail.com
In-home education and support.

Legal, Government & Financial Services

Department of Housing and Urban Development – Nebraska
Residential Service
1616 Capitol Avenue Suite 329
Omaha, NE 68102

Tel: (402) 492 3100
Email: NE_webmanager@hud.gov
Website: http://www.hud.gov/local/index.
cfm?state=ne&topic=offices

Nebraska Advocacy Services
Advocacy Service
134 South 13th Street Suite 600
Lincoln, NE 68508
Tel: (402) 474 3183
Toll Free: Toll Free: (800) 422 6691
Email: info@nebraskaadvocacyservices.org
Website: http://www.nebraskaadvocacyservices.org

Nebraska Department of Education Transition Services
Nebraska Department of Education
6949 South 110th Street
Omaha, NE 68128
Contact: Rita Hammit
Tel: (402) 595 2092
Website: http://ndetransition.site.esu9.org/

Nebraska Department of Education – Vocational Rehabilitation
Vocational Rehabilitation program
P.O. Box 94987
Lincoln, NE 68509
Tel: (402) 471 3644
Email: marketingteam.vr@nebraska.gov
Website: http://www.vr.ne.gov/index.html
https://www.facebook.com/NebraskaVR

Nebraska Department of Health and Human Services Home and Community Based Waiver
Nebraska Department of Health & Human Services
P.O. Box 95026,
Lincoln, Nebraska 68509-5026
Tel: (402) 471 6035
(800) 254 4202
Email: DHHS.Helpline@nebraska.gov
Website: http://dhhs.ne.gov/Pages/hcs_programs_
ad-waiver.aspx

Nebraska Early Development Network
301 Centennial Mall South P.O. Box 94987
Lincoln, NE 68509-4987
Tel: (402) 471 2463
Website: http://edn.ne.gov/

Nebraska Family Helpline
Toll Free: (888) 866 8660
Website: http://dhhs.ne.gov/behavioral_health/Pages/
nebraskafamilyhelpline_index.aspx

Nebraska Medicaid Program
Medical Service
301 Centennial Mall South

Lincoln, NE 68509
Tel: (402) 471 6035
Email: DHHS.Helpline@nebraska.gov
Website: http://dhhs.ne.gov/medicaid/Pages/med_
medprog.aspx

Office of Early Childhood
301 Centennial Mall South P.O. Box 94987
Lincoln, NE 68509-4987
Tel: (402) 471 4319
Contact: jan.thelen@nde.ne.gov
Website: http://www.education.ne.gov/oec

PTI Nebraska
3135 North 93rd Street
Omaha, NE 68134
Tel: (402) 346 0525 Voice & TDD
Toll Free: Toll Free: (800) 284 8520
Email: Info@pti-nebraska.org
Website: http://www.pti-nebraska.org

Community and Recreation Services

Arc of Lincoln/Lancaster County
Legal Resource
Arc of Lincoln/Lancaster County
5609 S 49th Street Suite 5
Lincoln, NE 68516
Tel: (402) 421 8866
Email: arcoflincoln@windstream.net
Website: http://www.arclincoln.org
https://www.facebook.com/thearcoflincoln?ref=br_tf

The Arc of Nebraska
Residential Service
215 Centennial Mall South Suite 508
Lincoln,NE 68508
Tel: (402) 475 4407
Email: pat@arc-nebraska.org
Website: http://www.arc-nebraska.org/
https://www.facebook.com/pages/The-Arc-of-
Nebraska/167646211703

Autism Action Partnership
14301 FNB Parkway Suite 115
Omaha, NE 68154
Tel: (402) 763 8830
Email - Gail Durkin: gdurkin@autismaction.org
Website: http://www.autismaction.org

Promotes autism awareness and provides resource to families and professionals in Nebraska and southwest Iowa.

Autism Center of Nebraska, Inc. (ACN)
Employment Service
9012 Q Street

Omaha, NE 68127
Tel: (402) 315 1000
Email: RFerdinand@ACNomaha.org
Website: http://acnomaha.org/

Provides a variety of residential, vocational, pre-vocational and educational services.

Autism Family Network
PO Box 67053
Lincoln, NE 68506
Tel: (402) 421 0874
Website: http://www.autismfamilynetwork.org/

The Autism Society of Nebraska
PO Box 83559
Lincoln, NE 68501
Tel: (877) 375 0120
Email: autismsociety@autismnebraska.org
Website: http://www.autismnebraska.org
https://www.facebook.com/AutismSocietyNebraska

Blue Rivers
Transportation Service
612 Grant St. Room 24
Beatrice, NE 68310
Tel: (402) 223 1352
Website: http://www.answers4families.org/family/
eldercare/transportation/blue-rivers-area-agency-aging-
transportation

Blue Valley Mental Health Center: Beatrice
Adult Day Care Program
1121 N. 10th St.
Beatrice, NE 68310
Tel: (402) 228 3386

Eastern Nebraska Community Office of Retardation and Developmental Disabilities (ENCOR)
Adult Day Program
900 S. 74th Plaza, Suite 200
Omaha, NE 68114
Tel: (402) 444 6500
Email: ckoontz@enhsa.com
Website: http://www.encor-dd.org

Goodwill Industries of Greater Nebraska
1804 S. Eddy
Grand Island, NE 68801
Tel: (308) 384 7896
Website: http://www.goodwillne.org/
https://www.facebook.com/goodwillgreatne

Higher Opportunities Through The Power of Employment
Employment Service
1645 N Street Suite A

Lincoln, NE 68508
Tel: (402) 441 4371
(888) 902 2822
Email: agreen@mha-ne.org
Website: http://www.mha-ne.org/hope/
https://www.facebook.com/mhanehope

Mosaic
Adult Day Program
National Supports Office
4980 S. 118th St.
Omaha, NE 68137
Tel: 877.3MOSAIC
Email: info@mosaicinfo.org
Website: http://www.mosaicinfo.org/
https://www.facebook.com/mosaicpossible

Nebraska APSE (Association of People Supporting Employment)
Employment Service
2127 E 23rd St.
Fremont, NE 68025
Tel: (402) 340 3497
Email: spirtg@northstarservices.net
Website: http://nebraskaapse.org/
https://www.facebook.com/pages/Nebraska-
APSE/148941103610

Nebraska Yellow Pages for Kids
Website: http://www.yellowpagesforkids.com/help/
ne.htm

Find educational consultants, psychologists, educational diagnosticians, health care providers, academic therapists, tutors, speech language therapists, occupational therapists, coaches, advocates, and attorneys. You will also find special education schools, learning centers, treatment programs, parent groups, respite care, community centers, grassroots organizations, and government programs.

NEVADA

Doctors, Clinics, Hospitals, and Other Health Services

Academic & Psychological Testing & Tutoring Services
APTS
7473 W. Lake Mead Blvd Suite 106
Las Vegas NV 89128
Tel: (702) 375 6505
Website: http://www.aptsofsnv.com

Autism Enlightenment
Dr. Nancy Sylvanie
Horizon Medical Center

2610 W. Horizon Ridge Pkwy #201-A
Henderson, NV 89012
Tel: (702) 492 6959
Email: artymom@msn.com
Website: http://www.autismenlightenment.com

Carl W. Ruggiero, DDS
Pediatric dentist
2145 Green Vista, Drive Suite #110
Sparks, NV 89431
Tel: (775) 331 9477
Email: was1@charterinternet.com

Foundation for Positively Kids
Positively Kids at Child Haven
701 N Pecos at Bonanza
Las Vegas, NV 89101
Tel: (702) 262 0037
Website: http://www.positivelykids.org/home.aspx

Lloyd B. Austin, DDS
850 "I" Street Suite A
Sparks, NV 89431
Tel: (775) 358 5330
Website: http://dentistryforchildrenreno.com/

Mary A. Grant, O.D.
2755 E. Desert Inn Rd, #270
Las Vegas, NV 89121
Tel: (702) 836 3600
Email: marygrantod@aol.com

Provides vision and ocular health examinations as well as vision/cognitive/behavioral therapy for those with ASD.

The Nevada Clinic
3663 Pecos McLeod
Las Vegas, NV 89121
Tel: (702) 732 1400
Toll Free: (800) 641 6661
Email: info@nevadaclinic.com
Website: http://www.nevadaclinic.com/page.php?p=1

Nourishing Spectrum
9811 W Charleston Blvd Suite 2197
Las Vegas, NV 89117
Tel: (702) 265 5549
Email: carey@nourishingspectrum.com
Website: http://www.nourishingspectrum.com
https://www.facebook.com/nourishingspectrum/
timeline?ref=page_internal

Holistic health coach practice specializing in counseling for families with children with ASD, including diet modification, GFCFSF diets, healthy recipes, and other services.

Summerlin Pediatric Dentistry
653 N. Town Center Dr. Suite 104
Las Vegas NV 89144
Tel: (702) 838 9013
Email: DrHoban@summerlinpediatricdentist.com
Website: http://www.AutismDentist.com
https://www.facebook.com/summerlinpediatricdentistry

Therapy Services

Achievable Behavior Strategies, LLC
9163 W. Flamingo Rd, Ste 100
Las Vegas, NV 89147
Tel: (702) 250 4891
Email: Justin@AchievableBehaviorStrategies.com
Website: http://www.AchievableBehaviorStrategies.com

Provides applied verbal behavior therapy and positive behavioral supports.

Achievement Therapy Center
6760 W. Quail Ave
Las Vegas, NV 89118
Tel: (702) 220 5514
Email: achievementtc@aol.com
Website: http://otformychild.com/#/home

Private OT practice specializing in Sensory Integration Therapy (SI), Neurodevelopmental Therapy and Oral Motor and Feeding Therapy.

Autism Care West
2110 E. Flamingo Rd., Ste 317
Las Vegas, NV 89119
Tel: (702) 326 5996
Email: info@autismcarewest.com
Website: http://www.autismcarewest.com

Specializes in the Home Program and Applied Behavior Analysis but providing support at many levels.

Behavioral Learning Solutions
P.O. Box 60811
Boulder City, NV 89006
Phone (702) 610 2076
Email: blsolutionsaba@yahoo.com
Website: http://blsolutionsaba.org
https://www.facebook.com/
BehavioralLearningSolutions

Provides services based Applied Behavior Analysis to children with autism and related learning disabilities.

Beug Behavioral Intervention and Consulting Services
9732 STATE ROUTE 445 #118
Sparks, NV 89441
Tel: (775) 843 7574
Email: jackie.beug@bbics.net
Website: http://www.bbics.net

Brain Solutions, Inc
8515 Edna Ave Suite 110
Las Vegas, NV 89117
Tel: (702) 340 2248
Email: info@BrainSolutionsInc.com
Website: http://www.brainsolutionsinc.com/
Facebook: https://www.facebook.com/
brainsolutionsnv?ref=bookmarks

Uses programs such as Tomatis®, Cellfield and Interactive Metronome to improve memory, attention, self-control and processing, and reduce anxiety.

Campbell Center for Autism
Sterling Park
7530 W. Sahara Ave. Suite 104
Las Vegas, NV 89117
Tel: (702) 260 2360
Email: jcampbell@campbellcenterforautism.com
Website: http://www.campbellcenterforautism.com

Services include ABA intervention, social skills programs, parent training, IEP consultation, typical sibling support groups, and community training.

CARE – Collaborative Autism Resources and Education
CARE, LLC
57 Meadowhawk Lane
Las Vegas, NV 89135
Tel: (702) 685 6713
Email: TRV1@cox.net
Website: http://educatorscare.com

The Gateway Center Las Vegas
74 N. Pecos Suite C
Henderson, NV 89074
Tel: (702) 778 4500
Email: info@gatewaycenterlasvegas.com
Website: http://gatewaycenterlasvegas.com/

Combines Applied Behavior Analysis, speech therapy, occupational therapy, neuropsychological assessment, and psychiatric treatment.

Dr. Melissa Kalodner
10120 S. Eastern Ave, Suite 225
Henderson, NV 89052
Tel: (702) 492 1232
Website: http://drkalodner.com/index.html

My Left Foot Children's Therapy
3030 S Jones Blvd., Suite 105
Las Vegas, NV 89146
Tel: (702) 360 1137
Email: Therapy@MLFChildrensTherapy.com
Website: http://www.mlfchildrenstherapy.com

Provides Physical Therapy, Occupational Therapy, Speech Therapy, Feeding Therapy, Aquatic Therapy,

Adaptive Swimming Lessons, and Group Classes for Children with Special Needs including: Yoga, Tae Kwon Do, Sensory Classes, and Social Classes.

N.E.A.T. Nevada Equine Assisted Therapy
P.O. Box 19935
Reno, NV 89511
Tel: (775) 473 5548
Email: NEATinfo@yahoo.com
Website: http://www.NevadaEquineAssistedTherapy.com
https://www.facebook.com/pages/
NEAT/218791952876

Nevada Behavioral Solutions
6889 S. Eastern Avenue
Las Vegas, NV 89032
Tel: (702) 900 0629
Email: info@nevadabehavioralsolutions.com
Website: http://www.nevadabehavioralsolutions.com/

Note-Able Music Therapy Services
McKinley Arts & Culture Center 925 Riverside Dr.,
Suites 1, 6 & 7
Reno, NV 89503
Tel: (775) 324 5521
Email: manal@note-ables.org
Website: http://note-ables.org
https://www.facebook.com/
NoteAbleMusicTherapyServices

Play and Learn Pediatric Occupational Therapy
3900 W. Charleston Blvd. #130
Las Vegas, NV 89102
Tel: (702) 250 7872
Email: bwburnett@playandlearnot.com
Website: http://www.playandlearnot.com

Provides evaluation and treatment to children ages birth through 12, including sensory integration therapy, therapeutic listening, and Handwriting Without Tears.

Proactive Autism Solutions
6767 W. Charleston Blvd. Suite 150
Las Vegas, NV 89146
Tel: (702) 754 6133
Email: info@proactiveautismsolutions.com
Website: http://www.proactiveautismsolutions.com

Provides ABA-based services.

Rescue My Speech
1510 W. Horizon Ridge Suite 160
Henderson, NV 89052
Tel: (702) 566 8255
Email: speech@rescuemyspeech.com
Website: http://www.rescuemyspeech.com
Facebook: https://www.facebook.com/
RescueMySpeech

Speech Therapy Center of Excellence, Inc
5552 S. Fort Apache Road Suite 120
Las Vegas, NV 89148
Tel: (702) 641 8255
Email: info@speechtherapycenterlv.com
Website: http://www.speechtherapycenterlv.com

Speech Works by Elissa
Las Vegas, NV 89101
Tel: (702) 733 8255
Email: info@speechworksbyelissa.com
Website: http://speechworksbyelissa.com/index.html

Southwest Autism & Behavioral Solutions
3027 E. Sunset Road Suite #108
Las Vegas, NV 89120
Tel: (702) 270 3219
Email: vfessenden@southwestbehavior.com
Website: http://www.southwestbehavior.com
https://www.facebook.com/pages/Southwest-Autism-Behavioral-Solutions/169341643106675

Southwest Autism & Behavioral Solutions provides direct ABA services to children and adolescents with ASD, including discrete trial teaching, picture exchange communication system, verbal behavior, incidental teaching, and functional behavior plans.

Summit Autism Services
848 N. Rainbow Blvd #2717
Las Vegas, NV 89107
Tel: (866) 610 2517
Email: info@summitautism.com
Website: http://www.summitautism.com

Provides ABA-based services to children with autism and other developmental disabilities.

Synapse Music Therapy
Las Vegas, NV 89128
Tel: (630) 392 1404
Email: bihinz@gmail.com
Website: http://www.synapsemusictherapy.com
https://www.facebook.com/synapsemusictherapylasvegas?fref=ts

Schools and Educational Services

Association of University Centers on Disabilities
Nevada University AUCD
University of Nevada 1664 N. Virginia St.
Reno, NV 89557
Tel: (775) 784 1110
Email: aucdinfo@aucd.org
Website: http://www.aucd.org
https://www.facebook.com/AUCDnetwork?ref=ts

Explore Knowledge Academy
5871 Mountain Vista St.
Las Vegas, NV 89120
Tel: (702) 870 5032
Email: info@ekacademy.org
Website: http://www.ekacademy.org/
https://www.facebook.com/exploreknowledgeacademy

Explore Knowledge Academy is a K-12, Project based Charter school in Las Vegas, NV.

Newton Learning Center
700 Greenbrae Drive
Sparks, NV 89431
Tel: (775) 358 0808
Email: rebeccaj@secondstart.org
Website: http://www.secondstart.org/newton_learning_center_northern_nevada.aspx
https://www.facebook.com/pages/Second-Start-Learning-Disabilities-Programs-Inc/124486539841?ref=bookmarks

A social-cognitive school for students on the Autism Spectrum.

Wahoe County School District
425 East Ninth Street
Reno, NV 89512
Tel: (775) 348 0200
Email: communications@washoeschools.net
Website: http://www.washoeschools.net/washoeschools
https://www.facebook.com/WashoeCountySchoolDistrict

Legal, Government & Financial Services

Desert Regional Center
1391 South Jones Boulevard
Las Vegas, NV 89146
Tel: (702) 486 6200
Website: http://mhds.nv.gov/

Law Offices of Benjamin Nadig, Chtd.
324 S. 3rd Street Suite 1
Las Vegas, NV 89101
Tel: (702) 545 7592
Email: nadigbenlaw@gmail.com
Website: http://www.benjaminnadig.com

Nevada Bureau of Vocational Rehabilitation
1370 South Curry Street
Carson City, NV 89703
Tel: (775) 684 4040
Email: detradmn@nvdetr.org
Website: http://detr.state.nv.us/Rehab%20Pages/voc%20rehab.htm

Nevada Department of Health and Human Services
1100 E. William Street Suite 101
Carson City, NV 89701
Tel: (775) 684 3600
Website: https://dhcfp.nv.gov/index.htm

Nevada Disability, Advocacy & Law Center
NDALC Las Vegas
2820 West Charleston Boulevard #11
Las Vegas, NV 89102
Tel: (702) 257 8150
Toll Free: (888) 349 3843
Website: http://www.ndalc.org

Nevada Early Intervention Services – Project ASSIST
Daniel Dinnell – State Family Resource Coordinator
Information & Referral Specialist
Department of Health and Human Services
IDEA Part C Office
Early Childhood Special Education Library
4126 Technology Way, Suite 100
Carson City, Nevada 89706
Email: ddinnell@dhhs.nv.gov
Toll Free: (800) 522 0066

Office of Special Education, Elementary and Secondary Education, and School Improvement Programs
700 E. Fifth Street Suite 113
Carson City, NV 89701
Tel: (775) 687 9200
Email: rfitzpatrick@doe.nv.gov
Website: http://nde.doe.nv.gov/SpecialEducation.htm

Special Care
PO Box 12838
Las Vegas, NV 89112
Tel: (248) 613 1198
Email: rsheffield@finsvcs.com
Website: http://www.massmutual.com/specialcare
Financial planning services.

Community and Recreation Services

Amplify Life, Home of Camp Lotsafun
3660 Baker Lane, Suite 103
Reno, NV 89509
Tel: (775) 827 3866
Email: info@AmplifyLife.org
Website: http://www.amplifylife.org
https://www.facebook.com/camp.lotsafun.9

Provides recreational, therapeutic, and educational programs for children, teens, and adults with developmental and cognitive disabilities. Hosts recreational camps, as well as community day programs and events in the Northern Nevada and Northern California area.

The Arc in Nevada
3983 S. McCarran Blvd #311
Reno, NV 89502
Toll Free: (800) 433 5255 Ext 3260
Email: perez@thearc.org
Website: http://www.thearcnevada.org
https://www.facebook.com/thearcnevada

Asperger's Syndrome/High Functioning Autism Support Group
72 N. Pecos Road Suite C
Henderson, NV 89012
Tel: (702) 421 1356
Email: aspergerhfagrp@aol.com
Website: http://aspergerhfagrp.com

Families for Effective Autism Treatment (FEAT) of Southern Nevada
7055 Windy St. Suite B
Las Vegas, NV 89119
Tel: (702) 368 3328
Email: help@featsonv.org
Website: http://www.featsonv.org
https://www.facebook.com/FEATsonevada

Provides information on treatment resources for families with children diagnosed with autism, autism spectrum disorder (ASD), and related disorders.

Family Ties of Nevada
Las Vegas: 6130 Elton Avenue, Suite 100
Las Vegas, NV 89107
(702) 740 4200
Email: info@familytiesnv.org
Website: http://www.familytiesnv.org

Goodfriends
10139 Donald Weese Ct
Las Vegas, NV 89129
Tel: (702) 818 5120
Email: GoodfriendsLV@hotmail.com
Website: http://www.meetup.com/LasVegas-Goodfriends/

Goodwill of Southern Nevada
1280 W. Cheyenne Ave
Las Vegas, NV 89030
Tel: (702) 214 2000
Website: http://www.sngoodwill.net/
https://www.facebook.com/GoodwillofSouthernNevada

Provides education, employment and training for people with disabilities and other barriers to employment, and to maximize the quality of life for each individual served.

Grant a Gift Autism Foundation
8550 West Desert Inn Road Suite 102-343
Las Vegas, NV 89117
Tel: (702) 564 2453
Email: info@grantagiftautismfoundation.org
Website: http://www.grantagiftfoundation.org/
https://www.facebook.com/GrantaGift?fref=ts

Programs include navigation & service coordination of a broad range of resources for families, community care assistance program, social/life skills groups, TeenWorks a vocational work Program as well as a sibling social support group.

JUSTin HOPE Foundation
P.O. Box 13383
Reno, NV 89507
Tel: (775) 453 9262
Email: justinhopefoundation@gmail.com
Website: http://www.justinhope.org/

Provides medical equipment, supplies and/or opportunities otherwise not available.

Nevada PEP – Parents Encouraging Parents
Nevada PEP
7211 W. Charleston Blvd.
Las Vegas, NV 89117
Tel: 702.388.8899
Email: pepinfo@nvpep.org
Website: http://www.nvpep.org
https://www.facebook.com/nvpep

Nevada Yellow Pages for Kids
Website: http://www.yellowpagesforkids.com/help/nv.htm

Find educational consultants, psychologists, educational diagnosticians, health care providers, academic therapists, tutors, speech language therapists, occupational therapists, coaches, advocates, and attorneys. You will also find special education schools, learning centers, treatment programs, parent groups, respite care, community centers, grassroots organizations, and government programs.

Northern Nevada Autism Network
c/o Dr Dean Ward
618 Idaho Street #3
Elko, NV 89801
Tel: (775) 753 9243
Email: info@nnan.org
Website: http://www.nnan.org/

Northern Nevada Center for Independent Living
999 Pyramid Way
Sparks, NV 89431
Tel: (775) 353 3599

Email: info@medtech-services.com
Website: http://www.nncil.org

Opportunity Village
6300 W. Oakey Boulevard
Las Vegas, NV 89146
Tel: (702) 259 3700
Website: http://www.opportunityvillage.org

Provides vocational training, community employment, day services, advocacy, arts and social recreation.

Sport-Social
7055 Windy St. Suite B
Las Vegas, NV 89119
Tel: (702) 485 5515
Email: Info@LVSportSocial.com
Website: http://www.lasvegasautism.com
https://www.facebook.com/sportsocial

Using ABA-based methods, teaches social skills to children and young adults through instruction in action sports, team sports, and the arts.

Trinity West
Stephanie Pohl
240 S. Rock Blvd.
Suite 133
Reno, NV 89502
Tel: (775) 857 2500
Email: spohl@trinity-services.org
Website: http://www.trinity-services.org/default.aspx
https://www.facebook.com/trinityservices

VSA Arts of Nevada
250 Court Street
Reno, NV 89501
Tel: (775) 826 6100, ext. 3#
Email: info@vsanevada.org
Website: http://www.vsanevada.org
https://www.facebook.com/pages/VSA-Nevada/155714231111759

Statewide program that provides children and adults with disabilities, the opportunity to experience the visual and performing arts first hand through participation in arts festivals, art workshops, classroom art residencies, training workshops and a variety of special events.

NEW HAMPSHIRE

Doctors, Clinics, Hospitals, and Other Health Services

Cedarcrest Center for Children with Disabilities
91 Maple avenue
Keene, NH 3431

Tel: (603) 358 3384 or (603) 358 3389
Website: http://www.cedarcrest4kids.org
Facebook: https://www.facebook.com/CedarcrestCenter

Center for Integrative Medicine
81 Hall Street
Suite 1
Concord, NH 03301
Tel: (603) 228 7245
Website: www.cfim.org

Individualized, integrative healthcare.

Core Physicians
7 Holland Way
Exeter, NH 03833
Tel: (603) 580 7939
Website: http://www.corephysicians.org/services/
primary-care-children-infants/
Facebook: https://www.facebook.com/CorePhysicians

Dartmouth-Hitchcock Medical Center
1 Medical Center Drive
Lebanon, NH 03756
Tel: (603) 650 5000
Website: http://www.dhmc.org
Facebook: https://www.facebook.com/
DartmouthHitchcock

Gail Vanark, MSN FNP-BC
3 Overlook Drive
Suite 1Amherst, NH 03031
Tel: (603) 673 7910
Website: www.preventivemedicinenh.com

Hampstead Hospital Developmental Disorders Program
218 East Road
Hampstead, NH 03841
Tel: (603) 329 5311
Email: info@hampsteadhospital.com
Website: http://www.hampsteadhospital.com/
developmental_disorders.htm

Heather Tallman Ruhm, MD
13 Torrey Road
Nashua, NH 03063
Tel: (603) 889 0508
Website: www.cfim.org

Nashua Dentistry for Children
155 Kinsley Street
Nashua, NH 03060
Tel: (603) 889 2164
Email: info@nashuadocs.com
Website: http://www.nashuadocs.com

Seacoast Child Development Clinic
University of New Hampshire-Institute on Disability/
UCED
55 College Road, 103 Pettee Hall
Durham, NH 03824
Tel: (603) 862 0561
E-mail: Seacoast.Clinic@unh.edu
Website: http://www.seacoastclinic.unh.edu/

Therapy Services

ABA4Autism, Inc.
P.O. Box 944
Milford, NH 03054
Tel: (603) 554 1820
Contact Name: Dawn Faucher
Email: dawn.faucher@aba4autism.net
Website: http://www.aba4autism.net
Facebook: https://www.facebook.com/ABA4AutismNH

Applied Behavioral Associates, LLC
Norcross Circle, PO Box 1304
North Conway, NH 03860
Tel: (603) 356 6616
Email: info@aba4kids.org
Website: http://www.aba4kids.org/

Autism Bridges
360 Route 101 Suite 11
Bedford, NH 03110
Tel: (603) 471 2522
Email: info@autismbridges.com
Website: http://www.autismbridges.com
Facebook: https://www.facebook.com/AutismBridges

Specializes in ABA therapy for children diagnosed with ASD and related disorders.

Becket Family of Services
P. O Box 58
Plymouth, NH 03264
Tel: (855) 536 1102
Email: jeff.caron@becket.org
Website: http://www.becket.org

Capital Kids OT
124 Hall Street Suite H
Concord, NH 03301
Tel: (603) 228 9160
Email: lynne@capitalkidsot.com
Website: http://www.capitalkidsot.com
Facebook: https://www.facebook.com/CapitalKidsOccu
pationalTherapy?fref=ts

Provides OT treatment focusing on sensory processing, fine and gross motor coordination and ADL's while using ABA techniques, Social Stories and PECS.

The Carriage Barn
PO Box 5
Kingston, NH 03857
Tel: (603) 378 0140
Website: http://carriage-barn.org

Equine-assisted therapy programs, including riding and therapeutic carriage driving activities for individuals of all ages with disabilities.

Constellations Behavioral Services
200 Griffin Rd. Suite 5
Portsmouth, NH 03801
Tel: (800) 778 5560
Email: info@constellationsbehavioral.com
Website: http://www.constellationsbehavioral.com

Works with schools and parents to develop and implement ABA programs.

Erin Neely, Psy.D.
370 Portsmouth Ave.
Greenland, NH 03840
Tel: (603) 531 1177
Email: erin@drerinneely.com
Website: http://www.drerinneely.com

Provides treatment for children with developmental disorders from preschool age through their early teens using a variety of modalities including visual aids, play therapy, social stories, Social Thinking curriculum, cognitive behavioral techniques, anxiety management, educational planning support, and behavior modification.

Portsmouth Music and Arts Center
973 Islington Street
Portsmouth, NH 03801
Tel: (603) 431 4278
Email: katie@pmaconline.org
Website: http://www.pmaconline.org

Music Therapy and Art Therapy.

Greater Nashua Mental Health Center at Community Council
100 West Pearl Street
Nashua, NH 03060
Tel: (603) 889 6147
Toll Free: (800) 762 8191
Email: contact@gnmhc.org
Website: http://www.gnmhc.org/
Facebook: https://www.facebook.com/pages/Greater-Nashua-Mental-Health-Center-at-Community-Council/277501002266097

Hands On Personal Education (HOPE) Behavioral Services, LLC
Portsmouth, NH 03801

Tel: (603) 812 5521
Email: hope.b.c.info@gmail.com
Website: http://www.hopebehavioralconsulting.com

Behavioral consulting for children and their families.

The Institute of Professional Practice, Inc.
6 Chenell Drive - Suite 100
Concord, NH 03301
Tel: (603) 224 8085 X1820
Email: info@ippi.org
Website: http://www.ippi.org
Facebook: https://www.facebook.com/IPPI.NH

Provides in-home ABA, 2 center-based programs, and some adult services.

Joshua Gear, MD
Psychiatrist
20 Ladd Street Suite 402
Portsmouth, NH 03801
Tel: (603) 610 0235
Email: info@joshuagearmd.com
Website: http://www.joshuagearmd.com

Psychiatric evaluation and treatment for children, adolescents and adults.

Manchester Community Music School
2291 Elm St
Manchester, NH 03104
Tel: (603) 644 4548
Email: info@mcmusicschool.org
Website: http://www.mcmusicschool.org
Facebook: https://www.facebook.com/mcmusicschool

Providing music therapy in both 1:1 and group sessions to individuals on the Autism Spectrum. Adaptive music lessons are also provided.

Monadnock Family Services
64 Main Street, Suite 301
Keene, NH 03431
Tel: (603) 357 4400
Website: http://www.mfs.org/

Northern Human Services
87 Washington Street
Conway, NH 03818
Tel: (603) 447 3347
Website: http://www.northernhs.org/

Positive Reinforcement (PR) ABA Therapy, Inc.
373 South Willow St Suite 266
Manchester, NH 03103
Tel: (877) 315 8080
Email: info@prabatherapy.com
Website: http://www.prabatherapy.com

The Rhythm Tree Music Therapy
16 Oak Street
Exeter, NH 03833
Tel: (603) 793 1941
Contact Name: Ryan Judd, MA, MT-BC
Email: ryan@therhythmtree.com
Website: http://www.ryanjudd.net
Facebook: https://www.facebook.com/
TheRhythmTreeMusic

Sara J. Lang OTR/L
7 Boomhower Rd.
Woodsville, NH 03785
Tel: (603) 986 8240
Email: sara@tracetherapeutics.com
Website: http://www.tracetherapeutics.com

Sonatina Music Therapy
130 Central Ave Suite 203
Dover, NH 03820
Tel: (603) 978 4808
Email: info@sonatinamusictherapy.com
Website: http://www.sonatinamusictherapy.com

Services include, individual music therapy sessions, group music therapy sessions, workshops for parents, caregivers & professionals, and music therapy assisted childbirth serves.

Speech Therapy Solutions, Inc.
224 Main Street Suite 2D
Salem, NH 03079
Tel: (603) 893 8550
Email: info@speechtherapysolutions.com
Website: http://www.speechtherapysolutions.com
Facebook: https://www.facebook.com/
speechtherapysolutions

Providing speech, occupational, physical therapy, and academic tutoring.

Stephen Quinlan, LICSW
53 Washington Street
Suite LL116
Dover, NH 03820
Tel: (603) 952 4161
Email: quinlan@gmail.com
Website: http://www.stephenquinlan.net

Swing for the Stars Pediatric Therapy Center
2 Pillsbury Street, Suite 404
Concord, NH 3301
Tel: (603) 228 7827
Email: info@swingforthestars.com
Website: http://www.swingforthestars.com
Facebook: https://www.facebook.com/SwingfortheStars

Provides occupational therapy and speech therapy services to children ages birth to 18, including treating sensory processing disorders and ASD.

Training Wheels Occupational Therapy
1360 South St
Portsmouth, NH 3801
Tel: (603) 501 0897
Email: molly@trainingwheelsnh.com
Website: http://www.trainingwheelsnh.com
Facebook: https://www.facebook.com/pages/Training-Wheels-Occupational-Therapy/285187118159613?sk=wall&filter=12

Occupational therapy for children with Sensory Integration difficulties, Autism Spectrum Disorders, and sensory, motor and developmental delays. Specializing in toddlers and preschoolers, sensory diets, and Therapeutic Listening.

West Central Behavioral Health
9 Hanover Street, Suite 2
Lebanon, NH 03766
Tel: (603) 448 0126
Website: http://www.wcbh.org/home.php?msg=RS

Wings and Hooves Therapeutic Riding, Inc.
PO Box 336
East Kingston, NH 03038
Tel: (603) 642 3722
Email: riding@wingsandhooves.org
Website: http://www.wingsandhooves.org
Facebook: https://www.facebook.com/
WingsandHooves

Schools and Educational Services

Birchtree Center
2064 Woodbury Avenue Suite 204
Newington, NH 03801-2808
Tel: (603) 433 4192
Website: http://www.birchtreecenter.org

NFI North-The Braford School
252 Route 103
Braford, NH 3221
Tel: (603) 938 2556
Email: anngratton@nafi.com
Website: http://www.nfinorth.com/nafinfi/Programs/
BehavioralHealth/BradfordSchoolNH.aspx

A fully licensed special education middle/high school serving boys and girls, offering individualized programs and clinical services.

Hampshire Country School
122 Hampshire Road
Rindge, NH 03461

Tel: (603) 899 3325
Email: office@hampshirecountryschool.net
Website: http://www.hampshirecountryschool.org

A boys-only boarding school, primarily offering middle school classes.

The Hunter School
768 Doetown Road PO Box 600
Runmey, NH 03266
Tel: (603) 786 9427
Email: info@hunterschool.org
Website: http://www.thehunterschool.org

The Hunter School is a therapeutic day and residential school for boys and girls with ADHD, Aspergers Syndrome and related conditions.

Lakeview NeuroRehabilitation Center
244 Highwatch Road
Effingham, NH 03882
Tel: (603) 539 7451
Toll Free: (800) 473 4221
Contact Name: Kim Giles, LICSW, Director of Admissions
Email: kgiles@lakeviewsystem.com
Website: http://www.lakeviewsystem.com/
https://www.facebook.com/lakeview

Serving youth and adults with neurological diagnoses providing a Special Education Accredited School that serves youth with ASD from age 8 to 22, as well as Psychiatry, Neurology, Neuropsychology, ABA, Physical Therapy, Occupational Therapy & Speech Therapy.

Monarch School of New England
61 Eastern Avenue P.O Box 1921
Rochester, NH 3886
Tel: (603) 332 2848
(603) 330 0566
Contact Name: Gail Henderson
Email: ghenderson@monarchschoolne.org
Website: http://www.monarchschoolne.org
Facebook: https://www.facebook.com/MonarchSchool
NewEngland?rf=158168664214629

Parker Academy
2 Fisk Road
Concord, NH 3301
Tel: (603) 410 6240
Email: contact@parkeracademy.com
Website: http://www.parkeracademy.com
Facebook: https://www.facebook.com/
parkereducationNH

Parker Academy is a private day school for middle and high school students.

Seacoast Learning Collaborative
87 State Route 27
Brentwood, NH 03833
Tel: (603) 679 2021
Email: rdiamontopoulos@slconline.org
Website: http://slconline.org/

SLC offers day programs serving elementary to high school aged students.

START Hospitality Program at Great Bay Community College
320 Corporate Drive
Portsmouth, NH 03801
Tel: (603) 427 7651
Email: ktotten@ccsnh.edu
Website: http://greatbay.edu/btcstart
Facebook: https://www.facebook.com/greatbaycc

START (Skills, Tasks, And Results Training), is a one-year classroom and internship curriculum for students over 18 years of age with special needs interested in the Hospitality Industry.

Wediko Children's Services
11 Bobcat Blvd.
Windsor, NH 03244
Tel: (603) 478 5236
Website: http://www.wediko.org
Facebook: https://www.facebook.com/
WedikoChildrensServices

Legal, Government & Financial Services

Ann N. Butenhof, CELA
Attorney
149 Hanover Street Suite 300
Manchester, NH 03101
Tel: (603) 296 0428 or (603) 296 0430
Email: ann@butenhofbomster.com
Website: http://www.butenhofbomster.com/

Legal services with respect to Medicaid eligibility rules, other public benefits programs, special needs trusts, long-term care planning and estate planning.

Cooper, Cargill, Chant P.A
Attorney
110 Pleasant Street PO Box 157
Berlin, NH 03570
Phone (603) 752 5200
Email: info@coopercargillchant.com
Website: http://www.coopercargillchant.com

Department of Housing and Urban Development
275 Chestnut St. 4th Floor
Manchester, NH 03101

Tel: (603) 666 7510
Email: NH_webmanager@hud.gov
Website: http://www.hud.gov/local/index.
cfm?state=nh&topic=offices

Disabilities Rights Center
64 N Main Street, Suite 2
Concord, NH 03301-4913
Tel: (603) 228 0432
Toll Free: (800) 834 1721
Email: advocacy@drcnh.org
Website: http://www.drcnh.org

Drummond Woodsum
100 International Drive Suite 340
Portsmouth, NH 03801
Tel: (603) 433 3317
Email: info@dwmlaw.com
Website: http://www.dwmlaw.com

Special education legal services.

Bureau of Special Education
101 Pleasant Street
Concord, NH 3301
(603) 271 2178
Contact Name: Ruth Littlefield
Email: rlittlefield@ed.state.nh.us
Website: http://www.education.nh.gov/instruction/
special_ed/

John S. Kitchen
Advocate
15 Dartmouth Street Suite 203
Auburn, NH 03032
Tel: (603) 669 6541
Email: johnjklaw@metrocast.com
Website: http://www.johnkitchenlawoffices.com/index.
html

Practice areas include probate, trust, gift and estate taxation and disability law.

Hamblett & Kerrigan, PA
20 Trafalgar Square, Suite 505
Nashua, NH 03063
Tel: (603) 883 5501
Toll Free: (800) 649 9503
Email: info@nashualaw.com
Website: http://www.nashualaw.com
Facebook: https://www.facebook.com/pages/Hamblett-
Kerrigan-PA/445201365539601?ref=stream

Special education and family law.

New Hampshire Hospital (NH Department of Health & Human Services)
36 Clinton Street
Concord, NH 03301

Tel: (603) 271 5300
Toll Free: (800) 852 3345 x 5300
Website: http://www.dhhs.nh.gov/dcbcs/nhh/index.htm

New Hampshire Vocational Rehabilitation
21 S. Fruit Street Suite 20
Concord, NH 03301
Tel: (603) 271 3471
Email contact: Lisa.Hatz@doe.nh.gov
Website: http://education.nh.gov/career/vocational/

Community and Recreation Services

Children's Museum of NH Autism Partnership Program, Exploring Our Way
6 Washington Street
Dover, NH 03820
Tel: (603) 742 2002
Email: paula@childrens-museum.org
Website: http://www.childrens-museum.org
http://www.childrens-museum.org/cmnh2010/
programs/content.aspx?id=420
Facebook: https://www.facebook.com/
ExploringOurWay

Concord Regional Arc, Inc.
P.O. Box 1173
Concord, NH 03302-1173
Tel: (603) 228 8279

Crotched Mountain (CM) Foundation
One Verney Dr.
Greenfield, NH 03047
Tel: (603) 547 3311
Email: info@crotchedmountain.org
Website: http://www.crotchedmountain.org

Provides specialized education, rehabilitation, community and residential support services.

Early Education and Intervention Network
2 Delta Drive
Concord, NH 03301
Tel: (603) 228 2040
Email: info@eeinnh.org
Website: http://www.eeinnh.org

Farmsteads of New England (FNE), Inc.
213 Center Road
Hillsborough, NH 03244
Tel: (603) 464 2590
Email: info@farmsteads-ne.org
Website: http://www.farmsteads-ne.org
Facebook: https://www.facebook.com/
farmsteadsofnewengland?fref=ts

Gateways Community Services
144 Canal St.
Nashua, NH 03064
Tel: (603) 882 6333
Email: info@gatewayscs.org
Website: http://www.gatewayscs.org/default.htm

Granite State Independent Living (GSIL)
21 Chenall Drive
Concord, NH 03301
(800) 826 3700
Email: info@gsil.org
Website: http://www.gsil.org
Facebook: https://www.facebook.com/
GraniteStateIndependentLiving

Greengard Center for Autism
PO Box 6596
Portsmouth, NH 03802
Tel: (603) 501 0686
Email: greengardcenter@gmail.com
Website: http://www.greengardcenter.org
Facebook: https://www.facebook.com/GreengardCenter

Day and residential programs for young adults with autism.

Inside Out Skill Development, LLC
112 North Policy Street
Salem, NH 03079
Tel: (603) 401 0842
Email: Nate@inside-out-development.com
Website: http://www.inside-out-development.com/

Lakes Region Community Services
635 Main Street
Laconia, NH 3249
Tel: (603) 524 8811
Email: info@lrcs.org
Website: http://www.lrcs.org
Facebook: https://www.facebook.com/pages/Lakes-Region-Community-Services/138925762841545

Early Intervention Program and Day Program serving the Lakes Region of NH.

Moore Center Services
195 McGregor St. Suite 400
Manchester, NH 03102
Tel: (603) 206 2700
Email: info@moorecenter.org
Website: http://www.moorecenter.org
Facebook: https://www.facebook.com/themoorecenter

New England Handicapped Sports Association
PO Box 2135
Newbury, NH 3255
Tel: (603) 763 9158

Email: info@nehsa.org
Website: http://www.nehsa.org
Facebook: https://www.facebook.com/
groups/38082022470/?fref=ts

NH Family Ties
Toll Free: (800) 499 4153 x241
Website: http://www.nhfamilyties.org/
Facebook: https://www.facebook.com/pages/
NH-Family-Ties/109319742481521?sk=info&tab=
overview

Parent Information Center (PIC)
54 Old Suncook Road
Concord, NH 03301
Tel: (603) 224 7005
Toll Free: (800) 947 7005
Website: http://www.parentinformationcenter.org

Plowshare Farm Lifesharing Community
32 Whitney Drive
Greenfield, NH 03047
Tel: (603) 547 2547
Email: info@plowsharefarm.org
Website: http://plowsharefarm.org

The River Center
Parent Support Group
46 Concord Street
Peterborough, NH 03458
Email: 4dininos@comcast.net
Website: http://www.rivercenter.us/

Yavneh Family Camp for Families Affected by Autism
PO Box 200
W. Nottingham, NH 03291
Tel: (617) 559 8860
Contact Name: Debbie Sussman, Director
Email: Debbie@campyavneh.org
Website: http://www.campyavneh.org
Facebook: https://www.facebook.com/CampYavneh?ref=ts

NEW JERSEY

Doctors, Clinics, Hospitals and Other Health Services

Advocare Atrium Pediatrics
301 Old Marton Pike West Suite 1
Marlton, NJ 08053
Tel: (856) 988 9101
Contact Name: Therese Zeitz
Email: tzeitz@challc.net
Website: http://www.advocareatriumpediatrics.com

Atlantic Integrative Medical Associates
Center for Well Being 101 Madison Ave, Suite 202
Morristown, NJ 07960
Tel: (973) 971 4686
Website: www.atlantichealth.org

The Autism Center
New Jersey Medical School
Behavioral Health Sciences Building F-level
Newark, NJ 07103
Tel: (973) 972 8930 or (973) 972 9422
Website: http://www.umdnj.edu/autismcenter

Center for Neurological and Neurodevelopmental Health (CNNH)
250 Haddonfield-Berlin Rd Suite 105
Gibbsboro, NJ 08026
Tel: (856) 346 0005
Contact Email: info@thecnnh.org
Website: http://www.theCNNH.org

Children's Specialized Hospital
313 South Avenue
Fanwood, NJ 07023
Toll Free: 888 CHILDREN (244 5373)
Contact Name: Jill Harris, Ph.D. Coordinator of Autism Center of Excellence Locations
Email: jharris@childrens-specialized.org
Website: http://www.childrens-specialized.org

Delaware Valley Pediatrics
132 Franklin Corner Road
Lawrenceville, NJ 08648
Tel: (609) 896 4141
Contact Name: Dr. Halvorsen
Website: http://www.delvalpeds.com

Dentistry for Special Needs Children
368 Lakehurst Road Suite 305
Toms River, NJ 08755
Tel: (732) 473 1123
Contact Name: Dr. Elisa Velazquez
Email: evdmd@yahoo.com
Website: http://www.oceanpediatricdental.com

Developmental Disabilities Center (DDC) at Morristown Medical Center
100 Madison Ave.
Morristown, NJ 07960
Tel: (973) 971 4095 Medical Appointments
Tel: (973) 971 5302 Mental Health Appointments
Website: www.atlantichealth.org

Developmental Pediatrics of Central Jersey
1806 Highway 35 Suite 107
Oakhurst, NJ 07755
Tel: (732) 660 0220
Contact Name: Alison Smoller, D.O.
Email: drsmoller@developmentalpediatricsnj.com
Website: http://www.developmentalpediatricsnj.com

Georges Ghacibeh, MD
255 West Spring Valley Avenue
Ste 205
Maywood, NJ 07607
Tel: (201) 546 8510
Website: www.progressiveneurology.com

A pediatric and adult neurology practice focusing on seizures and epilepsy, behavioral neurology and autism, and sleep disorders.

Hopewell Pharmacy and Compounding Center
1 West Broad StreetHopewell, NJ 08525
Tel: (800) 792 6670 or (609) 466 1960Fax: (800) 417 3864 or (609) 466 8222
Email: info@hopewellrx.com
Website: www.hopewellrx.com

Compounding pharmacy.

James Neubrander, MD
Road to Recovery Clinic
485A Route 1 South, Ste. 320
Iselin, NJ 08830
Tel: (732) 726 1222

Provides biomedical treatments, hyperbaric oxygen therapy, neurofeedback and QEEG, and other modalities for treating patients with ASD and other health conditions.

JFK Medical Center
65 James Street
Edison, NJ 08818
Tel: (732) 321 7000
Contact Name: Patricia Munday, Ed.D.
Website: http://www.jfkmc.org

Jodie A. Dashore OTD, MS (Pediatric Neurology), OTR/L, SIC, NDTC, TLPC, BOMC, BCHHP
Integrative NeuroSensory Associates, LLC
11 Burlington Drive
Marlboro, NJ 07746
Tel: (732) 772 1989
Fax: (732) 333 4526
Email: jdashore2@yahoo.com
Website: www.mysptc.com

Functional medicine and sensory integration practice.

K. Hovnanian Children's Hospital at Jersey Shore University Medical Center
1945 Route 33
Neptune, NJ 07753
Tel: (732) 776 4178
Website: http://www.khovnanianchildrenshospital.com

Laura Lagano, MS RD CDN
Laura Lagano Nutrition LLC
931 Bloomfield Street
Hoboken, NJ 07030
Tel: (917) 829 0250
Website: www.lauralagano.com
Individualized nutritional plans.

Ocean Pediatric Dental
368 Lakehurst Rd, Ste 305
Toms River, NJ 08755
Tel: (732) 473 1123
Contact Name: Dr Velaszuez
Email: EVDMD@yahoo.com
Website: http://www.oceanpediatricdental.com

Pediatric Dentistry of Wayne
Dr. Patrick Dinicola
330 Ratzer Road
Wayne, NJ 07470
Tel: (973) 696 6002

St. Joseph's Hospital & Medical Center
703 Main Street
Paterson, NJ 07501
Tel: (973) 754 2510
Website: http://www.stjosephshealth.org

Stuart Freedenfeld, MD
Stockton Family Practice
56 South Main Street
Stockton, NJ 08559
Tel: (609) 397 8585
Website: www.stocktonfp.com
Providing a wide variety of treatments for autism and many other conditions.

Tender Smiles
122 Professional View Drive
Freehold, NJ 07728
Tel: (732) 625 8080
Contact Name: Surbhi Alaigh
Email: tendersmiles4kids@yahoo.com
Website: http://www.tendersmiles4kids.com

Total Life Center
Peta Cohen MS RD
11 North Dean Street
Englewood, NJ 07631

Tel: (201) 541 7601
Website: www.totallifecenter.com
Individualized nutritional and related interventions for children and adults.

Therapy Services

Angelfish Therapy
Tel: (203) 545 0024
Fax (203) 321 2138
Email: Info@AngelfishTherapy.com
Website: www.angelfishtherapy.com

Aquatic therapy, swim lesson and summer camps with many locations in Connecticut, Massachusetts, New York, and New Jersey.

Bergen Pediatric Therapy Center
354 Old Hook Road Suite 104
Westwood, NJ 07675
Tel: (201) 722 4700
Email: Info@bergenpediatrictherapy.com
Website: http://www.BergenPediatricTherapy.com

Children's Wellness & Developmental Center, LLC
2006 Highway 71 Suite 6
Spring Lake Heights, NJ 07762
Tel: (732) 919 1335
Contact Name: Kerri D'Onofrio, MSN, APN, BC
Contact Email: kdonofrio1@gmail.com
Website: http://www.cwdcenter.com

ChildWorks Therapy Center
32 Gibraltar Drive
Morris Plains, NJ 07950
Tel: (862) 219 5678
Contact Name: Neala Schuster
Email: ChildWorksLLC@aol.com
Website: http://www.ChildWorksTherapyCenter.com

Classic Rehabilitation, Ltd.
745 Poole Ave located at YMCA
Hazlet, NJ 07731
Tel: (732) 367 1888
Contact Name: Marc Lubet
Email: info@classicrehab.com
Website: http://www.classicrehab.com

Creative Speech Solutions, LLC
151 Summit Avenue
Summit, NJ 07901
Tel: (908) 598 0228
Contact Name: Cynthia Marrapodi, MS, CCC-SLP
Email: cynthia@creativespeechsolutions.com
Website: http://www.creativespeechsolutions.com

A multi-disciplinary therapy center including speech-language pathologists, occupational therapists, music therapists and a nutritionist.

Crossroads Center of NJ
Jackie DeVries MS AIBT
947 Linwood Avenue
Suite 2N
Ridgewood, NJ 07450
Tel: (201) 253 0345
Website: www.crossroadscenterofnj.com

Providing neurofeedback and other wellness therapies for those with ASD and others.

NJ ABC's: Autism Behavioral, Communication and Sensory Integration Services
3100 Quakerbridge Road #28 located in Lakeview Child Center
Mercerville, NJ 08619
Tel: (732) 987 4141
Contact Name: Sara Stern, BCBA
Email: aba@njabcs.org
Website: http://www.njabcs.org

Behavior Assessment, Functional Behavior Assessment, Applied Behavior Analysis (ABA), Social Skills Training, Speech Therapy, Occupational Therapy, Sensory Integration, Parent Training, School-based services, Educational Workshops for parents and professionals.

Pediatric Rehabilitation of North Jersey
60 Owens Drive Suite 115
Wayne, NJ 07470
Tel: (973) 956 2900
Email: info@pediatricrehab.net
Website: http://www.pediatricrehab.net

Provides speech, OT, and PT services for children 0–18.

Schools and Education Services

ACELERO Learning
142 Atkins Avenue
Asburg Park, NJ 07712
Tel: (732) 988 7736 x6107
Contact Name: Toni Harrison
Email: tharrison@acelero.net
Website: http://www.acelero.net

Alpine Learning Group
777 Paramus Road
Paramus, NJ 07652
Tel: (201) 612 7800
Website: www.alpinelearninggroup.org

Bergen Center for Child Development
140 Park Street
Haworth, NJ 07641
Tel: (201) 385 4857
Website: www.bergencenter.com

The Community School
11 West Forest Avenue
Teaneck, NJ 07666
Tel: (201) 837 8070
Website: www.communityschool.k12.nj.us

The Forum School
107 Wyckoff Avenue
Waldwick, NJ 07463
Tel: (201) 444 5882
Website: www.theforumschool.com

Devereux: New Jersey
286 Mantua Grove Road Bldg. #4
West Deptford, NJ 08066
Tel: (856) 423 8919
Website: http://www.devereuxnj.org

Durand Academy & Community Services
230 N. Evergreen Avenue
Woodbury, NJ 08096
Tel: (856) 845 0666
Contact Name: Tom Ryan Education Administrator & Principal
Email: t.ryan@durandac.org
Website: http://www.durandac.org

Kingsway Learning Center
144 Kings Highway West
Haddonfield, NJ 08033
Tel: (856) 428 8108
Contact Name: Stefanie Mis
Email: smis@kingswaylearningcenter.org
Website: http://www.kingswaylearningcenter.org

Princeton Child Development Institute (PCDI)
300 Cold Soil Rd
Princeton, NJ 08450
Tel: (609) 924 6280
Email: info@pcdi.org
Website: http://www.pcdi.org

Rutgers, The State University of New Jersey
151 Ryders Ln.
New Brunswick, NJ 08901
Tel: (732) 932 4500
Contact Name: Sandra Harris, PhD, Executive Director
Email: sharris@rci.rutgers.edu
Website: http://dddc.rutgers.edu

SEARCH Day Program
73 Wickapecko Drive
Ocean, NJ 07712
Tel: (732) 531 0454
Contact Name: Karen Rauch
Email: info@searchdayprogram.com
Website: http://www.searchdayprogram.com

Legal, Government, and Not-for-profit Services and Organizations

Alisa Jacobson Esq.
Special Education Attorney

431 Margiasso Ct.
Rivervale, NJ 07675
Tel: (201) 573 0061

ASDworld
221 Union St.
Ridgewood, NJ 07450
Tel: (646) 701 1080
Contact Name:
Rick Colosimo
Email: rick@asdworld.com
Website: http://www.asdworld.com

Lawyer-parent representing children with an ASD to secure educational rights and improve financial and estate planning. Licensed to practice in NJ, NY, and CA.

Barger & Gaines
555 Route One South Suite 340
Iselin, NJ 08830
Tel: (908) 242 3635
Email: info@bargergaines.com
Website: http://bargergaines.com

Education attorneys advocating for the rights of special needs students and adults in public and private schools.

Carole Ann Geronimo Family Law
Carole Ann Geronimo Family Law
686 Godwin Avenue Suite LL
Midland Park, NJ 07432
Tel: (201) 512 4400
Email: cageronimolaw@yahoo.com

Special education law.

Freeman Law Offices, LLC
Main Office:
103 Carnegie Center, Suite 101
Princeton, New Jersey 08540
Tel: (888) 383 3037
Fax: (609) 228 6909

Offices also located at:
4400 Route 9 South, Freehold, New Jersey 07728
19 Chestnut Street, Haddonfield, NJ 08033

Website: www.freemanlawoffices.com

Law firm specializing in meeting the legal needs of those with disabilities. Areas of practice include special education, issues with respect to college and graduate school and disabilities, adult services, health insurance, estate planning, and guardianship.

Hinkle, Fingles & Prior
Attorneys at law

147 Columbia Turnpike Suite 106
Florham Park, NJ 07932
Tel: (215) 860 2100
Email: legal@hinkle1.com
Website: http://www.hinkle1.com

Specializing in disability and elder law.

Disability Rights New Jersey
210 South Broad Street 3rd Floor
Trenton, NJ 08608
Tel: (609) 292 9742
Toll Free: (800) 792 8600
Contact Name: Sarah Wiggins Mitchell
Website: http:// http://www.drnj.org/

Rachelle H. Milstein, Esq., Special Education Attorney
45 Nottingham Drive
Watchung, NJ 07069
Tel: (908) 561 1977
Contact Name: Shelly Milstein
Contact Email: smilstein@milsteinlaw.com
Website: http://www.milsteinlaw.com

Special Needs & Beyond
1800 Route 34 Bldg. 2, Suite 201
Wall, NJ 07719
Tel: (732) 922 6300
Contact Name: Linda Blum
Email: linda.blum@margfinancial.com
Website: http://www.specialneedsandbeyond.com

Special needs financial planning.

Community and Recreation Services

Advancing Opportunities
1005 Whitehead Road Extension, Suite 1,
Ewing, New Jersey 08638
Toll Free: (888) 322 1918
Website: http://www.advopps.org/
Facebook: https://www.facebook.com/AdvancingOppo rtunities?ref=stream&fref=nf

Arts Unbound (AU)
544 Freeman Street
Orange, NJ 07050
Tel: (973) 675 2782
Contact Name: Margaret Mikkelsen, Executive Director
Email: mmikkelsen@artsunbound.org
Website: http://www.artsunbound.org

Asperger Syndrome Education Network (ASPEN)
Lutheran Church of the Good Shepherd
Glen Rock, NJ 07452
Tel: (732) 321 0880
Email: info@aspennj.org
Website: http://www.aspennj.org

Birchwood Medical Day Care Service
115 Evergreen Pl
East Orange, NJ 07018
Tel: (973) 676 2600 x 118
Contact Name: Rosa Ibanez
Website: http://www.birchwoodadc.com

Has a day program for people over 18 with developmental disabilities.

CARING & Its Affiliates
407 West Delilah Road
Pleasantville, NJ 08232
Tel: (609) 484 7050
Email: info@caringinc.org
Website: http://www.caringinc.org

The Center For Family Support
205 Robin Road Suite 122
Paramus, NJ 07652
Tel: (201) 262 4021 or (201) 262 4047
Contact Name: Barbara Greenwald
Email: bgreenwald@cfsny.org
Website: http://www.cfsny.org

The Center for Vocational Rehabilitation
15 Merdian Rd
Eatontown, NJ 07724
Tel: (732) 544 1800 ext 224
Contact Name: Jaime Zicha
Email: jzicha@cvrus.org
Website: http://www.cvrus.org

The Citizen Advocacy Program
55 High Street
Mt. Holly, NJ 08060
Tel: (609) 267 5880
Contact Name: Lorraine Travaglione, Director
Website: http://www.arcnj.org

The Daniel Jordan Fiddle Foundation (DJF)
P.O. Box 1149
Ridgewood, NJ 07451
Tel: (201) 444 4141
Email: info@djfiddlefoundation.org
Website: http://www.djfiddlefoundation.org

Department for Persons with Disabilities (DPD)
1 Catholic Charities Way PO Box 2539
Oak Ridge, NJ 07438
(973) 406 1100
Email: info@dpd.org
Website: http://www.dpd.org
Facebook: https://www.facebook.com/DPDCC

Friends Of Cyrus (FOC)
401 Creek Road
Delanco, NJ 08075
Tel: (856) 255 5630
    (201) 909 8787
Contact Name: Kamelia Kameli, MA, LNHA, COO, Executive Director
Contact Email: kamelia@friendsofcyrus.com
Website: http://www.friendsofcyrus.com

Mom2Mom: A 24/7 Peer Counselor Helpline for Mothers of Children With Special Needs
Statewide, NJ
Toll Free: 877-914-MOM2
Contact Name: Cherie Castellano
Email: castelch@umdnj.edu
Website: http://www.mom2mom.us.com
FB: http://on.fb.me/WL1QV0

Mom2Mom is a free, confidential, 24/7 peer counseling helpline for N.J. mothers of children with special needs, specifically autism. Spanish-language counselors are available.

Mt. Bethel Village
130 Mt Bethel Road
Warren, NJ 07059-5129
Tel: (908) 757 7000
Contact Name: Carolann Garafola
Email: cgarafola@mtbethelvillage.com
Website: http://www.mtbethelvillage.com
Facebook: http://www.mtbethelvillage.com/#

New Horizons in Autism
671 Batchelor St.
Toms River, NJ 08757
(732) 918 0850
Contact Name: Michele Goodman, Executive Director
Email: goodman@nhautism.org
Website: http://www.nhautism.org

New Jersey All People Equal
661 Upper Mountain Ave United States
Little Falls, NJ 07424
Contact Name: Matthew Schinelli
Email: mschinelli3@gmail.com
Website: http://njape.org/

New Jersey Self-Advocacy Project
44 Stelton Road Suite 110
Piscataway, NJ 08854
Tel: (732) 926 8010
Contact Name: Takeena Thomas, Director

Quest Autism Programs, Inc.
691 Wyckoff Avenue
Wyckoff, NJ 07481
Tel: (201) 425 8397
Contact Name: Toli Anastassiou
Email: info@questnj.org
Website: http://www.questnj.org

Quest Autism Programs is a community-based day program based on ABA principles.

SAIL Adult Day Program at the Bergen County YJCC
605 Pascack Road
Washington Township, NJ 07676
Tel: (201) 666 6610 x 5822
Contact Name: Kimberly LoCicero
Email: klocicero@yjcc.org
Website: http://www.yjcc.org/index.php?option=com_content&view=article&id=128

Salem County Center for Autism (SCCA), Inc.
193 North Broadway
Pennsville, NJ 08070
Tel: (856) 678 9400
Contact Name: Stephanie Snyder-Phipps
Email: FamilyAdvisor@SalemCntyCenterforAutism.org
Website: http://www.SalemCntyCenterforAutism.org

Visitation Home Day Program
PO Box 11242
Hamilton, NJ 08620
Tel: (609) 838 1187
Contact Name: Denise Reil, Executive Director
Email: denise@visitationhome.org
Website: http://visitationhome.org

NEW MEXICO

Doctors, Clinics, Hospitals, and Other Health Services

CDD Early Childhood Evaluation Program (ECEP)
2300 Menaul NE

Albuquerque, NM 87107
Tel: (505) 272 9846
Toll Free: (800) 337 6076
Name: Phyllis Shingle
Email: pshingle@salud.unm.edu
Website: http://www.cdd.unm.edu/ECEP/

The Early Childhood Evaluation Program (ECEP) provides evaluations for children ages birth to three.

Sandia Pediatric Dentistry
7007 Wyoming Blvd NE Suite C-2
Albuquerque, NM 87109
Tel: (505)200-3516
Contact Name: Danen Sjostrom DDS
Email: info@sandiapediatricdentistry.com
Website: http://www.sandiapediatricdentistry.com

Dental care for children with Autism and special needs.

Sandra Lynn Whisler, MD FAAP
Sandra Lynn Whisler, MD FAAP
3751 Highway 528
Albuquerque, NM 87114
Tel: (505) 272 2900
Contact Name: Sandra Lynn Whisler
Specializes in Children with Disabilities

Young Children's Health Center
306 A San Pablo SE
Albuquerque, NM 87108
Tel: (505) 272 4071 or (505) 272 9242
Contact Name: Javier Aceves, MD FAAP
Website: http://www.hospitals.unm.edu

Therapy Services

Autism Communication Consultants
2521 San Pedro NE Suite F
Albuquerque, NM 87110
Tel: (505) 881 4618
Contact Name: Charlotte Scott
Email: autismcc@gmail.com
Website: http://www.autismcc.com

Behavior Change Institute (BCI)
6565 Americas Parkway Northeast Suite 200
Albuquerque, NM 87110
Tel: (505) 273 7799
Toll Free: (866) 273 2451
Contact Name: Kelly Weingart
Email: kweingart@behaviorchangeinstitute.com
Website: http://www.behaviorchangeinstitute.com

Provides adaptive skill building; behavior support planning; case management; early intervention services; functional behavior assessments, parent coaching &

consultation; school-based ABA Therapy; school consultation; and social skills development.

Bright Futures: Autism & Early Intervention, LLC
1225 Parkway Drive
Santa Fe, NM 87507
Tel: (505) 471 4505
Contact Name: Zoe Migel, MS, LISW, LSSW
Email: Zoe@BrightFuturesAEI.com
Website: http://www.BrightFuturesAEI.com

Clinical, Forensic and Neuropsychological Associates of New Mexico
3228 Los Arboles, N.E. Building 1-230
Albuquerque, NM 87107
Tel: (505) 331 2829
Contact Name: Maxann Shwartz, Ph.D., LLC
Email: drmax@nmpsych.com
Website: http://www.nmpsych.com

Early Intervention & Children's Services Family Infant Toddler Program
810 San Mateo, PO Box 26110
Santa Fe, NM 87502-6110
Tel: (505) 476 8973
Contact Name: Andy Gomm
Email: andrew.gomm@state.nm.us
Website: http://nmhealth.org/ddsd/nmfit/

Provides early intervention services to infants, toddlers who have or are at risk for developmental delays and families in New Mexico.

ExplorAbilities, Inc.
5006 Copper NE
Albuquerque, NM 87108
Tel: (505) 268 7988
Contact Name: Erin Moody
Email: explorabilities@gmail.com
Website: http://www.explorabilitiestherapy.com

Gallien Therapy Services, Inc.
1809 Indian Wells
Alamogordo, NM 88310
Tel: (575) 437 1967
Contact Name: Pam Gallien, MS, CCC-SLP
Email: info@gallientherapy.com
Website: http://www.gallientherapy.com

Gisela Wutzler
1939 Cherokee Rd. NW`
Albuquerque, NM 87107
Tel: (215) 5272453
Contact Name: Gisela Wutzler
Email: gisela.wutzler@gmail.com

Provides music therapy.

Jump Start Autism Center (JAC)
8500 Washington St. Northeast Suite A-1
Albuquerque, NM 87113
Tel: (505) 828 1550
Contact Name: Brian R. Lopez, PhD, Clinical Child Psychologist, Executive & Clinical Director
Email: blopez@jumpstartaba.com
Website: http://www.jumpstartaba.com

Provides comprehensive diagnostic evaluations and treatment, including ABA (center-, home-, and school-based), SLP, OT, parent training, and school consultation.

Stimulating Minds Autism Clinic, LLC
6100 Seagull St NE Suite B202
Albuquerque, NM 87109
Tel: (505) 433 4670
Contact Name: Jeanne Duggins
Email: info@stimulatingmindsautism.com
Website: http://www.stimulatingmindautism.com

Tresco, Inc.
1800 Copper Loop
Las Cruces, NM 88005
Toll Free: (888) 316 8528
Website: http://www.trescoinc.org

Provides early intervention services and support to children birth to three and their families; respite and personal care services for any age; supported employment and volunteer placement and training programs; residential living support services; and community participation and recreational activities.

Wonder Stage Learning
11600 Academy
Albuquerque, NM 87111
Toll Free: (888) 763 3167
Name: Jamie Ragsdale
Email: Jamie@WonderStageLearning.com
Website: http://www.wonderstagelearning.com/

Offers phone-based and in-person consulting and in-home ABA services, skilled child care, and tutoring.

Schools and Educational Services

Bernalillo Academy
Gibson Blvd., SE Suite 'A'
Albuquerque, NM 87108
Tel: (505) 924 6347
Contact Name: Yvonne Gurule, MSE
Email: yvonne.gurule@bernalilloacademy.org
Website: http://bernalilloacademy.org

A residential treatment center for boys and girls ages 5–17 offering ABA, individual, family, and equine therapy.

Lovington Preschool
Lovington Preschool
1000 South 1st Street
Lovington, NM 88260
Tel: (575) 739 2705
Contact Name: Kimberly Hess
Email: HessKG@valornet.com

Mission School of New Mexico
Po Box 91165
Albuquerque, NM 87199
Tel: (505) 341 0555

A private school for students in grades 1–12.

Pathways Academy
5651 Jefferson Street Northeast
Albuquerque, NM 87109
Tel: (505).341.0555
Website: http://pathwaysacademynm.org

Legal, Government & Financial Services

Albuquerque Therapeutic Recreation Program
Loma Linda Community Center 1700 Yale SE
Albuquerque, NM 87106
Tel: (505) 764 1525
Contact Name: Maggie Silva
Email: MaggieSilva@cabq.gov
Website: http://www.cabq.gov

Behavioral Health Services Division
37 Plaza La Prensa
Santa Fe, NM 87504
Tel: (505) 476 9266
Website: http://www.hsd.state.nm.us/bhsd/

Disability Rights New Mexico
Protection and Advocacy System
Disability Rights New Mexico
1720 Louisiana Blvd., N.E. Suite 204
Albuquerque, NM 87110
Tel: (505) 256 3100
Toll Free: (800) 432 4682
Contact Name: James Jackson
Email: nmpalonjose@yahoo.com
Website: http://www.drnm.org/

New Mexico Criminal Law Offices
1008 5th St. Northwest
Albuquerque, NM 87102
Tel: (505) 200 2982
Contact Name: Jack Mkhitarian

Email: newmexicocriminallaw@yahoo.com
Website: http://www.newmexicocriminallaw.com

Criminal defense attorneys specializing in defending clients with special needs and that suffer from wide ranges of disabilities.

New Mexico Division of Vocational Rehabilitation
435 Saint Michaels Drive Building D
Sante Fe, NM 87505
Toll Free: (800) 224 7005
Email: rsmith@state.nm.us
Website: http://www.dvrgetsjobs.com/

Zuni Entrepreneurial Enterprises
Zuni Entrepreneurial Enterprises Zuni, NM 87327
Tel: (505) 782 5798
Email: larryalflen@zeeinc.org
Website: http://www.zeeinc.org

Provides effective and comprehensive vocational training, meaningful employment opportunities.

Community and Recreation Services

Family Voices
2340 Alamo SE, Suite 102
Albuquerque, NM 87106
Tel: (505) 872 4774
Toll Free: (888) 835 5669
Website: http://www.familyvoices.org

Las Cumbres Community Services
404 Hutner Street
Espanola, NM 87532
Tel: (505) 753 4123
Email: rosita.rodriguez@lascumbres-nm.org
Website: http://www.lascumbres-nm.org/supportedemployment.php

Supported employment programs.

Life Roots
1111 Menaul Blvd NE
Albuquerque, NM 87101
Tel: (505) 255 5501
Website: http://www.liferootsnm.org/adultcommunityservices.aspx

LifeROOTS Adult Services provide individuals with disabilities ages 18(+) comprehensive support and services including: day habilitation, supported employment, job coaching, career discovery, literacy education.

Mandy's Special Farm
Adult Residential Care Facility
346 Clark Rd SW
Albuquerque, NM 87105
Tel: (505) 873 1187
Contact Name: Rhonda Rhoades or Heidi Rishel
Email: heidi@mandysfarm.org
Website: http://www.mandysfarm.org

Mandy's Special Farm is a home, in a farm setting, that specializes in adult female autism.

Parents Reaching Out
1920 "B" Columbia Drive SE
Albuquerque, NM 87106
Tel: (505) 247 0192
Toll Free: (800) 524 5176
Email: prodreamaker1@aol.com
Website: http://www.parentsreachingout.org

RCI Inc.
Realizing Confidence & Independence
1111 Menaul NE
Albuquerque, NM 87107
Tel: (505) 255 5501 X1126
Contact Name: Dr. Joseph McCarty
Email: josephm@rci-nm.org
Website: http://www.rci-nm.org

NEW YORK

Doctors, Clinics, Hospitals, and Other Health Services

Aslani-Breit, DDS, PLLC
1655 Elmwood Ave, Ste. 120
Rochester, NY 14620
Tel: (585) 427 8620
Email: maslani@rochester.rr.com
Website: http://rockidssmile.com/

Dr. Barbara Kenner
39 East 78th Street
New York, NY 10075
Tel: (212) 327 4979

Neuropsychological testing, assessment and consultation services for individuals with ASD and other challenges.

Beth Israel Medical Center
Child Development, Department of Pediatrics
Asma Sadiq, MD, Director
10 Union Square East
New York, NY 10003

Tel: (212) 844 8324
Website: www.livewellnewyork.com/asma-sadiq-md

Providing comprehensive care for children with ASD and other developmental and neurodevelopmental disabilities. Board certified by the American Board of Pediatrics; the American Board of Pediatrics, Developmental-Behavioral; and the American Board of Pediatrics.

Bock Integrative Medicine
Kenneth Bock, MD
Michael Compain, MD
50 Old Farm Road
Red Hook, NY 12571
Tel: (845) 758 0001
Website: www.bockintegrative.com

Individualized biomedical treatments for ASD and other conditions.

Bronx-Lebanon Hospital Center
Bronx Care POE Clinic
2432 Grand Concourse
Bronx, NY 10458
Tel: (718) 518 5131 X7877
Contact Name: Josefina Rivera
Website: http://www.bronxcare.org/our-services/pediatrics/other-initiatives

Center for Visual Management
Melvin Kaplan OD FCOVD
150 White Plains Road
Suite 410
Tarrytown, NY 10591
Tel: (914) 631 1070
Website: www.autisticvision.com

Providing evaluation, assessment and vision therapy.

Child Mind Institute
445 Park Avenue (entrance on 56th Street)
New York, NY 10022
Tel: (212) 308 3118
Email: info@childmind.org
Website: www.childmind.org

Provides clinical services for children and adolescents with a variety of challenges, including ASD, and provides parents with resources and information. Also is engaged in collaborative research.

The Child Study Center
Tel: (212) 263 6622
Email: services@aboutourkids.org
Website: www.aboutourkids.org

Among its services, the Child Study Center provides assessment and a wide range of treatment options for children with a variety of special needs and their families, including individual and group therapy, parenting training, medication treatment, and other specialized programs.

Children's Evaluation and Rehabilitation Center
The Children's Hospital at Montefiore
3415 Bainbridge Avenue
Bronx, NY 10467
Tel: (718) 741 2450

Early Childhood Center
1731 Seminole Avenue
Bronx, NY 10461

Rose F. Kennedy Center
1410 Pelham Parkway South
Bronx, NY 10461
Tel: (718) 430 8500

Fisher Landau Center for the Treatment of Learning Disabilities (Rousso)
1165 Morris Park Avenue
Bronx, NY 10461
Tel: (718) 430 3900

Website: www.cham.org/services/child/

Comprehensive diagnostic and treatment options for children with developmental disabilities.

Comprehensive Epilepsy Center
Orrin Devinsky, MD
NYU Langone Medical Center
223 East 34th Street, Ground Floor
New York, NY 10016
Tel: (646) 558 0803
Fax: (646) 385 7164
Website: www.med.nyu.edu/biosketch/od4
Pediatric neurologist

Developmental Behavioral Pediatrics of New York
Marilyn C. Agin, MD FAAP MA/CCC-SLP
107 West 90th Street, Townhouse H
New York, N.Y. 10024
Tel: (212) 274 9180
Fax: (212) 219 3688
Email: aysha@dbpny.com
Website: www.dbpny.com

Provides comprehensive developmental evaluations and recommendations.

The Developmental Neuropsychiatry Program
635 West 165th Street Room 635
New York, NY 10032

Tel: (212) 342 1600
Contact Name: Agnes Whitaker, MD, Maureen McSwiggan-Hardin
Email: cdnp@childpsych.columbia.edu
Website: columbiapsychiatry.org/disorders/autism

The Developmental Neuropsychiatry Program (DNP) is a clinical program designed to evaluate and treat children, adolescents, and adults with a wide variety of developmental conditions that affect social interaction and adjustment.

Geri Brewster, RD MPH CDN
140 West 30th Street, Suite 4E
New York, NY 10001
Phone: (914) 864 1976
Email: scheduling@geribrewster.com

Providing comprehensive nutritional treatments, NAET, and other modalities for individuals (including children) with ASD as well as others.

Giuseppina Feingold, MD
Valley Health & Hyperbarics
28A Indian Rock Route 59
Suffern, NY 10901
Tel: (845) 208 3624
Website: www.valleyhyperbarics.com

Integrative biomedical treatment for autism and other conditions. Also offers hyperbaric oxygen therapy.

Golisano Children's Hospital
Strong Memorial Hospital
601 Elmwood Ave.
Rochester, NY 14642
Website: http://www.urmc.rochester.edu/childrens-hospital

Kirch Developmental Services Center
Website: www.urmc.rochester.edu/childrens-hospital/developmental-disabilities/services/kirch.aspx

Comprehensive evaluation and treatment for children with ASD and other conditions.

Dr. Joseph Shapiro
Center for Unlimited Vision
128 W. 13th St
New York, NY 10011
Tel: (212) 255 2240
Email: visiondoc88@aol.com
Website: http://www.centerforunlimitedvision.com

Provides functional vision testing and vision therapy.

Kara Gross Margolis, MD
New York-Presbyterian
Morgan Stanley Children's Hospital

Columbia University Medical Center
3959 Broadway Fl 7th
New York, NY 10032
Tel: (212) 305 5903
Fax: (212) 342 5756
Email: kjg2133@columbia.edu
Website: www.cumc.columbia.edu/pediatrics/division/
gastroenterology-hepatology-and-nutrition/faculty
Pediatric gastroenterologist.

The Kelberman Center
1601 Armory Dr.
Utica, NY 13501
Tel: (315) 797 6241
Website: http://www.kelbermancenter.org

Provides evaluation and diagnosis; individualized education and services; social and life skills enhancement; innovative practices, training and research.

Lawrence B. Palevsky, MD
Tel: (631) 262 8505
Email: info@drpalevsky.com
Website: www.drpalevsky.com/services.asp

Holistic pediatrician providing comprehensive wellness care incorporating conventional and holistic approaches. Has extensive experience in working with families with ASD and other chronic health conditions.

Mary Coyle, D.I. Hom.
1133 Broadway
Room 1015
New York, NY 10010
Tel: (212) 255 4490
Email: wellnessny@realchildcenter.com
Website: www.realchildcenter.com

Holistic treatment for children with ASD and others uses homeopathy, homotoxicology and other modalities.

Maya Shetreat-Klein, MD
6003 Riverdale Avenue
Bronx, NY 10471
Tel: (718) 514 1576
Website: www.brainmending.com

Dr. Shetreat-Klein is a board-certified pediatric neurologist providing an integrative approach to neurological, behavioral, cognitive, and chronic health challenges in children, including children with ASD.

McCarton Center for Developmental Pediatrics
350 East 82nd Street
New York, NY 10028
Tel: (212) 996 9019
Fax: (212) 996 9047

Email: schedulingcoordinator@mccartoncenter.com
Website: www.mccartoncenter.com

Comprehensive evaluation and treatment of children with developmental challenges, including ASD.

Michael W. Elice, MD
AIM Integrative Medicine
Woodbury
80 Crossways Park Drive
Woodbury, New York 11797

Manhattan
211 E70th St.
New York, New York 10021
Tel: (516) 802 5028
Email: drelice@aimintegrative.com
Website: http://www.aimintegrativemedicine.com/

A facility dedicated to the children and adults with autism, allergy, immune and metabolic (AIM) problems.

Morton Teich, MD
930 Park Avenue
New York, NY 10028
Tel: (212) 988 1821
Website: www.mountsinai.org/profiles/morton-m-teich

Specializing in allergy and immunology.

Mt. Sinai Child Development Department Faculty Practice Associate
5 East 98th Street
10th Floor
The Mount Sinai Health System
New York, NY 10029
Tel: (212) 241 6710
Website: www.mountsinaifpa.org/patient-care/
practices/pediatrics-child-development

Diagnosis and comprehensive treatment for ASD and medical and developmental conditions.

New York-Presbyterian
Phyllis and David Komansky Center for Children's Health
Jennifer Cross, MB, ChB and others
505 East 70th Street
Helmsley Tower, 3rd Floor
New York, NY 10021
Tel: (646) 962 4303
Fax: (646) 962 0259
Website: weillcornell.org/jfcross

Comprehensive diagnostic evaluation and treatment for ASD.

Pediatric Assessment, Learning & Support
Tel: (212) 481 1664
Email: nypalsdoc@gmail.com
Website: www.nypals.com

Pediatric neuropsychological and other assessments and evaluations as well as therapy and other supports.

Pediatric Gastroenterology Resources of New York
Arthur Krigsman, MD
148 Beach 9th Street, Suite 2B
Far Rockaway, NY 11691
Tel: (718) 327 2200, ext. 101
Fax: (718) 732 2094
Website: www.autismgi.com

Treatment for gastrointestinal disorders in children with ASD and others.

Pierre Fontaine, RSHom CCH, CEASE certified
Homeopathic Services
192 Lexington Avenue
Suite 248
New York, NY 10016
Tek: (212) 334 7360
Website: www.homeopathicservices.com

Treats children with ASD and others experiencing health challenges using homeopathic modalities.

Seaver Autism Center
Tel: (212) 241 0961
Email: theseavercenter@mssm.edu
Website: icahn.mssm.edu/research/centers/seaver-autism-center

Provides diagnostic assessments, genetic testing, and treatments for children, adolescents and adults with ASD or suspected of having ASD. Treatment includes individual and group therapy, social skills treatments (including using a CBT approach), therapy supports for families, medication, service coordination, community outreach, including workshops, lectures and conferences.

Sidney Baker, MD
71 Ferry Road
Sag Harbor, NY 11963
Tel: (631) 725 9547
Website: www.autism360.org

Biomedical Interventions for individuals with ASD and other chronic health conditions.

Stephen Cowan MD
Center for Health & Healing
491 Lexington Avenue
Mt Kisco, NY 10549

Tel: (914) 864 1976
Website: www.stephencowanmd.com

Pediatrician and developmental pediatrician with a holistic treatment approach to children with special needs.

Steven M. Wolf, MD
Mount Sinai Beth Israel
10 Union Square East, Suite 5G
New York NY 10003
Tel: (212) 844 6944
Website: www.docnet.org/physicians/phys_bios.aspx?phys_id=99

Pediatric neurology.

Total Kids Developmental Pediatric Resources
Developmental Pediatric Services
Contact: Dr. Mark Freilich
Tel: (212) 787 2148
Fax: (646) 536 8729
Email: info@totalkidsny.com

Occupational Therapy Services
Contact: Anna Friedman, MS, OTR
Phone: (212) 787 2148
Fax: (646) 536 8729
Email: annaf@totalkidsny.com

Website: www.totalkidsny.com

Developmental pediatrician who provides comprehensive evalautions and recommendations. Observes children in multiple environments in assessing.

Therapy Services

ABA Psychologist and Associates
Airmont, NY 10952
Tel: (845) 290 0365
Contact Name: Dr. Nursel Kahya, BCBA-D
Email: nkahya@abapsychologist.com
Website: http://www.abapsychologist.com

Provides ABA-based programs in a variety of settings.

Angelfish Therapy
Tel: (203) 545 0024
Fax (203) 321 2138
Email: Info@AngelfishTherapy.com
Website: www.angelfishtherapy.com

Aquatic therapy, swim lesson and summer camps with many locations in Connecticut, Massachusetts, New York, and New Jersey.

Atlas Foundation for Autism
252 West 29th Street, 3rd Floor
New York, NY 10001
Tel: (212) 256 0846
Email: info@atlasforautism.org
Website: www.atlasforautism.org

Provides a wide range of services including: educational programming, afterschool, social groups, ST, OT, Solisten®, HANDLE®, workshops, professional development, parent training, play sessions, overnights, music and art sessions, yoga and recreation groups, and more for individuals with ASD, their families and other professionals.

Dr. Bobby Newman
100 West Park Avenue Office 210D
Long Beach, NY 11561
Tel: (516) 448 5042
Contact Name: Bobby Newman
Email: Bcba001@yahoo.com
Website: http://www.Room2grow.org

Performs initial evaluations, as well as functional analyses and behavior treatment plan design.

Bridge Kids of New York, LLC
Tel: (516) 526 5658
Email: info@bridgekidsny.com
Website: www.bridgekidsNY.com

Bridge Kids of New York, LLC provides a multidisciplinary approach to treatment and offers a variety of services, such as evaluations and consultations, parent education and advocacy, professional training and supervision, and supportive services for children.

Brooklyn Letters
Brooklyn, NY 11215
Tel: (347) 394 3485
Contact Name: Craig Selinger
Email: craig@brooklynletters.com
Website: http://www.brooklynletters.com

The Center for Small Jewels
3 The Boulevard
New Rochelle, NY 10801
Tel: (914) 632 9109
Contact Name: Cheryl Small Jackson
Email: Cheryl@csjinc.com
Website: http://www.csjinc.com

The Cody Center for Autism and Developmental Disabilities
5 Medical Drive
Port Jefferson Station, NY 11776

Tel: (631) 632 3070
Website: http://www.stonybrookmedicalcenter.org/codycenter

Crossroads Unlimited (CU), Inc.
1207 Castleton Ave.
Staten Island, NY 10310
Tel: (718) 420 6330
Contact Name: Lea Graham
Website: http://www.cuiny.org

Destiny's Ride Equestrian Center, LLC
300 New Concord Road
East Chatham, NY 12075
Tel: (518) 822 0562
Contact Name: Jodie O'Connell-Ponkos
Email: joconnell@destinysride.org
Website: http://www.destinysride.org

Equine therapy.

GallopNYC Giving Alternative Learners UpLifting Opportunities, Inc.
540 President Street, 3rd Floor Brooklyn, NY 11215
Tel: (646) 233 4507
Email: info@gallopnyc.org
Website: www.gallopnyc.org

Providing therapeutic riding, hippotherapy and equine assisted therapy at various locations in the New York City area. Also has a transition job skills program.

Hallowell New York City
117 West 72nd Street, Third Floor
New York, NY 10023
Tel: (212) 799 7777
Email: info@hallowellcenter.org
Website: www.hallowellnyc.com/

Offers assessment and treatment for ADHD and many other conditions and provides a wide range of treatment options that can be tailored to meet patient needs, including: Cognitive Behavioral Therapy, psychotherapy, Cogmed Working Memory Enhancement, Neurofeedback, Integrated Listening Systems, Sensory Optimizing Programs, Coaching, medication and medication management, and more.

Handicapped Children's Association of Southern New York
18 Broad St.
Johnson City, NY 13790
Tel: (607) 798 7117
Contact Name: Stephen M. Sano
Email: hca1serves@aol.com
Website: http://www.hcaserves.com

The Holistic Learning Center
Susan Varsames MA Ed, and others
222 Westchester Avenue
Suite 103
White Plains, NY 10604
Tel: (914) 793 9100
Website: www.holisticlc.com

The center provides evaluations as well as wide range of traditional and alternative treatment modalities to individualize treatment for a child with ASD and the family, including ABA, social groups, sensory integration, speech therapy, nutritional services, craniosacral therapy, listening therapy, Reiki and many others.

HorseAbility
223 Store Hill Rd On the College of Suny Old Westbury
Old Westbury, NY 11568
Tel: (516)-333-6151
Contact Name: Barbara Hotchkin
Email: LessonManager@HorseAbility.org
Website: http://www.HorseAbility.org

Equine facilitated programs.

Hudson Valley Young Achievers
60 Erie Street
Goshen, NY 10924
Tel: (845) 294 1882
Contact Name: Adrienne Maviglia
Email: hvyngachvrs@aol.com
Website: http://www.hudsonvalleyyoungachievers.com

Jane Gatanis, MA OR/L
145 4th Avenue
New York, NY 10003
Tel: (212) 674 6610
Website: www.janegatanis.com

Specializes in manual therapy and healing arts, including craniosacral therapy.

Lauren Tobinh-Puente, PhD
525 East 12th Street CFNew York, NY 10009
Tel: (917) 838 9274
Email: services@drtobingpuente.com
Website: www.drtobingpuente.com

Specializes in evaluating and treating children, including those with ASD. She uses the DIR model and other treatment modalities in treating children.

New York Pediatric Speech and Language Services, LLC
Tel: (914) 939 6400
Email: rozuckerman@optonline.net
Website: www.newyorkspeech.com

Evaluation and treatment of speech and language issues. Therapy includes individual and group settings, as appropriate.

Rusk Rehabilitation
NYU Langone Main Campus
530 First Avenue (at 30th Street), 9th Floor
New York, NY 10016

Also additional locations depending on treatment.
Tel: (212) 263 1999 or (212) 598 6000
Email: Rusk.Info@nyumc.org
Website: rusk.med.nyu.edu

Offers a variety of treatment including speech therapy, augmentative communication, feeding, occupational therapy, physical therapy, and others for many conditions in pediatric and other patient populations.

Spoonful of Speech
1234 West Broadway Suite 106
Hewlett, NY 11557
(516) 432 4234
Contact Name: Jennifer Kerr / Lirit Malekan
Email: spoonfulofspeech@gmail.com
Website: http://www.spoonfulofspeech.com

Services children ages 5-21 with speech, language, social and feeding difficulties.

Steven H. Blaustein, PhD
17 East 97th St.
New York, NY 10029
Tel: (212) 876 0357

Speech and language evaluations and therapy.

Thera-sitters
New York, Westchester, and the Hamptons
NY
Tel: (617) 794 7455
Contact Name: Kristen Weiss, M.Ed., BCBA
Email: therasitters@gmail.com
Website: http://therasitters.weebly.com/

Therasitters combines methods of ABA with babysitting services.

Theracare
Multiple locations across New York and New Jersey
Contact: www.theracare.com/tc/contact/
Website: hwww.theracare.com/tc/

Provides early intervention and preschool aged therapeutic services and service coordination. Autism-specific services include ABA therapy and the Academy for Young Minds program.

Theraplay
251 E 77th St. Lower Level
NY, NY 10075
Tel: (212)-288-1450
Contact Name: Kim Sullivan
Email: kim@Theraplaynyc.com
Website: http://www.Theraplaynyc.com

Theraplay is a multidisciplinary sensory gym offering pediatric therapy services including; Occupational Therapy, Physical Therapy, Speech Language Pathology, Children's Play Therapy, Nutrition, Counseling.

Theresa Revans-McMenimon, MS, LMHC, LMFT
70 Bedford Road
Pleasantville, NY 10570
Tel: (914) 769 7557
Email: trevans@optonline.net
Website: http://www.frmh.org

Watch Me Grow Children's Sensory Gym & Speech-Language Center
162 West 72nd Street, 5th Floor
New York, NY 10023
Tel: (212) 721 0208
Fax: (212) 721 4247

And
525 East 12th Street CF
New York, NY 10009
Tel: (212) 721 5220
Fax: (212) 982 9816

Email: info@WatchMeGrowNYC.com
Website: watchmegrownyc.com

Provides OT, ST, and PT as well as therapy evaluations and other services and programs, including summer programming, in two locations in NYC. Provides services through EI, CPSE, CSE and private pay.

Westchester Therapy Solutions
690 North Broadway
White Plains, NY 10603
Tel: (914) 686 3116
Contact Name: Susie Culhane
Email: info@wtstherapy.com
Website: http://www.westchestertherapysolutions.com/

Provides occupational and physical therapy to children with ASD at home or in their clinic. Expertise in Sensory Integration, motor coordination, fine motor skills, and play skills.

Schools and Educational Services

Aaron School
Elementary/Middle School:
309 East 45th Street

New York, NY 10017
Tel: (212) 867 5443

High School:
42 East 30th Street
New York, NY 10016
Tel: (212) 867 9594
Website: www.aaronschool.org

AHRC Middle/High School at the Regina Pacis School
1201 66th Street
Brooklyn, NY 11219
Tel: (212) 780 2532
Website: www.ahrcnyc.org

Anderson School
4885 Rt. 9, PO Box 367
Staatsburg, NY 12580
Tel: (845) 889 4034
Website: www.andersonschool.org

Andrus Children's Center – The Orchard School
1156 North Broadway
Yonkers, NY 10701
Tel: (914) 965 3700
Website: www.andruschildren.org

Association for Metro-Area Autistic Children (AMAC)
25 West 17th Street
NY, NY 10011
Tel: (212) 645 5005
Website: http://www.amac.org

Early intervention through young adult ABA-based educational services.

Atlas Foundation for Autism
252 West 29th Street, 3rd Floor
New York, NY 10001
Tel: (212) 256 0846
Email: info@atlasforautism.org
Website: www.atlasforautism.org

Provides a wide range of services including: educational programming, afterschool, social groups, ST, OT, Solisten®, HANDLE®, workshops, professional development, parent training, play sessions, overnights, music and art sessions, yoga and recreation groups, and more for individuals with ASD, their families and other professionals.

Birch Family Services
104 West 29th Street, Third Floor
New York, NY 10001
Tel: (212) 616 1800
Fax: (212) 741 6739
Website: www.birchfamilyservices.org

Provides education, habilitation, and residential services at a number of locations to people with ASD and other special needs and support for their families. Also provides training to professionals working with those with ASD and other special needs.

Bridges to Adelphi Program
Division of Student Affairs, Adelphi University
University Center, Room 302
Garden City, NY 11530
Tel: (516) 877 3665
Email: admissions@adelphi.edu
Website: http://students.adelphi.edu/sa/bridges/

A supplemental support program for students at Adelphi University with neuro-social and non-verbal disorders.

Block Institute School
376 Bay 44th Street
Brooklyn, NY 11214
Tel: (718) 946 9700

Brooklyn Autism Center Academy (BAC)
57 Willoughby St. Floor 3
Brooklyn, NY 11201
Tel: (718) 554 1027
Email: info@brooklynautismcenter.org
Website: http://www.brooklynautismcenter.org

Provides ABA-based educational programs.

Brooklyn Blue Feather Elementary School
2335 Gerritsen Avenue
Brooklyn, NY 11229
Tel: (718) 834 0597
Website: www.ahrcnyc.org

Brookville Center for Children's Services
189 Wheatley Road
Brookville, NY 11545
Tel: (516) 626 1000
Website: www.ahrcnyc.org

Center for Developmental Disabilities
72 South Woods Road
Woodbury, NY 11796
Tel: (516) 921 7650
Website: www.centerfor.com

Center for Discovery
PO Box 840
Harris, New York 12742
Tel: (845) 794 1400
Website: www.thecenterfordiscovery.org/

Provides educational, health, and residential services for individuals with ASD and other conditions from age 5 through adulthood and offers a wide range of clinical, social, creative arts and recreational programming.

The Child School/Legacy High School
587 Main Street
Roosevelt Island, NY 10044
Tel: (212) 223 5055
Website: www.thechildschool.org

Clear View School Day Treatment Program
480 Albany Post Road
Briarcliff Manor, NY 10510
Tel: (914) 941 9513
Website: www.clearviewschool.org

College Support Program
4500 Harlem Road
Amherst, NY 14226
Tel: (716) 839 2620
Website: http://www.collegesupportprogram.org

College & University Support Services (CUSP)
Albany, NY 12206
Tel: (315) 203 3913
Contact Name: Stephen Motto
Email: steve@cuspservices.com
Website: http://www.cuspservices.com

CUSP provides individualized coaching and mentoring programs to improve organizational skills, self advocacy, effective communication and job readiness skills.

Developmental Disabilities Institute (DDI)
99 Hollywood Drive
Smithtown, NY 11787
Tel: (631) 366 2900
Website: www.ddiinfo.org

Devereux New York
12 Schuman Rd.
Millwood, NY 10546
Tel: (914) 941 1991
Website: http://www.devereuxNY.org

Provides occupational and physical therapy to children with ASD at home or in their clinic. Expertise in Sensory Integration, motor coordination, fine motor skills, and play skills.

Eden II Programs
150 Granite Ave.
Staten Island, NY 10303
Tel: (718) 816 1422
Email: info@eden2.org
Website: http://www.eden2.org

Eden II Program on LI/Genesis School
270 Washington Avenue
Plainview, NY 11803
Tel: (516) 937 1397
Website: www.eden2.org

Elija Foundation
665 N. Newbridge Rd.
Levittown, NY 11756
Tel: (516) 433 4324
Website: http://www.elija.org

The ELIJA School
100 Periwinkle Road
Levittown, NY 11756
Tel: (516) 216 5270
Website: www.elija.org

Esther Ashkenas Central Park Early Learning Center
Central Park, West
Manhattan, NY
Website: schools.ahrcnyc.org/sponsor/eacpelc/

Preschool providing education and therapeutic services for children 3-5 with ASD and other developmental challenges, offering a variety of classrooms to meet learners' needs, including integrated classrooms.

Ferncliff Manor—SAIL
1154 Saw Mill River Rod
Yonkers, NY 10710
Tel: (914) 968 4854
Website: www.sailatferncliff.com

Franziska Racker Centers
3226 Wilkins Road
Ithaca, NY 14850
Tel: (607) 272 5891 X332
Contact Name: Dr. Karen Fried
Email: karenfcl@rackercenters.org
Website: http://www.rackercenters.org

ABA-oriented preschool services, birth-to-three diagnostic services, school-age ABA-oriented consultation, adult residential services and other services.

The Gateway Schools
211 W 61st Street
New York, NY 10023
Tel: (212) 777 5966
Website: www.gatewayschool.org

Gersh Academy
21 Sweet Hollow Road
Huntington, NY 11743
Tel: (631) 385 3342

254-04 Union Turnpike
Glen Oaks, NY 11004
Tel: (718) 343 5303
Website: www.gershacademy.org

Gillen Brewer
410 East 92 Street
New York, NY 10128
Tel: (212) 831 3667
Website: www.gillenbrewer.com

The Hagedorn Little Village School
750 Hicksville Road
Seaford, NY 11783
Tel: (516) 520 6000
Contact Name: Roberta Cooperman
Email: Roberta.Cooperman@littlevillage.org
Website: http://www.littlevillage.org/

Provides educational and therapeutic services for children birth through elementary school with developmental disabilities year-round, including diagnostic evaluations and treatment, early intervention, a preschool, and an elementary school.

The Hallen School
97 Centre Avenue
New Rochelle, NY 10801
Tel: (914) 636 6600
Contact Name: Stephanie Dalbey
Email: Sdalbey@thehallenschool.net
Website: http://www.thehallenschool.net

Special education school serving students ranging from 5 to 21 years of age with ASD.

HASC—Hebrew Academy for Special Children
3 locations serve school-age children:
321 Woodmere Blvd.
Woodmere, NY 11598
Tel: (516) 295 1340

555 Remsen Avenue
Brooklyn, NY 11236
Tel: (718) 495 3510 x 6220

14th Avenue
Brooklyn, NY 11219
Tel: (718) 331 1624
Website: www.hasc.net

Hawthorne Country Day School
5 Bradhurst Avenue
Hawthorne, NY 10532
Tel: (914) 592 8526

Manhattan Annex:
156 William Street
New York, NY 10031
Tel: (212) 281 6531
Website: www.hawthornecountryday.org

The Hawthorne Country Day School educates children birth to 21 years old with special needs, including ASD.

Heartshare Elementary School
1825 Bath Avenue
Brooklyn, NY 11214
Tel: (718) 621 1614
Website: heartshare.org/programs/school

Karafin School
40-1 Radio Circle
Mount Kisco, NY 10549
Tel: (914) 666 9211
Website: www.karafinschool.com

League School
567 Kingston Avenue
Brooklyn, NY 11203
Tel: (718) 498 2500
Website: www.leaguecenter.org

Learning Spring Academy
247 East 20th Street
New York, NY 10003
Tel: (212) 239 4926
Website: www.learningspring.org

Manhattan Children's Center
124 West 95th Street
New York, NY 10025
Tel: (212) 749 4604, (646) 619 2629
Website: www.manhattanchildrenscenter.org

Provides ABA-based services to children ages 3 to 18.

The McCarton School
331 West 25th Street
New York, NY 10001
Tel: (212) 229 1715
Email: info@mccartonschool.org
Website: http://www.mccartonschool.org

The McCarton School provides an educational program for children with ASD by using an integrated one-to-one model of therapy of ABA, speech and language therapy, motor skills training, and peer interaction.

The Mosaic School
1309 Wantagh Avenue
Wantagh, NY 11793
Tel: (516) 765 3696
Contact Name: Lauretta Murdock

Email: mosaiclm@aol.com
Website: http://www.themosaicschool.org

School for students with autism, ages 5–18 using ABA principles.

The Neighborhood Charter School of Harlem
132 West 124th St.
New York, NY 10027
Email: info@ncsharlem.org
Website: http://www.ncsharlem.org

New Life School
831 Eagle Avenue
Bronx, NY 10456
Tel: (718) 665 2760
Website: thenewlifeschool.org

New Frontiers in Learning (NFIL)
80 Broad St Suite 1702
New York, NY 10004
Tel: (646) 558 0085
Contact Name: Samantha Feinman, M.S.Ed, PhD, Director
Email: sfeinman@nfil.net
Website: http://www.nfil.net

New York Center for Autism Charter School
433 East 100th Street
New York, NY 10029
Tel: (212) 860 2580
Fax: (212) 860 2960
Website: www.nycacharterschool.org

Small ABA-based charter school for children with ASD.

New York Center for Child Development
328 East 62nd St.
New York, NY 10065
Tel: (212) 752 7575
Contact Email:
Email: info@nyccd.org
Website: http://www.nyccd.org

New York Child Learning Institute
123-14 14th Avenue
College Point, NY 11356
Tel: (718) 445 0752
Website: www.nycli.org

Ongoing Academic and Social Instructional Support (OASIS) Program at Pace
Pace University School of Education,
163 William St. 16th Floor
New York, NY 10038
Tel: (212) 346 1891
Website: http://www.pace.edu/school-of-education/centers/tara/oasis

Pathways School
291 Main Street
Eastchester, NY 10709
Tel: (914) 779 7400
Website: www.pathwaysschool.com

**Phyllis L. Susser School for Exceptional Children –
Birch Family Services**
71-64 168th Street
Flushing, NY 11365
Tel: (718) 591 8100
Website: www.birchfamilyservices.org/education/
susser.html

Quality Services for the Autism Community (QSAC)
253 West 35th Street
New York, NY 10001
Tel: 718 7 AUTISM
Contact Name: Kevin Mattivi
Email: kmattivi@qsac.com
Website: http://www.qsac.com

REACH Academy (Greenburgh-Northcastle Schools)
1700 Old Orchard Road
Valhalla, NY 10595
Tel: (914) 693 3030
Website: www.greenburghnorthcastleschools.com

Reach for the Stars Learning Center
3300 Kings Highway
Brooklyn, NY 11234
Tel: (718) 677 0797

Rebecca School
40 East 30th Street
New York, NY 10016
Tel: (212) 810 4120
Contact Name: Elizabeth O'Shea
Email: eoshea@rebeccaschool.org
Website: http://www.rebeccaschool.org

Rebecca School is a therapeutic day school for children ages 4 to 21, promoting the education and development of children with neurodevelopmental delays of relating and communicating, including autism spectrum disorders. The school uses the DIR/Floortime model and a variety of therapeutic modalities.

**School for Language and Communication
Development**
Elementary/Middle School:
100 Glen Cove Avenue
Glen Cove, NY 11542
Tel: (516) 609 2000

Middle School:
70-24 47th Avenue
Woodside, NY 11377
Tel: (718) 476 7163

High School:
87-25 136 Street
Richmond Hill, NY 11418
Tel: (718) 291 2807
Website: www.slcd.org

Shema Kolainu-Hear Our Voices
4302 New Utrecht Avenue
Brooklyn, NY 11219
Tel: (718) 686 9600

Bronx Office:
1600 Parkview Ave, Suite B
Bronx, NY 10461
Tel: (718) 829 7744
Website: www.hear-our-voices.org

Shield Institute
144-61 Roosevelt Ave.
Flushing, NY 11563
Tel: (718) 939 8700 X1170
Contact Name: Mary McKillap
Email: mmckillop@shield.org
Website: http://www.shield.org

St. Dominic's School
500 Western Highway
Blauvelt, NY 10913
Tel: (845) 359 3400
Website: www.stdominicshome.org/stdominicsschool.
html

St. Francis de Sales School for the Deaf
260 Eastern Parkway
Brooklyn, NY 11225
Tel: (718) 636 4573
Website: www.sfdesales.org

The Successful Learning Center
P.O. Box 2116
Monroe, NY 10949
Tel: (845)-662-1322
Contact Name: Melinda Placanica
Email: info@successfullearningcenter.com
Website: http://www.successfullearningcenter.com
Website: http://access2college.com

The Successful Learning Center provides collegiate-based learning opportunities for adults with developmental disabilities.

Summit Educational Resources
150 Stahl Road
Getzville, NY 14068
Tel: (716) 629 3400
Contact Name: Mary Pat Sperrazza
Email: info@summited.org
Website: http://www.summited.org

Summit School Children's Residence Center
339 North Broadway
Upper Nyack, NY 10960
Tel: (845) 358 7772
Website: www.summitnyack.com

Variety Child Learning Center
47 Humphrey Drive
Syosset, NY 11791
Tel: (516) 921 7171
Toll Free: (800) 933 8779
Website: http://www.vclc.org

Vocational Independence Program (VIP)
NYIT 300 Carlton Ave.
Central Islip, NY 11722
Tel: (631) 348 3354
Contact Name: Dr. Ernst Van Bergeijk, Associate Dean
& Executive Director
Email: evanberg@nyit.edu
Website: http://www.nyit.edu/vip

Westchester Exceptional Children's School
520 Route 22
North Salem, NY 10560
Tel: (914) 277 5533
Website: www.wecschool.org

Legal, Government & Financial Services

ACCES-VR
1 Commerce Plaza Room 1609
Albany, NY 12234
(800) 222 5627
Email: accesadm@mail.nysed.gov
Website: http://www.acces.nysed.gov/vr/

Advocates for Autism
333 Birch Street
Vestal, NY 13850
Tel: (607) 754 9694
Contact Name: Sally Colletti
Email: advocatesforautism@yahoo.com
Website: http://www.advocatesforautism.com

Advocates for Children of NY
151 West 30th Street 5th Floor
New York, NY 10001

Tel: (212) 947 9779
Email: aespada@advocatesforchildren.org
Website: http://www.advocatesforchildren.org

Barger & Gaines
116 Main St.
Irvington, NY 10533
Tel: (914) 902 5918
Email: info@bargergaines.com
Website: http://bargergaines.com
Education attorneys.

Center for Independence of the Disabled (CIDNY)
841 Broadway Suite 301 between 13th and 14th
New York, NY 10003
Tel: (212) 674 2300 or (212) 674 5619
Email: info@cidny.org
Website: http://www.cidny.org/
CIDNY provides a variety of services for people with disabilities in New York City, helping to navigate complex benefit programs.

Law Offices of Adam Dayan
100 Church Street 8th Floor
New York, NY 10007
Tel: (646) 845 7462
Email: adayan@dayanlawfirm.com
Website: http://www.dayanlawfirm.blogspot.com
Special education law.

Law Office of Andrew K. Cuddy
145 E. Genesee Street
Auburn, NY 13021
Tel: (716) 868 9103
Contact Name: Andrew K. Cuddy
Email: acuddy@cuddylawfirm.com
Website: http://www.cuddylawfirm.com
Special education law.

Law Offices of Lauren A. Baum, P.C.
61 Broadway, Suite 1060
New York, New York 10006
Tel: (212) 644 4414
Fax: (212) 644 8470
Special education law.

Law Offices of Neal Howard Rosenberg
9 Murray Street, Suite 4W
New York, NY 10007
Tel: (212) 732 9450
Email: info@nyedlaw.com
Website: www.nyedlaw.com
Special education law.

Law Office of Nicholas J. Agro, P.C.
1000 Main Street
Port Jefferson, NY 11777
Tel: (631) 642 2478
Contact Name: Nicholas Agro
Email: nick.agro@nyeducationlaw.com
Website: http://www.nyeducationlaw.com
Special education law.

Law Offices of Regina Skyer & Associates
276 5th Avenue, Suite 402
New York, NY 10001
Tel: (212) 532 9736
Fax: (212) 532 9846
Email: info@skyerlaw.com
Website: www.skyerlaw.com
Special education law.

Legal Services of Central New York, Inc
472 South Salina Street, Suite 300
Syracuse, NY 13202
Tel: (315) 703 6500
Contact Name: Beth Wallbridge
Email: bwallbridge@wnylc.com
Website: http://www.lscny.org

Legal Services of the Hudson Valley
4 Cromwell Place
White Plains, NY 10601
Tel: (914) 949 1305
Website: http://www.lshv.org

Littman Krooks LLP
655 Third Avenue
New York, New York 10017
Tel: (212) 490 2020

And
399 Knollwood Road
White Plains, NY 10603
Tel: (914) 684 2100

And
300 Westage Business Center Drive, Suite 400
Fishkill, NY 12524
Tel: (845) 896 1106
Website: www.littmankrooks.com

Legal issues relating to special needs including planning and special education.

Long Island Developmental Disabilities Services Office
415A Oser Avenue
Happauge, NY 11788
Tel: (631) 434 6000
Website: http://www.lifssac.com

Marna E. Solarsh, Esq.
670 White Plains Rd. Suite 121
Scarsdale, NY 10583
Tel: (914) 725 7070
Contact Name: Marna Solarsh
Email: msolarsh@earthlink.net
Website: http://www.marnasolarshlaw.com

Expertise in the areas of special education law, guardianship, special needs trusts and future planning.

Martin & Colin, PC
Lisa Colin, Esq.
44 Church St.
White Plains, NY 10601
Tel: (914) 771 7711
Email: info@martincolin.com
Website: martincolin.com

Provides legal services relating to special needs families including: matrimonial and custody issues for families with special needs children; personal injury, if a special needs child is injured in an accident or as a victim of a crime; also provides services as a Parent Coordinator assisting separated parents in coordinating parenting challenges; and Vaccine Exemption issues.

Mayerson & Associates
330 West 38th Street, Suite 600
New York, NY 10018
Tel: (212) 265 7200
Email: admin@mayerslaw.com
Website: mayerslaw.com
Special education law.

New York State Office of Mental Health
44 Holland Avenue
Albany, NY 12229

Office for People with Developmental Disabilities
4 Holland Avenue
Albany, New York 12229
Tel: (866) 946 9733
Contact: Acting Commissioner Kerry Delaney
Email: Commissioners.Correspondence.Unit@opwdd.ny.gov
Website: www.opwdd.ny.gov

Person Centered Care Services (PCCS)
1811 Victory Boulevard
Staten Island, NY 10314
Tel: (718) 370 1088 or (718) 370 1088 x2216
Contact Name: Cris Marchionne
Email: cmarchionne@pccsny.org
Website: http://www.pccsny.org/home

PCCS provides guidance and consultation to people with an intellectual or developmental disability and their families about sources of funding, benefits, and entitlements.

Stuart Flaum, ChSNC
1290 Avenue of the Americas
Suite 3410
New York, NY 10104
Tel: (888) 552-SNFP
Fax: (212) 202 4197
Email: sflaum@financialguide.com
Website: www.specialneedsfamilyplanning.com

Special needs family planning.

Thivierge & Rothberg PC
140 Broadway 46th Floor
New York City, NY 10005
United States
Tel: (212) 397 6360
Contact Name: Christina D. Thivierge
Email: christina@trspecialedlaw.com
Website: http://www.trspecialedlaw.com

Special education law.

Westchester County Department of Community Mental Health
112 East Post Road
White Plains, NY 10601
Tel: (914) 995 5220
Contact Name: Grant Mitchell, M.D., Commissioner
Website: http://www.westchestergov.com/MentalHealth

Wilcenski & Pleat, PLLC
5 Emma Lane
Clifton Park, NY 12186
Tel: (518) 881 1621
Email: lawyers@WPLawNY.com
Website: http://www.WPLawNY.com

Practice in the areas of special needs estate planning and trust and estate administration, traditional estate planning and trust and estate administration, and elder law.

Community and Recreation Services

14th St. Y
344 East 14th Street
New York, NY 10003
Tel: (212) 780 0800
Email: info@14streety.org
Website: www.14streety.org/kids/kol-special-needs-and-inclusion-programs/

The KOL program is for children 4-17 with special needs and includes a variety of opportunities in sports, swimming, the arts, technology, and other activities, as well as parent and professional workshops.

92nd Street Y
1395 Lexington Avenue
New York, NY 10128
Tel: (212) 415 5500
Website: www.92y.org/SpecialNeeds

Provides a variety of programs for children with special needs and others, including classes, afterschool programs, aquatics, camps, Jewish religious education.

Access Equestrian
787 S. Bedford Road
Bedford, NY 10506
Tel: (914)-552-5591
Contact Name: Denise Avolio
Email: diavolio@optonline.net
Website: http://www.accessequestrian.com

https://www.facebook.com/AccessEquestrian

ActionPlay
Toll Free: (844) 228 7529
Email: heather@actionplay.org
Website: actionplay.org

Offers a number of ways to involve those ASD in arts, education, and culture including workshops/programs for individuals with ASD, and consulting and training opportunities.

Adults & Children with Learning & Developmental Disabilities (ACLD)
807 South Oyster Bay Road
Bethpage, NY 11714
Tel: (516) 822 0028
Contact Name: Aaron Liebowitz, Executive Director
Website: http://www.acld.org

American Autism Association
192 Lexington Avenue Suite 245
New York, NY 10016
(877) 654 4483
Contact Name: Eduard Rozenfeld
Email: info@myautism.org
Website: http://www.myautism.org

The Arc of Monroe County
1000 Elmwood Ave.
Rochester, NY 14620
Tel: (585) 271 0660
Website: http://www.arcmonroe.org

Arc of Westchester
265 Saw Mill River Road
Hawthorne, NY 10532
Tel: (914) 949 9300

Email: info@westchesterarc.org
Website: http://www.westchesterarc.org

ARISE
635 James Street
Syracuse, NY 13203
Tel: (315) 472 3171
Website: http://www.ariseinc.org

Arts Horizons
2785 Frederick Douglass Blvd
New York, NY 10039
Tel: (212) 268 7219 X 108
Contact Name: Dena Malarek
Email: dena@artshorizons.org
Website: http://www.artshorizons.org

Arts Horizons is an education organization that brings professional artists to schools/ communities.

Atlas Foundation for Autism
252 West 29th Street, 3rd Floor
New York, NY 10001
Tel: (212) 256 0846
Email: info@atlasforautism.org
Website: www.atlasforautism.org

Provides a wide range of services including: educational programming, afterschool, social groups, ST, OT, Solisten®, HANDLE®, workshops, professional development, parent training, play sessions, overnights, music and art sessions, yoga and recreation groups, and more for individuals with ASD, their families and other professionals.

Autism Council of Rochester, Inc.
1023 Commons Way at Pieter's Family Life Center
Rochester, NY 14623
Tel: (585)-413-1681
Contact Name: Lawana Jones
Email: info@theautismcouncil.org
Website: http://www.theautismcouncil.org

Services include: advocacy, sibling support, and peer support groups, social and recreational programs, and Transition Services (Community Connections for volunteer and employment opportunities) for individuals that are aging out of school.

Autism Services, Inc.
4444 Byrant Stratton Way
Williamsville, NY 14221
Tel: (716) 631 5777 or 1 (888) AUTISM4
Contact Name: Veronica Federiconi
Email: vfedericoni@autism-services-inc.org
Website: http://www.autisticservices.org/

Birch Family Services
104 West 29th Street, Third Floor
New York, NY 10001
Tel: (212) 616 1800
Fax: (212) 741 6739
Website: www.birchfamilyservices.org

Provides education, habilitation, and residential services at a number of locations to people with ASD and other special needs and support for their families. Also provides training to professionals working with those with ASD and other special needs.

Center for Disability Services
314 South Manning Blvd.
Albany, NY 12208
Tel: (518) 437 5700
Contact Name: Christina Rajotte
Email: rajotte@cfdsny.org
Website: http://www.cfdsny.org

Center for Discovery
PO Box 840
Harris, New York 12742
Tel: (845) 794 1400
Website: www.thecenterfordiscovery.org/

Provides educational, health, and residential services for individuals with ASD and other conditions from age 5 through adulthood and offers a wide range of clinical, social, creative arts and recreational programming.

Continuing Developmental Services
860 Hard Rd
Webster, NY 14580
Tel: (585) 341 4600
Contact Name: Jennifer LeTendre
Email: jletendre@cdsunistel.org
Website: http://www.cdsunistel.org

Provides transitional and employment services.

City Access New York
1207 Castleton Avenue, 2nd FlStaten Island, NY 10310-1709
Tel: (718) 285 6548
Fax: (718) 442 7141
Website: www.CityAccessNY.org

Promotes access to educational, vocational and cultural programs for individuals of all abilities.

The Compass Project (at JCCA)
Jewish Child Care Association
45 Manetto Hill Road
Plainview, NY 11803
Tel: (516) 822 3535 X355
Contact Name: Evan Oppenheimer
Email: felixe@jccany.org

Website: http://www.jccany.org/site/
PageServer?pagename=programs_compass_splash

Compass Program provides information, advocacy assistance and college planning to families of Jewish adolescents and young adults with ASD and other learning disabilities transitioning into high school and college.

Crystal Run Village
601 Stony Ford Rd.
Middletown, NY 10941
Tel: (845) 692 4444
Contact Name: Elise Gold
Email: Elise_Gold@crvi.org
Website: http://www.crvi.org

Offers services in such areas as vocational training and placement, residential services, educational opportunities, recreational training and opportunities, and personal and domestic skills training.

Daytime Moon Creations
New York, NY
Contact Name: Jenna Gabriel
Email: jenna.gabriel@daytimemooncreations.org
Website: http://www.daytimemooncreations.org
Website: http://www.daytimemoonblog.wordpress.com

Offers extracurricular programs, in-school programs and an inclusive internship program.

Developmental Disabilities Institute (DDI)
99 Hollywood Drive
Smithtown, NY 11787
Tel: (631) 366 2950 or (631) 366 2900
Contact Name: David Bartash, Chairperson
Website: http://www.ddiny.org

Provides educational, residential, day habilitation and vocational services, as well as medical and dental services.

East End Disability Associates
32 Circle Drive
Shoreham, NY 11786-1321
Tel: (631) 369 7345
Email: info@eed-a.org
Website: http://www.eed-a.org

Provides supports and services for people with developmental disabilities.

Eric Chessen
Autism Fitness
Email: eric@autismfitness.com
Website: www.autismfitness.com

Either on-site or distance (via Skype or phone), consults with professionals and parents to develop/enhance fitness/PE programs for those with ASD.

Family Resource Network
46 Oneida Street
Oneonta, NY 13820
United States
Toll Free: (800) 305 8814
Tel: (607) 432 0001
Contact Email:
Email: familyrn@dmcom.net
Website: http://www.familyrn.org

F.E.G.S
Coram Supervised Individual Residential Alternative (IRA)
New York, NY 10013
Tel: (516) 496 7550 ext 211
Website: http://www.fegs.org

24-hour supervised residence for individuals with ASD who are no longer eligible for children's services.

Fountain House
425 W 47th St
New York, NY 10036
Email: fhinfo@fountainhouse.org
Website: http://www.fountainhouse.org

Gersh Experience
465 Payne Ave.
North Tonawanda, NY 14120
Tel: (716) 693 4509
Contact Name: Dustin Panian, Ed.D., MBA, Executive Director
Contact Email:
Email: dpanian@GERSHACADEMY.onmicrosoft.com
Website: http://www.gershexperience.com

GROW
P.O. Box 1692
White Plains, NY 10602
Tel: (914) 493 1318
Contact Email:
Email: info@grow-ny.org
Website: http://www.grow-ny.org

HeartShare Human Services of New York
12 MetroTech Center 29th Floor
Brooklyn, NY 11201
Tel: (718) 422 4200
Email: info@heartshare.org
Website: http://www.heartshare.org

A community-based organization providing a range of services to children and adults with developmental disabilities.

Helping Our Participants Exercise (HOPE) Fitness
2750 N. Jerusalem Rd
North Bellmore, NY 11710
Toll Free: (877) 396 4673
Email: Info@HOPEFitness.org
Website: http://www.HOPEFitness.org

Intrepid Sea, Air & Space Museum Complex
Pier 86W 46th St and 12th Ave
New York, NY 10036-4103
Tel: (877) 957 7447 or (212) 245 0072
Website: www.intrepidmuseum.org

Offers special programming for visitors with autism and other special needs.

JCC Manhattan
334 Amsterdam Ave
New York, NY 10023
Contact: Allison Kleinman, Director, Center for Special Needs
Tel: (646) 505 4367
Email: akleinman@jccmanhattan.org
Website: www.jccmanhattan.org/special-needs/

Provides programs for children and adults with a wide range of special needs covering a variety of social, recreational and educational activities. Also provides support and resources for families of individuals with special needs.

JCC on the Hudson
371 S. Broadway
Tarrytown, NY 10591
Tel: (914) 366 7898
Email: info@jcconthehudson.org
Website: http://jcconthehudson.org

Jewish Board of Family and Children's Services, Inc.
120 West 57th Street
New York, NY 10019
(888) 523 2769
Tel: (212) 582 9100
Website: http://www.jbfcs.org

JobPath
22 West 38th Street, 11th Floor
New York, NY 10018
Tel: (212) 944 0564
Email: info@jobpathnyc.org
Website: www.jobpathnyc.org/

Provides a variety of programs for employment, supported living, community supports, life coaching, and service coordination.

Keoni Movement Arts, Inc.
Dance Art New York (DANY) Studios
400 W 43rd St. Suite 27J

New York, NY 10036
Tel: (212) 643 9013 or (917) 747 9516
Contact Name: Paul Keoni Chun
Email: paul@KeoniMovementArts.org
Website: http://www.KeoniMovementArts.org

Keoni Movement Arts offers yoga, dance and gymnastics (Yo-Dan-Nastics™) classes for individuals with special needs.

Kids Enjoy Exercise Now (KEEN)
P.O. Box 5115
New York, NY 10185
Tel: (212) 768 6785
Contact Name: Maggie Harrison, Executive Director
Email: info@keennewyork.org
Website: http://www.keennewyork.org

One-to-one recreational opportunities for children and young adults with developmental disabilities at no cost to their families and caregivers.

Kid Esteem Center for Social Learning
175 S 11th St.
Lindenhurst, NY 11704
Tel: (631) 321 6675
Email: kidesteem@aol.com
Website: http://www.kidesteem.com

Lifespire
350 Fifth Avenue Suite 301
New York, NY 10118
Tel: (212) 741 0100
Email: info@lifespire.org
Website: http://www.lifespire.org

Lifestyles for the Disabled
930 Willowbrook Road Building 12-G
Staten Island, NY 10314
Tel: (718) 983 5351 or (718) 983 1952
Email: info@lfdsi.org
Website: http://www.lfdsi.org

Lifestyles for the Disabled provides the intellectually disabled with realistic work settings and experiences on Staten Island.

Life's Worc
1501 Franklin Avenue
Garden City, NY 11530
Tel: (516) 741 9000 X470
Contact Name: Florence Faga, Admissions Coordinator
Email: ffaga@lifesworc.org
Website: http://www.lifesworc.org

Provides a wide range of services to individuals with ASD and other challenges.

Maryhaven Center of Hope
51 Terryville Road
Port Jefferson Station, NY 11776
Tel: (631) 474 4120
Contact Name: Lewis Grossman, Executive Director
Website: http://maryhaven.chsli.org

The Meeting House
133 East 58th Street
New York, NY 10022
Tel: (212) 355 1908
Website: www.themeetinghouseafterschool.org

Provides a wide range of safe and supportive after-school program and additional events for children with special needs, including academic support, physical activities, visual arts, music and drama.

Mental Health Association of Nassau County
16 Main Street
Hempstead, NY 11550
Tel: (516) 489 2322
Contact Name: Steven Greenfielci, Executive Director
Website: http://www.mhanc.org

Museum Access Consortium
Website: museumaccessconsortium.org

Many museums and cultural institutions in New York City have programming for visitors with autism and other special needs. MAC provides a convenient central portal for visitors to learn about programs and activities for families with special needs at many of these institutions.

National Autism Association New York Metro Chapter
200 Cabrini Blvd., #66,
New York, NY 10033
Tel: (212) 977 7722
Email: Kim.MackRosenberg@naanyc.org
Website: www.naanyc.org and www.national
autismny.org

Local chapter of the National Autism Association, providing educational programs for parents and professionals, first responder training, workshops, family and children events, Helping Hand Grants, support for a Sensory Summer Program, advocacy, and more. Collaborates with many other local and national organizations.

New York Transit Museum
Boerum Place
Brooklyn, NY 11201
Tel: (718) 694 1600
Website: web.mta.info/mta/museum

Offers special programs for visitors with special needs in a fun and interactive museum environment.

On Your Mark
645 Forest Ave
Staten Island, NY 10310
Tel: (718) 720 9233
Contact Name: Dr. Joseph Coppolo Jr.
Email: drcoppolo@onyourmark.org
Website: http://www.onyourmark.org

Oswego Industries, Inc.
7 Morrill Place
Fulton, NY 13069
Tel: (315) 598 3108
Contact Name: Lisa Petrocci-Clay
Email: lclay@oswegoind.org
Website: http://www.oswegoindustriesinc.org

Provides vocational training, job assistance, and employment opportunities for individuals at many levels.

Parent Network of Western New York
1000 Main Street
Buffalo, NE 14202
Tel: (716) 332 4170
Email: info@parentnetworkwny.org
Website: http://www.parentnetworkwny.org
https://www.facebook.com/ParentNetwork

People, Inc.
1219 N. Forest Rd. PO Box 9033
Williamsville, NY 14231
Tel: (716) 634 8132
Website: http://www.people-inc.org

Provides a variety of services, including residential, employment, community outreach, health care and recreation programs.

Promoting Specialized Health and Care (PSHC)
56 Beach St.
Staten Island, NY 10304
Tel: (718) 720 2603
Email: info@PSCH.org
Website: http://www.PSCH.org

Quality Services for the Autism Community (QSAC)
253 West 35th Street
New York, NY 10001
United States
718 7 AUTISM
Contact Name: Kevin Mattivi
Email: kmattivi@qsac.com
Website: http://www.qsac.com

Ramapo For Children
Rhinebeck, NY 12572
Tel: (845) 876 8423

Contact Name: Karri Wolfe
Email: kwolfe@ramapoforchildren.org
Website: http://www.ramapoforchildren.org

Resources for Children with Special Needs (RCSN)
116 E. 16th St.
5th Floor
New York, NY 10003
(212) 677 4650
Email: info@resourcesnyc.org
Website: http://www.resourcesnyc.org/

Assists families in navigating and accessing services in New York City.

Riverstone Senior Life Services Open Door Program
99 Fort Washington Ave. at 163rd St
New York, NY 10032
Tel: (212) 927 5600 X118
Contact Name: Milagros Fermin, Program Director
Website: http://www.riverstonenyc.org/programs/open-door

Sinergia
2082 Lexington Avenue
New York, NY 10035
Tel: (212) 643 2840
Contact Name: Myrta Cuadra Lash
Email: cuadralash@sinergiany.org
Website: http://www.sinergiany.org

Assists Latinos and other underserved persons in accessing services in New York City.

Skills Unlimited, Inc.
405 Locust Avenue
Oakdale, NY 11769
(631) 567 3320
Contact Name: Bernie Ryan
Email: bryan@skillsunlimited.org
Website: http://www.skillsunlimited.org/index.html

Skills Unlimited offers a wide variety of employment related support free of charge to consumers seeking placement.

Sky Riding Long Island
989 Connetquot Ave.
Central Islip, NY 11743
Tel: (516) 241 2046
Contact Name: Nancy Tejo
Email: info@skyridingli.com
Website: http://www.SkyRidingLI.com

Therapeutic/adaptive horseback riding lessons for individuals with mental, physical and/or emotional developmental delays.

Springbrook
2705 State Highway 28
Oneonta, NY 13820
Tel: (607) 286 7171
Contact Name: Patricia Kennedy, Executive Director
Email: kennedyp@springbrookny.org
Website: http://www.springbrookny.org

Staten Island Mental Health Society (SIMHS)
669 Castelton Ave.
Staten Island, NY 10301
Tel: (718) 442 2225
Contact Name: Kenneth Popler, PhD, MBA, President/CEO
Email: helpkids@simhs.org
Website: http://www.simhs.org

Strokes of Genius
Tel: (917) 757 1019
Email: info@strokesofgeniusinc.org
Website: strokesofgeniusinc.org

Empowers individuals with ASD by providing a variety of educational art studio experiences and workshops focusing on the abilities of individuals with ASD, exhibits artwork, and provides a means for artists to make their work available for sale. Also provides training to professionals.

Super Soccer Stars – Shine Program for Children with Special Needs
606 Columbus Ave. New York, NY 10024
Tel: (212) 877 7171
Website: newyork.supersoccerstars.com/shine

Taconic Innovations, Inc.
115 South Macquesten Parkway
Mount Vernon, NY 12590
Tel: (914) 668 9041 ex 304
Contact Name: Sandy Ali
Email: Sandy@Taconicinnovations.com
Website: http://www.Taconicinnovations.com

Provides services and supports to children and adults with developmental disabilities in Dutchess, Columbia, Putnam, Ulster, Orange, Westchester counties, as well as the Bronx.

Tech Kids Unlimited
2 Metrotech Center, 8th Floor
Brooklyn, NY 11201
Contact Name: Keri Swisher, Program Coordinator
Email: keri@techkidsunlimited.org
Website: http://www.techkidsunlimited.org

Provides a wide range of programs for children with special needs to learn different aspects of technology. Includes after school, in-school, weekend and week-long programs.

Triform Camphill Community
20 Tri Form Rd.
Hudson, NY 12534
Tel: (518) 851 9320
Contact Name: Tim Paholak
Email: admissions@triform.org
Website: http://triform.org

Triform Camphill Community, in Hudson, New York, is a residential community for young adults with developmental disabilities.

WeeZee – The Science of Play
480 North Bedford Road
Chappaqua, NY 10514
Tel: (914) 752 2100
Website: www.weezeeworld.com

Offering a variety of options to participate, the facility creates sensory experiences designed to improve physical fitness, socialization and academic performance for children of all abilities.

Windmills and Tulips
PO Box 321
Purchase, NY 10577-0321
Tel: (917) 763 2732
Contact Name: Jennifer Schultz
Email: jennifer@windmillsandtulips.com
Website: http://www.windmillsandtulips.com

YAI Network
460 West 34th Street
New York, NY 10001
Tel: (212) 273 6100 or (212) 273 6182
Website: http://www.yai.org

Includes more than 450 programs and serves more than 20,000 people every day.

YogaShine: Yoga/Dance/Movement Therapy
7-11 Legion Drive
Valhalla, NY 10595
Tel: (914) 769 8745
Contact Name: Vitalah Gayle Simon, M.Ed., LCAT, ADTR, RYT-500
Email: yogashine@verizon.net
Website: http://www.yogashine.com

NORTH CAROLINA

Doctors, Clinics, Hospitals, and Other Health Services

Autism Answers
346 Wagner Dr Suite 206
Fayetteville, NC 28303

Tel: (910) 868 6868
Contact Name: Becky Givens
Email: becky@myautismanswers.org
Website: http://www.myautismanswers.org

Provides a multifaceted treatment model that combines medical, nutritional, and behavioral techniques in treating individuals with ASD.

Autism Education and Research Institute (AERI)
P.O. Box 31711
Raleigh, NC 27622
Tel: (1-866-727-AERI (2374)
Contact Name: Catherine Hughes, Director of Family Support Services
Email: support@aerionline.com
Website: http://www.aerionline.com

AERI provides psychological testing, training and consultation, autism services (throughout the lifespan), family-based mental health services, parent-child interaction therapy, trauma services, and transition services.

Black Mountain Center
932 Old U.S. 70
Black Mountain, NC 28711
Tel: (828) 259 6700
Email: bmntc.info@dhhs.nc.gov
Website: http://www.bmcnc.org/

Black Mountain Neuro-Medical Treatment Center provides services and supports to individuals and families affected by a variety of disabilities and health challenges.

The Carolina Institute for Developmental Disabilities (CIDD)
101 Renee Lynne Court
Carrboro, NC 27510
Tel: (919) 966 5171
Email: Info@cidd.unc.edu
Website: http://www.cidd.unc.edu

Offers a wide array of services for families across North Carolina.

CenterPoint Human Services
4045 University Parkway
Winston-Salem, NC 27106
Tel: (336) 714 9100
Toll Free: (888) 581 9988
Website: http://www.cphs.org

Crossroads Behavioral Healthcare
Elkin, NC 28621
Tel: (336) 835 1000
Email: Healthcare@crossroadsbhc.org

Dorothea Dix Hospital
820 South Boylan Avenue
Raleigh, NC 27699
Tel: (919) 733 5540
Contact Name: James W. Osberg, III, Ph.D., Director
Website: http://www.ncdhhs.gov/dsohf/services/dix/about-dix.htm

Duke Children's Hospital and Health Center
Duke Clinic 1-I 2301 Erwin Road
Durham, NC 27710
Tel: (919) 668 4000
Website: http://www.dukechildrens.org

Family Psychiatry and Psychology Associates
104-A Fountain Brook Circle
Cary, NC 27511
Tel: (919) 233 4131
Website: http://www.fppa.com

Provides individual, multidisciplinary, and/or a team approach, with a broad range of services to clients including assessment, psychotherapy and medication management.

Neurosensory Center Of Charlotte
14330 Oakhill Park LN.
Huntersville, NC 28078
Tel: (704) 746 3942
Email: timjackson@nsccharlotte.com

Sandhills Center for MH/DD/SAS
PO Box 9
West End, NC 27376-0009
Tel: (910) 673 9111
Toll Free: (800) 256 2452
Contact Name: Michael Watson
Email: michaelw@www.sandhillscenter.org
Website: http://www.sandhillscenter.org

Therapy Services

A New Leaf Therapeutic Services, PLLC
581 Executive Place Suite 500
Fayetteville, NC 28305
Tel: (910) 493 3555
Contact Name: Mackenzie Toland
Email: Mackenzie@fayettevillenewleaf.com
Website: http://www.fayettevillenewleaf.com

Provides ABA therapy and outpatient therapy to family members and siblings of children with ASD.

Autism Innovations, LLC
93 E. Trafalgar Ct.
Clayton, NC 27520
Tel: (919) 390 7771
Contact Name: Danielle Kelly, M.Ed., NBCT
Email: Dkelly@auinnovations.com
Website: http://Www.auinnovations.com

Provides structured social skills instruction and other interventions to individuals with ASD, sensory integration disorders, and emotional disabilities within the home setting.

Carolina Care Solutions, LLC
1409 East Blvd., Suite 102-A
Charlotte, NC 28203
Tel: (704) 770 1862
Contact Name: Amanda Peay
Email: apeay@carolinacaresolutions.com
Website: http://www.carolinacaresolutions.com

Carolina Pediatric Therapy
9 Summit Avenue Suite B
Asheville, NC 28803
Tel: (828) 670 8056
Website: http://www.CarolinaPeds.com

Licensed speech-language pathologists, occupational therapists, physical therapists, and early childhood interventionists.

Catherine Leister & Associates
11535 Carmel Commons Blvd, Suite 100
Charlotte, NC 28226
Tel: (704) 541 3737
Contact Name: Kimberly Binford
Email: kb@terrifictalkers.com
Website: http://www.terrifictalkers.com

Provides the highest quality speech, language, and communication services for children, ages 18 months to 18 years.

Clinical Psychology Services of Raleigh
Raleigh, NC 27601
Tel: (919) 673 9433
Contact Name: Virginia Fee, Ph.D.
Email: Virginia.fee.phd@gmail.com

Practice is entirely focused on ASD, with social/communication/behavior focus, using ABA, Denver Model, and Pivotal Response Training.

Collaborative Autism Treatment (CAT)-Campus
3209 Yorktown Ave
Durham, NC 27713
Tel: (919) 213 9841
Website: http://www.cat-campus.com

Community Counseling Services
1550 Tanglewood Dr
Hickory, NC 28601
Tel: (828) 381 5920
Contact Name: Mary Ruff
Website: http://www.ccs-sd.org

Cornerstone Family Services
10423 Ligon Mill Road
Wake Forest, NC 27587
Tel: (919) 630 4191
Contact Name: Suzanne Germann
Email: cornerstone@cfskids.com
Website: http://www.cfskids.com

Creative Consultants
Charlotte, NC
Tel: (919) 459 5472
Contact Name: Denise Freeman DeCandia
Email: denise@creativeconsultantsnc.com
Website: http://www.creativeconsultantsnc.com

Crossroads Counseling
425 7th Ave. SW
Hickory, NC 28602
Tel: (828) 327 6633
Website: http://www.crossroadscounseling.org

Crystal Coast Autism Center
5242 Hwy 70 W.
Morehead City, NC 28557
Tel: (252) 240 2255
Contact Name: Elizabeth Romera
Email: director@ccautismcenter.org
Website: http://www.ccautismcenter.org

A resource center with occupational and speech therapy.

Delta Behavioral Group, PLLC
Charlotte, NC 28237
Tel: (704) 931 8870 or (855) 201 5498
Contact Name: Marla O'Neill
Email: moneill@deltabehavior.com
Website: http://www.deltabehavior.com

Developmental Therapy Associates, Inc.
875 Walnut St, Suite #100
Cary, NC 27511
Tel: (919) 465 3966
Contact Name: Greg Stivland
Email: info@developmentaltherapy.com
Website: http://www.developmentaltherapy.com

Provides occupational therapy and speech/language therapy.

Dreamweavers Unlimited, Inc.
1010 E. Garrison Blvd
Gastonia, NC 28054
Tel: (704) 868 8551
Contact Name: Blayke Turrubiartes
Email: dwublayke@bellsouth.net
Website: http://www.dreamweaversnc.com

Exceptional Equestrians
300 Enola Rd.
Morganton, NC 28655
Tel: (828) 433 2291
Website: Http://www.jirdc.org/files/EEBrochure.pdf

A therapeutic horseback riding program for adults and children with disabilities.

Katie Brady, LCSW
3209 Yorktown Avenue
Durham, NC 27713
Tel: (919) 360 0408
Email: katie.brady.lcsw@gmail.com
Website: Http://katiebradylcsw.org/about/

Provides in-home therapy to individuals with ASD and their families, as well as social groups and consultation.

Lifespan ABA, Inc.
351 Wagoner Drive Suite 350
Fayetteville, NC 28303
Tel: (910) 493 3999
Contact Name: Sharonda Ferguson
Email: lifespan@lifespanabanc.org
Website: http://lifespanabanc.org

Provides applied behavior analysis therapy to children, adolescents, and adults with ASD.

May Center Services
Camp Lejeune, NC 28547
Tel: (910) 333 0814
Contact Name: Merry Rainey
Email: mrainey@mayinstitute.org
Website: http://www.mayinstitute.org

Committed to making ABA services accessible to military families who have children with autism spectrum disorders (ASD).

Pediatric Hands On Therapy
PO Box 1471
Belmont, NC 28012
Tel: (704) 747 3788
Contact Name: Freida Smith
Email: pediatrichandsontherapy@yahoo.com
Website: http://www.pediatrichandsontherapy.com

Occupational therapists focused on play-based therapy.

Riverwood Therapeutic Riding Center
6825 Rolling View Drive
Tobaccoville, NC 27050
Tel: (336) 922 6426
Contact Name: Kim Beauchamp
Email: rtrc@windstream.net
Website: http://www.riverwoodtrc.org

Therapeutic riding center, serving children and adults with disabilities.

Smoky Mountain Center
PO Box 127
Sylva, NC 28779
Tel: (828) 586 5501
Toll Free: (800) 849 6127
Contact Name: Tom McDevitt
Email: tom@smokymountaincenter.org
Website: http://www.smokymountaincenter.org

Coordinates prevention, treatment, and support services for individuals and families with developmental disabilities, and other needs.

Spectrum Support Services
25213 Burbage Circle
Cary, NC 27519
Tel: (919) 641 2826
Contact Name: Lamar R. Pittman, BA., QP
Email: lpittman23@hotmail.com

St. Gerard House (SGH)
620 Oakland Street
Hendersonville, NC 28791
Tel: (828) 693 4223
Email: info@stgerardhouse.com
Website: http://www.stgerardhouse.com

Offers evidence-based treatment for individuals with ASD and other challenges.

Weehabilitate - Pediatric Therapy
2200 E. Millbrook Rd.
Suite 117
Raleigh, NC 27604
Tel: (919) 880 5770
Contact Name: Nicole Parten, Owner/Director
Email: nicole@weehabilitate.com
Website: http://www.weehabilitate.com

WeeHabilitate Pediatric Therapy is a pediatric occupational therapy, speech therapy, and feeding therapy and also provides a preschool for special needs children ages 2-5.

Schools and Educational Services

Autism Consulting and Training, Inc.
PO BOX 53

Asheville, NC 28802
Tel: (305) 793 8280
Contact Name: Jennifer Strauss
Email: straussjen10@gmail.com
Website: http://www.autismconsultingandtraining.com

Autism Consulting and Training, Inc. provides in-home educational services to children on the Autism Spectrum in Miami, Florida and Asheville, North Carolina and sets up individualized programs.

Cyzner Institute
7022 Sardis Road
Charlotte, NC 28270
Tel: (704) 366 8260
Contact Name: Dr. Lisa Cyzner
Email: lcyzner@yahoo.com
Website: http://www.cyznerinstitute.com

An educational and therapeutic institute for children pre-school aged through 6th grade who have special needs.

Little Town Learning Center
402 S. Wright Street P.O. Box 487
Burgaw, NC 28425
Tel: (910) 259 3311
Contact Name: Angela Beacham
Email: abeacham@bizec.rr.com

Little Town Learning Center is a certified Developmental Day Center, serving children birth to 12 years of age.

Philips Academy of NC
3115 Providence Rd
Charlotte, NC 28211
Tel: (704) 365 4533
Contact Name: Deborah Hofland, Executive Director
Email: dhofland@philipsacademync.org
Website: Http://philipsacademync.org/

School for middle and high school students with complex language, learning and developmental disabilities and ASD, offering remediation, practical instruction, and community-based application.

The Stogner Scholarship for Autism
Tel: (336) 608 9418
Contact Name: Wendi Stogner
Email: wendi@scholarshipsforautism.org
Website: http://www.scholarshipsforautism.org

The Stogner Scholarship for Autism, Inc. is a 501(C)3 Non-Profit Organization dedicated to awarding scholarships to people diagnosed with ASD living in the state of North Carolina.

Talisman Transitions
1109 White Pine Drive
Hendersonville, NC 28739

Tel: (888) 458 8226 or (828) 697 1113
Contact Name: Sarah Marr
Email: smarr@talismanacademy.com
Website: http://www.talismanprograms.com
Website: http://www.talismanacademy.com

Talisman Transitions is a residential training program for young adults 18-24 that provides comprehensive and individualized preparation for college/vocational programs and independent living.

UNC-Charlotte Office of Disability Services
9201 University City Blvd
Charlotte, NC 28233-0001
Tel: (704) 687 4355
Contact Name: Kristin Kolin
Email: dissrvcs@uncc.edu
Website: http://www.ds.uncc.edu

The University of North Carolina at Greensboro - Beyond Academics
3607 MHRA Building
1111 Spring Garden St.
Greensboro, NC 27412
Tel: (336) 334 3905
Contact Name: Eric Marshburn
Email: e_marshb@uncg.edu
Website: http://beyondacademics.uncg.edu

Legal, Government & Financial Services

A Special Needs Plan
6000 Fairview Rd. Suite 400
Charlotte, NC 28210
Tel: (704) 557 9637 or (704) 557 9630
Contact Name: Andrew Spafford, Manager, Family and Organization Outreach
Email: Aspafford@aspecialneedsplan.com
Website: http://www.aspecialneedsplan.com

Special needs financial planning.

Department of Housing and Urban Development
1500 Pinecroft Road Suite 401
Greensboro, NC 27407
Tel: (336) 547 4000
Contact Name: Edward Ellis
Email: NC_webmanager@hud.gov
Website: http://www.hud.gov/local/index.cfm?state=nc&topic=offices

Disability Rights North Carolina
2626 Glenwood Avenue Suite 305
Raleigh, NC 27608
Tel: (877) 235 4210 or (919) 856 2195
Website: http://disabilityrightsnc.org

Division of Mental Health, Developmental Disabilities, and Substance Abuse Services
325 N. Salisbury Street
Raleigh, NC 27699
Tel: (919) 733 7011
Contact Name: Jim Jarrard, Acting Director
Website: http://www.ncdhhs.gov/mhddsas/index.htm

Division of Vocational Rehabilitation Services
21 Mail Service Center
Raleigh, NC 27699
Tel: (800) 689 9090
Website: http://www.ncdhhs.gov/dvrs

Insurance Resource Group, Inc
304 N. Church St
Concord, NC 28025
Tel: (704) 792 1204
Contact Name: Ted B. Banther
Email: tbanther@ctc.net

Estate Planning for Special Needs Families

The Moncrieffe Law Firm
107 Windel Drive, Suite 201
Raleigh, NC 27609
Tel: (919) 757 2642
Contact Name: Attorney Monica Moncrieffe
Email: info@moncrieffelaw.com
Website: http://www.moncrieffelaw.com

Special education law.

NC Division of Child Development
319 Chapanoke Rd
Raleigh, NC 27603
Tel: (919) 662 4499
Website: http://www.ncchildcare.net

Stacey Gahagan, Attorney
50101 Governors Drive, Suite 100
Chapel Hill, NC 27517
Tel: (919) 606 4119 or (919) 942 1430
Contact Name: Stacey Gahagan
Email: stacey@gahaganlaw.com
Website: http://www.gahaganlaw.com

Special education law.

Community and Recreation Services

3 Irish Jewels Farm
Tel: (919) 602 9883
Contact Name: Erin O'Loughlin
Email: Erin@3IrishJewelsFarm.org
Website: http://www.3IrishJewelsFarm.org

Aspie Travel
2103 Red Forest Road
Greensboro, NC 27410
Tel: (855) GO ASPIE (462-7743)
Contact Name: Jackie Longino
Email: jackie@aspietravel.com

Autism Center for Life Enrichment (ACLE)
810 Warren Street
Greensboro, NC 27401
Tel: (336) 333 0197
Contact Name: Latisha Dawson, Program Director
Website: Http://autismsociety-nc.org/

Autism Foundation of the Carolinas
PO Box 12671
Charlotte, NC 28220
Contact Name: Lori Schleicher
Email: info@autismcarolinas.org
Website: http://autismcarolinas.org

Autism Services of Mecklenburg County (ASMC), Inc.
2211-A Executive St.
Charlotte, NC 28208
Tel: (704) 392 9220
Email: info@asmcinc.com
Facebook: https://www.facebook.com/ASMCInc

Offers residential and support services.

Autism Society of North Carolina
505 Oberlin Rd, Suite 230
Raleigh, NC 27605-1345
Tel: (919) 743 0204
(800) 442 2762
Contact Name: Tracey Sheriff, CEO
Email: tsheriff@autismsociety-nc.org
Website: http://www.autismsociety-nc.org

Bayada Nurses
8801 JM Keynes Dr.
Charlotte, NC 28262
Tel: (704) 688 2500
Contact Name: Erin McBride
Email: emcbride@bayada.com
Website: http://www.bayada.com

Beacon Transitions
836 3rd Ave. West
Hendersonville, NC 28739
Tel: (828) 388 5478 or (828) 713 9584
Contact Name: Kelly Stamey, MA
Email: kstamey@beacontransitions.com
Website: http://beacontransitions.com/

Beacon Transitions is an intentional living community where services help students achieve more independence.

Capabilities Fitness
117 W First Street
Lowell, NC 28098
Tel: (704)3015754 or 7047182032
Contact Name: Amber Gibson
Email: Amber@capabilitiesfitness.com
Website: Http://www.capabilitiesfitness.com/

Fitness programs for children and adults with disabilities.

Camp Lakey Gap
222 Fern Way
Black Mountain, NC 28711
Tel: (828) 669 8977
Contact Name: Elsa Berndt
Email: elsa.berndt@yahoo.com
Website: http://www.christmount.org/camplakeygap

Therapeutic recreation using visually structured programming that is highly supervised, encouraging independence and socialization.

Child Care Resources Inc.
4600 Park Road, Suite 400
Charlotte, NC 28209
Tel: (704) 376 6697
Email: mailbox@childcareresourcesinc.org
Website: http://www.childcareresourcesinc.org

Creative Supports, Inc.
Charlotte, NC 28202
Tel: (704) 426 3806
Contact Name: Anna Quinlivan
Email: anna@creativesupportsinc.org
Website: http://www.creativesupportsinc.org

DanceAbilities Academy
1385 E. Garrison Blvd.
Gastonia, NC 28054
Tel: (704) 867 1140
Contact Name: Tess Walters
Email: danceabilities@mail.com
Website: http://www.DanceAbilitiesAcademy.org

Offers free dance, karate, yoga, gymnastics, cheerleading, and wheelchair classes and other services to children and adults with a variety of disabilities.

Developmental Disabilities Resources, Inc.
9929 Albemarle Road, Suite 4-A
Charlotte, NC 28227
Tel: (704) 573 9777 or (866) 313 9777
Email: ddrweb@ddrinc.org
Website: http://www.ddrinc.org

Easter Seals North Carolina
2315 Myron Dr.
Raleigh, NC 27607

Tel: (919) 783 8898
Toll Free: (800) 6662 7119
Email: info@nc.eastersealsucp.com
Website: http://www.nc.easterseals.com

Exceptional Children's Assistance Center (ECAC)
907 Barra Row, Suites 102/103
Davidson, NC 28036
Tel: (704) 892 1321
Toll Free: (800) 962 6817
Email: ecac@ecacmail.org
Website: http://www.ecac-parentcenter.org

First in Families of North Carolina
3109 University Drive
Durham, NC 27707
Tel: (919) 251 8368
Email: info@fifnc.org
Website: http://www.fifnc.org

Full Spectrum Farms
3101 Old Cullowhee Road
Cullowhee, NC 28723
Tel: (828) 293 2521
Contact Name: Harold Watson, Executive Director
Email: harold@fullspectrumfarms.org
Website: http://www.fullspectrumfarms.org

Provides a farm community to adults with ASD where individuals can live and work.

GHA
213 N. Second St.
Albemarle, NC 28001
Tel: (704) 982 9600
Contact Name: Dawn Allen
Website: Http://www.ghaautismsupports.org/

iCan House
862 W. Fourth Street
Winston-Salem, NC 27101
Tel: (336) 723 0050
Contact Name: Kim Shufran
Email: kim@icanhouse.com
Website: http://www.iCanHouse.com

The iCan House is a resource center for families with children on the autism spectrum.

Independent Opportunities, Inc.
9216 University City Blvd
Charlotte, NC 28213
Tel: (704) 547 8521
Contact Name: Greg J. Krypel
Email: GregKrypel_IOI@bellsouth.net
Website: http://www.chooseioi.com

IQuOLIOC
141 Thomas Humphrey Road
Jacksonville, NC 28546-9700
Tel: (910) 355 2000
Contact Name: Tammy Cleveland
Email: tammycleveland@iquolioc.org
Facebook: Website: http://www.facebook.com/pages/IQuOLIOC-Inc/120397467981136?sk=wall

IQuOLIOC (Improving Quality Of Life In Our Community) Eagles Nest Retreat offers Residential Support for young adults. Also provides Respite, Therapeutic Day & Travel Camps, ABA/Floortime, Sensory Integration, Social Skills Training, Volunteerism, Home and Community Based Waiver Program (NC CAP MR/DD) for children and adults.

Irene Wortham Center
916 W. Chapel Road
Asheville, NC 28803
Tel: (828) 274 7518
Website: http://www.iwcnc.org/index.php?option=com_content&task=view&id=10&Itemid=12

Supported employment program.

J. Iverson Riddle Developmental Center
300 Enola Road
Morganton, NC 28655
Tel: (828) 433 2731
Website: http://www.jirdc.org

Provides comprehensive residential care to citizens from 34 counties in the western portion of the state.

Journey Camp, A Sensory-Smart Camp for Sensational Kids
2300 Austin Traphill Road
Elkin, NC 28621
Tel: (336) 366 7416
Contact Name: Jennifer Blackburn Bracey
Email: jennifer@soulcompass.com
Website: http://www.soulcompasscenter.com

Kids with Autism Making Progress in Nature (KAMPN)
1255 Wildcat Ridge
Deep Gap, NC 28618
Tel: (828) 264 0054
Email: kampn4autism@gmail.com
Website: Http://kampn4autism.appstate.edu/

An overnight camping experience for children with autism and their families.

National Inclusion Project
PO Box 110104
RTP, NC 27709
Tel: (919) 314 5540
Website: Http://www.inclusionproject.org/

New Hope ASD Consulting
1202 Braxton Bragg Ct.
Hillsborough, NC 27278
Tel: (919) 260 1077
Contact Name: Casey Palmer
Email: newhopeasdconsulting@yahoo.com

North Carolina Council for Exceptional Children
3924 Laurel Grove Road
Winston-Salem, NC 27127
Contact Name: Charmion Rush
Email: charsingl@yahoo.com
Website: http://nccec.coe.ecu.edu

Outstanding Autism Support and Instructional Services (OASIS)
3114 Randall Pkwy. Suite 4
Wilmington, NC 28403
Tel: (910) 769 4586
Contact Name: Kim Reinhardt, Program Coordinator
Email: Kim.Reinhardt.@oasisnc.org
Website: http://www.oasisnc.org

Parker Autism Foundation
5290 Cambridge Bay Drive
Charlotte, NC 28269
Tel: (704) 819 4952
Contact Name: Shelley Reilley
Website: http://www.parkerautismfoundation.org

Saving Grace Farm
565 Trexler Loop
Salisbury, NC 28144
Tel: (704) 638 2339 or (704) 798 5955
Contact Name: Janna Griggs
Email: janna@savinggracefarm.com
Website: http://savinggracefarm.com

Provides services to people with special needs through interactions with horses.

ShineLight
2825 Arlington Ave.
Fayetteville, NC 28303
Tel: (910) 323 1335
Email: info@shine-light.org
Website: http://www.shine-light.org

Stanly County Partnership For Children
1000 North First Street, Suite 8
PO Box 2165
Albemarle, NC 28002
Tel: (704) 982 2038
Website: http://www.stanlypartnership.org

Trusted Parents
1914 JN Pease Place
Charlotte, NC 28262
Tel: (980) 229 7253
Contact Name: Nikia Bye
Email: nikiabye@trustedparents.org
Website: http://www.trustedparents.org

Wake County Grandparents Support Group
505 Oberlin Rd. Suite 230
Raleigh, NC 27605
Tel: (919) 865 5058 or (919) 280 0603
Contact Name: Maureen Morrell
Email: mmorrell@autismsociety-nc.org.
Website: http://wakecountyautismsociety.org/

Walkin' Roll Activities League, Inc.
PO Box 334
Claremont, NC 28610
Tel: (828) 228 0616
Website: http://www.walkinroll.org

Sports activities for those with various challenges, including physical challenges.

Wings of Eagles Ranch
4800 Thunderbolt Road
Concord, NC 28025
Tel: (704) 784 3147
Website: http://www.wingsofeaglesranch.org

Provides therapeutic horseback riding, high and low rope adventures, and other outdoor activities.

NORTH DAKOTA

Doctors, Clinics, Hospitals, and Other Health Services

Dakota Boys and Girls Ranch- Western Plains Residential Center
1227 N. 35th St
Bismarck ND, 58501
Tel: (701) 221 5304 or (701) 261 9040
E-mail: a.reuschlein@dakotaranch.org
https://www.dakotaranch.org/

Provides treatment programs for boys and girls in grades 9 through 12.

Dakota Clinic
401 3rd Street SE
Jamestown, ND 58401
Tel: (701) 253 5300
Toll Free: (800) 247 0159
Contact Name: Myra J Quanrud, MD FAAP
Website: http://www.innovishealth.com

Jamestown Hospital
419 5th Street NE
Jamestown, ND 58401
Tel: (701) 252 1050
Website: http://www.jamestownhospital.com

Prairie Therapy
3120 4th Ave. Northwest
Minot, ND 58703
Tel: (701) 839 1311
Contact Name: Kelly Drevecky, OTR/L
Email: kelly@prairietherapy.com

A pediatric outpatient clinic that works extensively with patients with ASD, Sensory Processing challenges, and related challenges.

Saint Sophie's Psychiatric Care
3000 North 14th St. Suite 2A
Bismarck, ND 58503
Tel: (701) 751 8008
Website: http://www.st-sophies.com

Assessment, diagnostics, individual therapy, and group therapy/skills training for those with ASD.

Tioga Medical Center
810 Welo Street
Tioga, ND 58852
Tel: (701) 664 3305
Website: http://www.tiogahealth.org

Therapy Services

Changing Behavior
Fargo, ND 58103
Tel: (701).238.3930
Contact Name: Alee S.
Email: changingbehavior@live.com
Website: http://www.youcangrowtoday.com

Providing individualized behavioral therapy services as well as school consultations.

Heart of Behavior, LLC
Fargo, ND 58102
Tel: (218) 329 5609
Contact Name: Crystal Henderson, M.S., BCBA, LABA
Email: crystal@heartofbehavior.com
Website: http://www.heartofbehavior.com

North Dakota Autism Center, Inc.
4733 Amber Valley Parkway Suite 200
Fargo, ND 58104
Tel: (701) 277 8844
Contact Name: Darcy Kasprowicz
Email: dkasprowicz@ndautismcenter.org
Website: http://ndautismcenter.org

Schools and Educational Services

Little Coyotes Preschool; Wilkinson School
42 University Avenue
Williston, ND 58801
Tel: (701) 572 2346 or (701) 572 1580
Website: http://nationalautismnetwork.com/directory/12187-little-coyotes-preschool/

Legal, Government & Financial Services

Department of Housing and Urban Development
657 2nd Avenue North Room 366
Fargo, ND 58108
Tel: (701) 239 5136
Contact Name: Joel Manske
Email: ND_webmanager@hud.gov
Website: http://www.hud.gov/local/index.cfm?state=nd&topic=offices

Developmental Disabilities Unit–Early Intervention
1237 W. Divide Avenue Suite 1A
Bismarck, ND 58501
Tel: (701) 328 8936
Toll Free: (800) 755 8529
Contact Name: Debra Balsdon, Part C Coordinator
Email: sobald@state.nd.us
Website: http://www.nd.gov/dhs/services/disabilities/earlyintervention

This program is designed to identify children at risk in the earliest stages.

Division of Vocational Rehabilitation
1237 West Divide Avenue, Suite 1B
Bismarck, ND 58501
Tel: (701) 328 8950
Contact Name: Russ Cusack
Email: rcusack@nd.gov
Website: http://www.nd.gov/dhs/dvr/

Guardianship Association of North Dakota
5201 Bishops Boulevard, Suite B
Fargo, ND 58104
Tel: (701) 235 4457
Email: dbyzewski@catholiccharitiesnd.org
Website: http://www.gand.org

North Dakota Protection & Advocacy Project
400 E. Broadway, Suite 616
Bismarck, ND 58501
Tel: (701) 328 2950
Toll Free: (800) 472 2670
Contact Name: Teresa Larson
Email: Beckatpa@aol.com

Website: http://www.ndpanda.org

The Protection & Advocacy Project (P&A) advocates for the legal rights of North Dakotans with disabilities.

Pathfinder Parent Center

1600 2nd Ave. Southwest
Minot, ND 58701
Tel: (701) 837 7500
Toll Free: (800) 245 5840
Email: info@pathfinder-nd.org
Website: http://www.pathfinder-nd.org

Community and Recreation Services

ADA Paratransit

867 48th St
Grand Forks, ND 58201
Tel: (701) 746 2600
Website: http://www.grandforksgov.com/government/bus/dial-a-ride

ADA-Para transit is a transportation service provided to those who cannot, for physical or cognitive reasons, ride the City Bus system in Grand Forks, ND and East Grand Forks, MN.

Anne Carlsen Center

701 3rd Street NW PO Box 8000
Jamestown, ND 58402
Tel: (701) 252 3850
Toll Free: (800) 568 5175
Contact Name: Eric Monson
Email: eric.monson@annecenter.org
Website: http://www.annecenter.org

Bethel Kids

2702 30th Ave. South
Fargo, ND 58103
Tel: (701) 232 4476
Contact Name: Pastor Gary Seifers
Email: garysiefers@bethelfc.com
Website: http://www.bethelfc.com/ministries/bethel-kids

Family Voices of North Dakota

PO Box 163 312 2nd Ave. W
Edgeley, ND 58433
Tel: (888) 522 9654
Contact Name: Donene Feist
Email: fvnd@drtel.net
Website: http://www.fvnd.org

A statewide health information and education center for families who have children with a special health need or disability from birth to age 26 and for the professionals that serve them.

Horses Helping Humans

Triple H Miniature Horse Rescue
4747 22nd Ave.
Mandan, ND 58554
Tel: (701) 220 4449
Contact Name: Alison Smith
Email: hhhmhr@mac.com
Website: http://www.horseshelpinghumans.net

Horses Helping Humans is a program offered through Triple H Miniature Horse Rescue and provides an equine-assisted activities program.

Pride, Inc.

1200 Missouri Ave.
Bismarck, ND 58504
Contact Name: Darcy Severson
Email: darcys@prideinc.org
Website: http://www.prideinc.org/

Red River Valley Asperger-Autism Network

P.O. Box 281
West Fargo, ND 58078
Tel: (701) 566 1675
Contact Name: JoAnne Vieweg
Email: jrview@cableone.net
Website: http://www.rrvan.org

OHIO

Doctors, Clinics, Hospitals, and Other Health Services

Ali Carine, DO
Dr. Carine Integrative Pediatrics

3300 Riverside Dr.
Upper Arlington, OH 43221
Tel: (614) 459 4200
Email: mail@drcarine.com
Website: www.drcarine.com

Dr. Carine and her team provide holistic, integrative pediatric care to address the needs of their patients; care includes primary pediatric care.

Allen Lewis, MD
Integrative Pediatrics of Ohio, LLC

1090 Beecher Crossing N
Suite C
Columbus, OH 43230
Tel: (614) 245 4750
Website: www.integrativepediatricsofohio.com

Dr. Cheryl Hammes
Integrative Wellness
4003 Broadview Rd.
Richfield, OH 44286
Tel: (330) 659 2320
Email: Drcheryl@drcheryl.info
Website: www.drcheryl.info

Provides integrative treatment for a variety of health concerns, including autism.

Deborah Nash, MD
Nash Integrative Medicine, Inc.
245 S. Garber Dr.
Tipp City, OH, 45371
Tel: (937) 877 1222
Website: www.uvmc.com/physician.aspx?phid=39266

Dr. Nash is a family physician providing integrative health care to patients.

Elizabeth Meuller, DDS, & Associates
9200 Montgomery Road, Suite 4B
Cincinnati, OH 45242
Tel: (513) 791 3660
Email: katy@outstandingdentalteam.com
Website: http://www.outstandingdentalteam.com

Pediatric dental services.

Lee-Silsby Compounding Pharmacy
3216 Silsby Road
Cleveland Heights, OH 44118
Tel: (800) 918 8831 or (216) 321 4300
Fax: (216) 321 4303
Email: contact@leesilsby.com
Website: www.leesilsby.com

Compounding pharmacy.

The Nisonger Center at The Ohio State University
1581 Dodd Drive
Columbus, OH 43210
Tel: (614) 292 0775
Website: http://nisonger.osu.edu

Offers services and resources, including autism spectrum disorder clinics, behavioral support services, family directed developmental clinics.

Noah Erickson, D.C., Med. Ac.
Dr. Noah's ARC
8261 Market Street
Boardman, OH 44512
Tel: (330) 726 3456
Website: www.Drnoahsarc.com

Providing biomedical treatments for children with ASD and other conditions, using epigenetics and nutrigenomics to individualize treatment.

Philip DeMio, MD
320 Orchardview Avenue
Suite 2
Seven Hills, OH 44131
Tel: (216) 901 0441

And
1347 Worthington Woods Blvd., Suite B
Worthington, OH 43085
Tel: (614) 436 2036
Website: www.drdemio.com

Comprehensive testing and biomedical treatment for children with ASD and other conditions.

Sensory Focus/The Vision Development Team
10139 Royalton Rd., Suite D
North Royalton, OH 44133
Tel: (440) 230 0923
Email: info@sensoryfocus.com
Website: http://www.sensoryfocus.com

Vision services and therapy for children and adults, focusing on those with special needs.

West Chester Chiropractic Center
8039 Cincinnati-Dayton Rd
West Chester, OH 45069
Tel: (513) 777 7575
Contact Name: Dr. Chris Coffman
Email: westchesterchiro@fuse.net
Website: http://www.westchesterchiro.com

Therapy Services

Achievement Centers for Children
15000 Cheerful Lane
Strongsville, OH 44136
Tel: (440)-238-6200
Contact Name: Cory Ramsey
Email: cory.ramsey@achievementctrs.org
Website: http://www.achievementcenters.org

Provides support, services, and programs including education and autism services, therapy, family support, recreation and adapted sports, and Therapeutic Horsemanship activities.

Autism Education and Research Institute (AERI)
3201 Belmont Street Suite 201
Bellaire, OH 43906
Toll Free: 1 (866) 727 AERI (2374) or
1(866) 501 AERI (2374)
Contact Name: Catherine Hughes, Director of Family Support Services
Email: support@aerionline.com
Website: http://www.aerionline.com

Autism Services for Kids
20920 Farnsleigh Rd
Shaker Heights, OH 44122
Tel: (216) 921 5251
Contact Name: Kate Vanderplough
Email: autismanswers@aol.com
Website: http://autismservicesforkids.com

Specializes in ABA, VB, and play therapy.

Behavioral Intervention Institute of Ohio
24865 Detroit Road Suite 3
Westlake, OH 44145
Tel: (866) 965 2446
Contact Name: Michele Murphy
Email: mmurphy@
behavioralinterventioninstituteofohio.com
Website: http://www.
behavioralinterventioninstituteofohio.com
https://www.facebook.com/
BehavioralInterventionInstituteOfOhio

BIIO provides intensive 1:1, 1:2, and group ABA services, as well as OT, ST, social skills groups, and IEP services.

Building Blocks Therapy, LLC
25221 Miles Rd. Suite F
Warrensville Heights, OH 44128
Tel: (216) 282 1234
Contact Name: Rechama Jacobovitch
Email: rechama@abacleveland.com
Website: http://www.buildingblockstherapy.org

Offers individualized in-home programs, school programs using Verbal Behavior, FBA functional behavior assessments, behavior intervention plans (BIP), advocacy, parent training. Also provides access to occupational therapy, speech therapy and other related services.

Central Ohio Behavioral Consulting
Marysville, OH 43040
Email: info@cobcllc.com
Website: http://www.cobcllc.com

Provides ABA-based behavior intervention services in the home, at school, and within the community as well as social skills groups, educational advocacy, and parent training.

Child and Family Psychological Associates
822 Portage Trail W
Cuyahoga Falls, OH 44221
Tel: (330)-923-9344
Contact Name: Michelle Matzke
Email: michellermatzke@gmail.com
Website: http://www.childandfamilypsychologists.com

Offers behavioral treatment, parent training, school consultation, and comprehensive assessments.

Chrysalis Autism Services
72 Cranston Court
Dayton, OH 45458
Tel: (937) 776 6272
Contact Name: Lisa Flake
Email: lflake@trumpetbehavioralhealth.com
Website: http://www.daytonautismservices.com

Provides ABA- and verbal behavior–based therapy.

Cincinnati Center for Autism (CCA)
305 Cameron Rd
Cincinnati, OH 45246
Tel: (513)-874-6789
Contact Name: Betsey Shanahan
Email: bshanahan@cincinnaticenterforautism.org
Website: http://www.cincinnaticenterforautism.org

Offers a variety of programs which address the communication, educational, social and behavioral needs of children with ASD.

4 Paws For Ability
253 Dayton Avenue
Xenia, OH 45385
Tel: (937) 374 0385
Email: karen4paws@aol.com
Website: http://www.4pawsforability.org

Trains and places service dogs.

Music Therapy Services, LLC
8447 Beechmont Ave
Cincinnati, OH 45255
Tel: (513) 474 6064
Contact Name: Mimi Sinclair
Email: msinclair@music-therapy-cincinnati.com
Website: http://www.music-therapy-cincinnati.com
http://www.facebook.com/musictherapycincinnati

New Day Counseling & Wellness, Inc.
4690 Belmont Ave.
Youngstown, OH 44505
Tel: (330) 759 7799
Contact Name: Amy Moore, CEO

Power of One Support Center Agency, Inc.
3220 Lowell Dr
Columbus, OH 43204
Tel: (614) 599 1729
Contact Name: PJ Richardson
Email: powerofone@wowway.com

Provides ABA in their center or at homes as well as respite care, play dates, social groups, and other services.

Step By Step Academy
445 E. Dublin-Granville Road
Worthington, OH 43085
Tel: (614) 436 7837
Contact Name: Jody McCague
Contact Email:
jmccague@stepbystepacademy.org
Website: http://www.stepbystepacademy.org

The Sensory Learning Program
3454 Oak Alley Court, Suite 209
Toledo, OH 43606
Tel: (419) 578 0057
Contact Name: Keri Porter
Email: kporter4sensorylearning@gmail.com
Website: http://www.sensorylearning-toledo.com

Schools and Educational Services

Autry Learning Center
8078-E Beechmont Ave
Cincinnati, OH 45255
United States
Tel: (513) 474 7407 or (614) 551 9745
Contact Name: Jennifer Day-Haeger
Email: autrylc@swohio.twcbc.com
Website: http://www.autrylearning.com

Provides one-on-one education and advocacy for students with ASD through individualized programs.

Defiance College–ASD Affinity Program
701 N. Clinton St.
Defiance, OH 43512
Tel: (419) 783 2365
Contact Name: Brad Harsha
Email: bharsha@defiance.edu
Website: http://www.defiance.edu/autism/affinity/program

Implements a range of services offering academic, social and residential support for qualifying students.

IDEA House Educational Services
1206 N Main Street
North Canton, OH 44720
Tel: (330) 760 4965
Contact Name: Angela Shumate
Email: shumate.ideahouse@gmail.com
Website: http://ihes.co

Kent State University
DeWeese Health Center Room 23
1500 Eastway Dr.
Kent, OH 44242
Tel: (330) 672 0722
Contact Name: Robert Baer

Email: rbaer@kent.edu
Website: http://www.kent.edu/sas

Ohio Coalition for the Education of Children with Disabilities (OCECD)
165 West Center St Suite 302
Marion, OH 43302-3741
Tel: (740) 382 5452 Voice & TDD
Toll Free: (800) 374 2806
Email: ocecd@gte.net
Website: http://www.ocecd.org

Ohio State University
150 Pomerene Hall
1760 Neil Avenue
Columbus, OH 43017
Tel: (614) 292 9218
Contact Name: Margo Vreeburg Izzo
Email: izzo.1@osu.edu
Website: http://www.ods.ohio-state.edu

Legal, Government & Financial Services

Disability Rights Ohio
50 West Broad Street Suite 1400
Columbus, OH 43215
Tel: (614) 466 7264
Toll Free: (800) 282 9181
Website: http://www.disabilityrightsohio.org

Advocates for the human, civil and legal rights of people with disabilities in Ohio.

Emily Lewis
5650 Blazer Parkway
Dublin, OH 43017
Tel: (614) 734 6270
Contact Name: Emily Lewis, Attorney at Law
Email: ejl@elewislaw.com
Website: http://www.elewislaw.com

Legal representation on issues relating to school law, student/parent advocacy, and disability law.

Hamilton County Developmental Disabilities Services
1520 Madison Road
Cincinnati, OH 45206
Tel: (513) 794 3300
Contact Name: Family Liaison
Email: lynne.calloway@hamiltondds.org
Website: http://www.hamiltondds.org

Hickman & Lowder Co.
1300 East 9th St, Ste 1020
Cleveland, OH 44114
Contact Name: Judith Saltzman, Attorney at Law

Email: JSaltzman@Hickman-Lowder.com
Website: http://hickman-lowder.com

Attorneys specializing in advocacy for special needs children.

Inclusion Advocates
9433 Montgomery Road, 2nd Floor
Cincinnati, OH 45242
Tel: (513) 834 8013
Contact Name: Ellen Mavriplis, Director
emavriplis@cinci.rr.com
Website: http://www.InclusionAdvocates.com

Special education advocacy services for children in the Greater Cincinnati/Northern Kentucky area.

Krugliak, Wilkins, Griffiths & Dougherty Company LPA
4775 Munson Street North west
Canton, OH 44719
Tel: (330) 497 0700 or (330) 497 4020
Email: jlile@kwgd.com
Website: http://www.kwgd.com/jennifer-lile

Practice areas include: Estate & Trust Planning, Elder Law Planning, Special Needs Planning and Probate Administration.

Law Office of Linda Fritz-Gasteier
1604 E Perkins Ave. #206
Sandusky, OH 44870
Tel: (419) 624 8133
Contact Name: Linda Fritz-Gasteier
Contact Email:
Email: lfglaw@bex.net
Website: http://www.gasteierlaw.com/index.html

Special education law.

Ohio Rehabilitation Services Commission
400 E. Campus View Blvd.
Columbus, OH 43235
United States
Toll Free: (800) 282 4536
Website: http://www.rsc.ohio.gov/

Stein, Chapin and Associates, LLC
32 West Hoster Street Suite 200
Columbus, OH 43215
Tel: (614) 360 2637
Toll Free: (888) 889 3586
Contact Name: David K Stein and Lance Chapin
Website: http://www.steinchapin.com

Community and Recreation Services

Abilities First Foundation
4710 Timber Trail DR
Middletown, OH 45044
Tel: (513) 423 9496
Contact Name: Bettie Roundtree
Email: bettie.roundtree@abilitiesfirst.org
Website: http://www.abilitiesfirst.org

Active Day
2100 Bethel Road
Columbus, OH 43220
Tel: (614) 538 8870
Contact Name: Carla Sandy
Email: csandy@activeday.com
Website: http://www.activeday.com

Medical adult day care centers.

The ARC of Ohio
1335 Dublin Rd. Suite 205C
Columbus, OH 43215
(614) 487 4720
Email: arcohio@rrohio.com
Website: http://www.thearcofohio.org/

Ardmore
Center for Autism
981 East Market Street
Akron, OH 44305
Tel: (330) 535 2601
Contact Name: Dan Hurd, Director of the Center for Autism Mike Noe, Coordinator of Autism Services
Email: dhurd@ardmoreinc.org
Website: http://www.ardmoreinc.org

Autism Society of Central Ohio
P.O. Box 272
Worthington, OH 43085
Tel: (614) 284 6323
Email: centralohioasa@gmail.com
Website: http://www.autismcentralohio.org

Autism Society of Northwest Ohio
4334 Secor Road Suite 1
Toledo, OH 43623
Tel: (419) 578 2766
Contact Name: Linell Weinberg
Email: asno.org@bex.net
Website: http://www.asno.org

Autism Society of Ohio
470 Glenmont Ave
Columbus, OH 43214
Tel: (614) 487 4726

Email: askASO@autismohio.org
Website: http://www.autismohio.org

Autism Center of Southeastern Ohio (ACSO)
1701 Colegate Drive
Marietta, OH 45750
Tel: (740)-373-3781 ext 54
Contact Name: Melissa Nething
Email: melissan@wcbdd.org
Website: http://www.AutismACSO.org

Bittersweet Farms
12660 Archibold-Whitehouse Rd.
Whitehouse, OH 43571
Tel: (419) 875 6986 X1209
Contact Name: Vicki Obee-Hilty, Executive Director
Email: vobee@bittersweetfarms.org
Website: http://www.bittersweetfarms.org

Provides residential, vocational, and recreational support to adults with ASD, allowing them to participate in farm-related activities that provide meaning and purpose.

Brandon's Place
26118 Broadway Ave.
Oakwood Village, OH 44146
Tel: (440) 232 9906
Email: info@brandonsplace.org
Website: http://www.brandonsplace.org

Provides recreational programming for individuals with autism of all ages and their families.

Cardinal Learning Center LLC
One North Commerce Park Drive Suite 113
Cincinnati, OH 45215
Tel: (513)-260-3193
Contact Name: Felicisa Evans
Email: CLCCincy@gmail.com
Website: http://www.cardinallearning.net/

Provides after-school care and summer enrichment programs, recreational, social, and community activies.

Cincinnati Recreation Commission
805 Central Ave Suite 800
Cincinnati, OH 45202
Tel: (513) 352 4028
Contact Name: Alayne Kazin
Email: alayne.kazin@cincinnati-oh.gov
Website: http://www.cincyrec.org/tr

The Cincinnati Recreation Commission's Division of Therapeutic Recreation offers leisure services for individuals with disabilities.

Clippard YMCA Learning Center/Train 4 Autism
8920 Cheviot Rd
Cincinnati, OH 45251

Tel: (513) 894 2006 or (513) 923 4466
Contact Name: David Martorano
Email: dmartorano@cincinnatymca.org
Website: http://www.train4autism.org
Website: http://www.cincinnatiymca.org/our-ys/branches/clippard-ymca

Columbus Special Hockey
Columbus, OH
Contact Name: Kelly Good
Email: kellymhabel@yahoo.com
Website: http://columbusspecialhockey.com

Columbus Chill Youth Hockey Association (CCYHA) partners with the American Special Hockey Association (ASHA) and USA Hockey to provide children and adults who have developmental disabilities with the opportunity to play ice hockey.

Families with ASD
5989 Meijer Dr. Suite 9
Milford, OH 45150
Tel: (513) 685 9750
Email: familieswithasd@yahoo.com
Website: http://www.familieswithasd.org/

Fieldstone Farm TRC
16497 Snyder Road P.O. Box 23129
Chagrin Falls, OH 44023
Tel: (440) 708 0013
Contact Name: Teresa Morris
Email: tmorris@fieldstonefarmtrc.com
Website: http://www.fieldstonefarmtrc.com

Fieldstone Farm is a Premier Accredited Center that offers horsemanship instruction for people with disabilities. For over 30 years our certified instructors have supported equestrians in learning all about horses.

Great Lakes Collaborative for Autism
2040 W. Central Avenue
Toledo, OH 43606
Tel: (419) 291 7031
Contact Name: Catina Harding, Executive Director
Email: catina@bex.net
Website: http://www.GreatLakesAutism.org

Hattie Larlham
9772 Diagonal Rd
Mantua, OH 44255
Contact Name: Ingrid Kanics
Website: http://hattielarlham.org

Hattie Larlham is a nonprofit organization that provides medical, residential, recreational and vocational services.

Hiram Farm Living and Learning Community
PO Box 1547
Hiram, OH 44234

Tel: (330) 569 3441
Contact Name: Kim Hummell
Email: kimmeehummell@yahoo.com
Website: http://www.hiramfarm.org

Serves adults with Asperger's Syndrome by offering them meaningful work on an organic farm.

Innovative Piano, Inc.
Westlake, OH 44145
United States
Tel: (443) 944 8237
Toll Free: (800) 997 7093
Contact Name: Amy
Website: http://www.innovativepiano.com

Provides piano instruction to individuals with developmental disabilities, using, among other things, ABA-based techniques.

Josiah's House, Inc.
981 Keynote Circle Dr. Suite 13
Brooklyn Heights, OH 44131
Tel: (216) 236 6960
Contact Name: Irene Jones, Founder/President
Email: irene@josiahhouseinc.org
Website: http://www.josiahshouseinc.org

An adult day/evening service for individuals with ASD and other disabilities. Services include: life skills, vocational training, personal hygiene, sign language, communication, and community activities.

New Hope Specialized Services
13951 Progress Parkway Suite A
North Royalton, OH 44133
Tel: (440) 628 8270
Contact Name: John Wallencheck
Email: info@nhssohio.com
Website: http://www.nhssohio.com
Email: https://www.facebook.com/NewHopeSpecializedServices?ref=hl

Offers both onsite and community based employment for individuals with developmental disabilities.

NREX Home Care, LLC
6164 Cleveland Ave
Columbus, OH 43231
Tel: (614) 8916594
Contact Name: Carrie McLaughlin
Email: inrexhomecare@gmail.com
Website: http://www.inrexhomecare.com

Ohio APSE
2979 Black Kettle Trail
Dublin, OH 43017
Tel: (614) 791 0575

Contact Name: Dee Marks
Email: deemarks@deeservices.net
Website: http://www.ohioapse.org/

Opportunities for Ohioans With Disabilities (OOD)
150 E. Campus View Blvd.
Columbus, Ohio 43235
Tel: (800) 282 4536 or (614) 438 1200
Website: http://www.ood.ohio.gov/

LEAP
2545 Lorain Ave
Cleveland, OH 44113
Tel: (216) 696 2716
Contact Name: Melanie Hogan
Email: mhogan@leapinfo.org
Website: http://www.leapinfo.org

Milestones
23880 Commerce Park #2
Beachwood, OH 44122
Tel: (216) 464 7600
Email: info@milestones.org
Website: http://www.milestones.org

Peace By Piece
18897 Detroit Extension
Lakewood, OH 44107
Tel: (216) 644 3296
Contact Name: David Fox
Email: Peacebypiececleveland@aol.com
Website: https://www.facebook.com/pages/Peace-By-Piece-Cleveland-Inc/517674238256627?sk=info&tab=page_info

Red Treehouse
Cleveland, OH 44106
United States
Tel: (216) 229 5758 X1126
Contact Name: Linda Kresnye
Email: lkresnye@rmhcleveland.org
Website: http://www.redtreehouse.org

REM Ohio, Inc.
2765 Maret St
Canton, OH 44705
Tel: (330) 456 3455 or (330) 456 3405
Contact Name: Joyce Burroughs
Email: joyce.burroughs@thementornetwork.com
Website: http://www.rem-oh.com

Offers day program services for adults with developmental disabilities.

RMS Autism Transition Center
7135 Hamilton Ave
Cincinnati, OH 45231

Tel: (513) 522 2400
Contact Name: Marisa Brandstetter
Email: MBrandstetter@teamrms.com

A day program for young adults with ASD facilitating the transition from childhood to adulthood.

Rose-Mary Center
19350 Euclid Ave
Euclid, OH 44117
Contact Name: Donna Cantlin
Website: http://www.clevelandcatholiccharities.org/rosemary.htm

Safe Haven Farms
5970 No Mans Rd
Middletown, OH 45042
Tel: (513) 422 4863
Contact Name: Dennis Rogers
Email: dennis.rogers@safehavenfarms.org
Website: http://www.safehavenfarms.org

Residential day and community services for individuals on the autism spectrum providing a variety of meaningful living, working, learning and leisure activities.

Sunshine Community
7223 Maumee Western Road
Maumee, OH 43537
Tel: (419)-865-0251
Email: eholland@sunshine.org
Website: http://www.sunshineincnwo.org/

Supported And Facilitated Environments (SAFE)
Youngstown, OH 44511
Tel: (330) 507 3893
Contact Name: Jen Gonda
Email: safeprograms@gmail.com
Website: http://www.safeprograms.org

West Toledo YMCA- Special Needs Swim Class
2110 Tremainsville Rd
Toledo, OH 43604
Tel: (419) 475 3496
Contact Name: Kathy LaFountain, Aquatics Director
Email: klafountain@ymcatoledo.org
Website: http://www.ymcatoledo.org/programs/aquatics/

OKLAHOMA

Doctors, Clinics, Hospitals, and Other Health Services

Indian Health Care Resource Center (IHCRC)
550 S. Peoria Avenue
Tulsa, OK 74120
Tel: (918) 588 1900

Website: http://www.ihcrc.org

Oklahaven Children's Chiropractic Center
4500 N. Meridian
Oklahoma City, OK 73112
Tel: (405) 948 8807
Contact Email:
Email: oklahaven@flash.net
Website: http://www.chiropractic4kids.com

Red Rock Behavioral Health Services
4400 North Lincoln Blvd.
Oklahoma City, OK 73105
Tel: (405)-424-7711
Email: christip@red-rock.com
Website: http://www.red-rock.com/

Smile Galaxy Pediatric Dentistry
9801 S Pennsylvania Ave.
Oklahoma City, OK 73159
Tel: (405) 692 1222
Website: http://www.SmileGalaxyKids.com

Tulsa Developmental Pediatric
4520 South Harvard Street Suite 200
Tulsa, OK 74135
Tel: (918) 743 3224 or (918) 743 2660
Contact Name: Richard Craig Irwin, MD FAAP
Website: http://www.tulsadevelopmental.com

Therapy Services

ABA-OK
515 S Santa Fe Ave. Suite 103
Edmond, OK 73003
Tel: (405)-458-0511
Contact Name: Jennifer Hancock
Email: info@abaoklahoma.com
Website: http://www.aba-ok.com

Addresses the behavioral and educational needs of individuals with ASD or other learning/developmental disabilities.

Able Kids Therapy
5970 E. 31st Street Suite F
Tulsa, OK 74135
Tel: (918) 622 6599
Email: ablekidstherapy@yahoo.com
Website: http://www.ablekidstherapy.com

Specializing in working with children who have problems with sensory information processing, gross and fine motor coordination, handwriting, communication (verbal and non-verbal), social and emotional abilities. Offers both individual and group therapy.

Aspire Oklahoma, LLC
2020 Willow Run St. Suite 100
Enid, OK 73703
Tel: (580) 823 8017
Sandra Reese-Keck
Email: aspireoklahoma@gmail.com
Website: http://www.aspireoklahoma.com

Uses ABA principles.

Autism Concepts Incorporated (ACI) Learning Centers
600 West 18th Street
Edmond, OK 73013
Toll Free: (800) 345 0448
Contact Name: Nancy Champlin, BCBA
Email: Autism@concepts.com
Website: http://www.acilearningcenters.com

Provides ABA with an emphasis on verbal behavior, for children with ASD and other developmental disabilities.

Can Do Kids Therapy
14 E Ayers
Edmond, OK 73034
Tel: (405) 513 8186
Contact Name: Dianna Persun, OTR Owner
Email: staff@stc-ok.com
Website: http://www.stc-ok.com

Provides OT and ST services as well as community events, free screenings, and parent education.

Full Circle Developmental Center
4101 NW 122nd St Suite C
Oklahoma City, OK 73120
Tel: (405) 562 9260 or (405) 260 9559
Contact Name: Billee Swallow
Email: info@fullcircleokc.com
Website: http://www.fullcircleokc.com

Green Country Behavioral Health Services, Inc.
619 North Main Street
Muskogee, OK 74401
Tel: (918)-682-8407
Website: http://gcbhs.org/

Project PEAK at University of Oklahoma Health Sciences Center
Autism Clinic 1100
N.E. 13th Street
Oklahoma City, OK 73117-1039
Tel: (405) 271 5700
Website: http://www.oumedicine.com/pediatrics/department-sections/developmental-behavioral-pediatrics/child-study-center/programs-and-clinical-services/school-support-services/autism-project-peak

A collaborative effort of the Child Study Center and the Oklahoma State Department of Education. Services are provided by an interdisciplinary team of certified special education teachers, speech/language pathologists, occupational therapists and psychologists.

TherapyWorks
7608 East 91st Street
Tulsa, OK 74133
Tel: (918) 663 0606
Contact Name: Brenda Hayman-Hensley
Email: bhensley@therapyworkstulsa.com
Website: http://www.therapyworkstulsa.com

Provides speech and occupational therapy.

Total Poss-Abilities
2917 NW 156th St
Oklahoma City, OK 73013
Tel: (405) 607 4440
Contact Name: Shannon Roberson, MOTR/L
Email: possabilities@coxinet.net
Website: http://www.totalposs-abilities.com

Offering children and their families outpatient clinical and natural environment based OT services, including therapy focusing on sensory processing challenges.

Tulsa Center for Child Psychology, PLLC (TCCP)
5110 South Yale Avenue Suite 103
Tulsa, OK 74135
Tel: (918) 779 7637
Contact Name: Dr. Walton
Email: drw@tc4cp.com
Website: http://www.tc4cp.com

Provides a full range of psychological services to children, adolescents and their families.

Schools and Educational Services

Child Development Laboratory-RISE Program
Oklahoma State University, College of Human Sciences
Department of Human Development and Family Science
110 Human Sciences West
Stillwater, OK 74078
Tel: (405) 744 7767
Contact Name: Dianna Ross
Email: dianna.ross@okstate.edu
Website: http://humansciences.okstate.edu/hdfs/cdl/

The Rise School is an inclusive preschool for children with and without developmental disabilities. OT, PT, ST, and music therapy using an integrated approach.

Children's New World
702 Garth Brooks Blvd
Yukon, OK 73099
Tel: (405) 354 5056
Website: http://www.childrensnewworld.com

Rose Rock Academy
3301 N. Martin Luther King Ave
Oklahoma City, OK 73111
Tel: (405)-548-1280
Contact Name: Ashley Talsma
Email: Ashley.Talsma@sequelyouthservices.com
Website: http://www.roserockacademy.org/

Inpatient residential treatment center for ASD addressing children Pre-K through grade 12.

Legal, Government & Financial Services

Holmes, Holmes & Neisent P.L.L.C.
501 NW 13th Street
Oklahoma City, OK 73103
Tel: (405) 235 8455
Website: http://www.medicaidoklahoma.com/index.asp

Legal services regarding financial planning and related issues.

Oklahoma Department of Mental Health and Substance Abuse Services
1200 NE 13th St. P.O. Box 53277
Oklahoma City, OK 73152
Tel: (405) 522 3908
Toll Free: (800) 522 9054
Website: http://ok.gov/odmhsas

Oklahoma Department of Rehabilitation Services (DRS)
3535 N.W. 58th Street Suite 500
Oklahoma City, OK 73112
Tel: (405) 951 3470
Email: dbowers@okdrs.gov
Website: http://www.okrehab.org/

Oklahoma Disability Law Center
2915 Classen Blvd. Suite 300
Oklahoma City, OK 73106
Tel: (405) 525 7755
Toll Free: (800) 880 7755
Contact Name: Kayla Bower
Website: http://www.oklahomadisabilitylaw.org

Oklahoma Early Access Autism Project
3901 NW 63rd Street, Suite 100
Oklahoma City, OK 73116
Tel: (405)-295-5273
Contact Name: Jeanne Chambers

Email: Jeanne-Chambers@ouhsc.edu
Website: http://www.EarlyAccessOK.org

The Oklahoma Early Access Autism Project partners with local communities to offer monthly autism screenings and awareness throughout the state.

SoonerCare
2400 N. Lincoln Blvd.
Oklahoma City, OK 73105
Tel: (405) 521 3646

SoonerCare, Oklahoma's Medicaid program, provides health care to children under the age of 19, adults with children under the age of 18, pregnant women and people who are older than 65 or have blindness or another disability.

SoonerStart
1000 NE 10th St., Room 904
Oklahoma City . OK 73117 Tel: (405) 271 8333
Contact Name: John M. Corpolongo, M.S., Director
Email: john@health.ok.gov
Website: http://ok.gov/sde/soonerstart

SoonerStart is Oklahoma's early intervention program. It is designed to meet the needs of families with infants or toddlers with developmental delays.

Community and Recreation Services

Tulsa Autism Foundation
6585 South Yale Suite 410
Tulsa, OK 74136
Tel: (918) 502 4678
Contact Name: Jennifer Sollars Miller
Email: jennifer@autismtulsa.org
Website: http://www.autismtulsa.org

Dale Rogers Training Center
2501 N Utah
Oklahoma City, OK 73107
Tel: (405) 946 4489
Email: dalerogers@drtc.org
Website: http://www.drtc.org

Provides paid vocational training for people with disabilities through various programs.

Developmental Wings
103 Eastland Road
Roland, OK 74954
(479) 221 2895
Contact Name: Jeff Edwards
Email: gjeffed@gmail.com
Website: http://www.developmentalwings.com

Provides services to people with autism and developmental disabilities and underserved populations.

Lawton Autism Support Group
Learning Tree Academy
1908 NW 38th Street
Lawton, OK 73501
Tel: (580) 591 2680
Contact Name: Sandy Jones
Email: sjones@lawtonps.org
https://www.facebook.com/LTAAutism

Lifestroke Aquatics
17425 Golden Hawk Ln
Edmond, OK 73012
Tel: (405) 315 2752
Contact Name: Melissa Andrade
Email: supernurse123@hotmail.com

Make Promises Happen
Central Christian Camp (CCC) 1 Twin Cedar Ln
Guthrie, OK 73044
Tel: (405) 282 2811
Toll Free: (800) 299 2811
Contact Name: James Wheeler, Executive Director
Email: James@CentralChristianCamp.org
Website: http://www.centralchristiancamp.org/make-promises-happen

Make Promises Happen (MPH), a program of Central Christian Camp, provides outdoor recreational opportunities for individuals 6 and older with special needs.

Oklahoma Autism Network
Tolbert Center for Developmental Disabilities,
Department of Rehabilitation Services
College of Allied Health University of Oklahoma
Health Sciences Center
1200 N Stonewall Ave.
Oklahoma City, OK 73117
Tel: (405) 271 2131 or (405) 271 7476
Contact Name: Judy Pluess, Family Services Coordinator
Email: judy-pluess@ouhsc.edu
Website: http://www.okautism.org

Sunbeam Family Services
616 NW 21st St
Oklahoma City, OK 73103
Tel: (405) 528 7721
Website: http://sunbeamfamilyservices.org/

Provides care for the poor and working poor in our community. Services include Counseling, Early Childhood Education, Foster Care and Senior Services.

TARC
2516 East 71st St., Suite A
Tulsa, OK 74136-5531
Tel: (918)-582-TARC (8272)
Toll Free: (800)-688-TARC (8272)

Contact Name: John F. Gajda, Executive Director
Email: jgajda@ddadvocacy.net
Email: tarc@ddadvocacy.net
Website: www.ddadvocacy.net

TOPSoccer
PO Box 1324
Harrah, OK 73045
Tel: (405) 788 6535
Contact Name: Ray Robinson
Email: Rayrobinson12a@comcast.net
Website: http://www.oksoccer.com/programs/topsoccer.aspx

TOPSoccer is a modified version of the game of soccer that was designed to provide opportunities for athletes with disabilities.

OREGON

Doctors, Clinics, Hospitals, and Other Health Services

Albertina Kerr's Children's Developmental Health Services
424 NE 22nd Avenue
Portland, OR 97232
Tel: (503)-228-6479
Website: http://www.albertinakerr.org/Youthamp;Family/ChildrensDevelopmentalHealthServices

Developmental/behavioral pediatrics provides evaluation and diagnosis and ongoing case management for children with ASD and other challenges.

Dr. Chris Chlebowski
739 N. Main St
Ashland, OR 97520
Tel: (503) 236 9609
Email: info@ashlandnaturalmedicine.com
Website: http://ashlandnaturalmedicine.com/

Children's Chiropractor who specializes in the use of homeopathy, herbal treatments, and dietary changes for children with autism.

Bluefish Dental
1429 SW 15th St.
Redmond, OR 97756
Tel: (541) 923 1300
Email: info@bluefishdental.com
Website: http://www.bluefishdental.com

Child Development & Rehabilitation Center (CDRC)
Portland:
Doernbecher Children's Hospital, 700 SW Campus Dr.
7th Floor

Portland, OR 97239
Eugene:
University of Oregon Campus
901 E.18th Avenue
Eugene, OR 97403
Tel: (503) 346 0640 or (877) 346 0640
Website: http://www.ohsu.edu/xd/health/child-development-and-rehabilitation-center

Specializes in diagnosis, assessment, and intervention related to disorders affecting development, including ASD.

Glenn Jarosz, ND
Flourish Natural Medicine
17685 SW 65th Ave.
Lake Oswego, OR 97035
Tel: (503)-747-2021

Naturopathic physician who practices integrative care including care for chronic health issues including ASD.

John A. Green III, MD
The Evergreen Center
516 High Street
Oregon City, OR 97045
Tel: (503) 722 4270
Website: www.childrenandautism.com

Providing biomedical and nutritional treatments for children with ASD and other conditions. The Evergreen Center offers a number of models of care to help it to reach as many families as possible.

Providence Neurodevelopmental Center for Children
Clinics in East & West Portland, Gresham & Newberg
830 NE 47th Ave
Portland, OR 97213
Tel: (503)-215-2233 (East Portland)
Tel: (503)-216-2339 (West Portland)
Website: http://www.ProvidenceOregon.org/pncc

Developmental needs, from infancy through adolescence. Our developmental pediatricians, psychologist, therapists, audiologists, dietitians and social workers collaborate on individualized programs for each child.

Valerie LaRosa, N.D.
Good Life Medicine Center
827 NE Alberta St.
Portland, OR 97211
Tel: (503) 477 6670
Website: http://www.drvalerielarosa.com

Provides primary family care as well as a focus on pediatric developmental conditions such as ASD and chronic health challenges.

Wendy Cohan, R.N.
Portland, OR
Tel: (503)-977-2342 or (503)-413-9369
Email: choosehealth@glutenfreechoice.com
Website: http://www.glutenfreechoice.com

Counseling, education, and support, and assistance in meal planning to people newly diagnosed with gluten intolerance.

Therapy Services

A Hope for Autism
2120 SW Jefferson Street, Suite 200B
Portland, OR 97201
Tel: (503) 516 9085
Contact Name: Robbin Sobotka-Soles, BCABA
Email: robbin@ahopeforautism.net
Website: http://www.ahopeforautism.org

Uses a variety of ABA-based treatment techniques for learning and generalization of skills.

Autism Behavioral Consulting (ABC)
129 NE 102nd Ave. Suite E
Portland, OR 97220
Tel: (360) 571 2432
Contact Name: Audra Jensen, M.ED.,BCBA, Executive Director
Email: info@autismabc.org
Website: http://www.autismabc.org

Individualized therapy programs for children using ABA as well as additional educational therapy, classroom observations and collaborative social activity.

Autism Research and Resources of Oregon (ARRO)
P.O. Box 4282
Portland, OR 97208-4282
Tel: (971) 258 2360
Contact Name: Kathleen Henley
Email: kathyh@arroautism.org
Website: http://arroautism.org

Includes medical, educational, psychological, social services, and/or vocational training aspects.

Barbara Avila Consulting
7739 SW Capitol Hwy, Suite 220
Portland, Oregon 97219
Tel: (503)-432-8760
Email: jonathansynergyac@gmail.com
Website: http://www.barbaraavilaconsulting.com

Bridgeway House
37770 Upper Camp Creek Rd.
Springfield, OR 97478
Tel: (541) 345 0805

Contact Name: Patricia Wigney, Executive Director
Email: bridgewayhouse@comcast.net
Website: http://www.bridgewayhouse.org

Offers treatments, therapies, counseling, education, instruction, training, advocacy, support, and resource information for children and their families of all income levels with ASD.

Cascade Behavioral Intervention
PO Box 1432
Bend, OR 97709
Tel: (541) 480 2570
Contact Name: Jenny Fischer, MS, BCBA
Email: jenny.fischer@mac.com
Website: http://www.cascadebehavior.com

Providing behavioral consultation using ABA principles; specialization in early intensive behavioral intervention for young children with ASD.

Dvortcsak Speech and Language Services, Inc.
818 SW 3rd Ave. #68
Portland, OR 97204
Tel: (503) 887 1130
Contact Name: Anna Dvortcsak
Email: anna@dslsi.com
Website: http://www.dslsi.com

Provides in-home speech and language services. SLPs have extensive ABA and Developmental Interventions training for children with ASD and also are trained to implement Project ImPACT.

Forward Stride
18218 SW Horse Tale Drive
Beaverton, OR 97007
Tel: (503) 590 2959
Contact Name: Bill Mitchell, Acting Executive Director
Email: bill@forwardstride.org
Website: http://www.forwardstride.org

Individualized programs rooted in Equine Assisted Activities and Therapies (EAAT).

Heart to Heart Speech Therapy, LLC
2855 Hayes St Suite 101
Newberg, OR 97132
Tel: (503) 901 5652
Contact Name: Jamie Davis
Email: Jamie.heart2heart@gmail.com
Website: http://www.Heart2heartspeech.com

The Joys of Living Assistance Dogs
P.O. Box 21804
Keizer, OR 97303
Portland, OR
Tel: (503) 551 4572
Contact Name: Theresa Green

Email: info@joydogs.org
Website: http://www.joydogs.org

Trains assistance dogs and places them with individuals needing assistance.

Mind and Minds Play and Skill Center
5291 NE Elam Young Pkwy. #130
Hillsboro, OR 97124
Tel: (503) 701 0353
Contact Name: Adely Mooso, Director
Email: mindandminds@yahoo.com
Website: http://www.mindandminds.com

Pathways for Potential
10151 SW Barbur Blvd, Ste 108
Portland, OR 97219
Tel: (503) 245 5249
Contact Name: Chris Marie Messina
Email: chris.m.messina@gmail.com
Website: http://www.pathwaysforpotential.com

Social skills groups coupled with behavioral therapy and academic support for children ages 3–12 with ASD.

Pediatric Therapy Services
532 N Main Ave
Gresham, OR 97030
Tel: (503) 666 1333 or (503) 516 3924
Contact Name: Jami Baillie
Email: jami@oregonpts.com
Website: http://www.oregonpts.com

Physical, occupational, and speech therapy practice.

Philippe Reisberg, MA
12 SE 14th Ave Suite 206
Portland, OR 97214
Tel: (503) 267 8040
Contact Name: Philippe Reisberg
Email: philippe@mentoredlearning.com
Website: http://www.mentoredlearning.com

Academic support including tutoring and coaching; Individual counseling for ADHD, autism, & developmental disabilities; family therapy and coaching for ADHD, autism, & developmental disabilities; parent coaching; individual counseling for anxiety and depression; and family therapy.

Portland Autism Center, LLC
1 Lincoln Center, 10300 SW Greenburg Road Suite 240
Portland, Oregon, OR 97223
Tel: (503) 206 6285
Contact Name: Karen McKibbin or Erin Moran
Email: info@portlandautismcenter.com
Website: http://www.portlandautismcenter.com

Quigong Sensory Training Institute
PO Box 92
McMinnville, OR 97128
Tel: (503) 474 0218
Contact Name: Kris Gabrielsen
Email: kris.reed@juno.com
Website: http://www.qsti.org

Teaches parents how to give a 15 minute Qigong massage to their child, once a day for at least five months, which may have a positive impact in areas such as sleep, aggression, transition, and social behaviors.

Self Express Music Therapy
8704 SW 9th Dr.
Portland, OR 97219
Tel: (971)-221-5428
Contact Name: Emily Ross
Email: emily@selfexpressmusic.com
Website: http://www.selfexpressmusic.com

Sensory KIDS, LLC
1425 N Killingsworth St
Portland, OR 97217
Tel: (503)-575-9402
Email: info@sensorykidsot.com
Website: http://www.sensorykidsot.com

Sensory KIDS is a pediatric therapy clinic specializing in sensory processing and regulatory disorders, providing Sensory Integration, DIR/Floortime, dance/movement therapy, mental health services, parent support groups, and comprehensive evaluations.

Sundstrom Clinical Services
8440 SE Sunnybrook Blvd
Clackamas, OR 97015
Tel: (503) 653 0631
CFlachsbart@sundstromclinic.com
Website: http://www.sundstromclinic.com

Schools and Educational Services

Columbia Regional Program
2600 S.E. 71st Ave.
Portland, OR
Tel: (503) 916 5730 or (503) 916 5348
Contact Name: Sandra Pemberton, supervisor
Website: http://www.crporegon.org

Services for students with ASD offered at several schools throughout Portland area. Free.

Disability Services at Oregon Tech
3201 Campus Dr.
Klamath Falls, OR 97601
Tel: (541) 851 5227
Contact Name: William Proebstel

Email: william.proebstel@oit.edu
Website: http://www.oit.edu/academics/ssc/disability-services

Legal, Government & Financial Services

Circle of Friends Advocacy
14407 SW Teal Blvd. # 99 D
Beaverton, OR 97008
Tel: (503) 524 9420
Contact Name: Joni Anderson
Email: purpleslp@msn.com
Website: http://www.circleoffriendsadvocacy.com

Special education advocates.

Fitzwater Meyer Hollis & Marmion, LLP
6400 SE Lake Rd. Suite 440
Portland, OR 97222
Tel: (503)-786-8191
Contact Name: Melanie Marmion, Esq.
Email: mmarmion@fitzwatermeyer.com
Website: http://www.fitzwatermeyer.com/welcome

Providing legal services in all areas of estate planning, administration, probates, guardianships/conservatorships and elder law.

KP Law, PC
5200 SW Meadows Road
Suite 150
Lake Oswego, OR 97035
Tel: (503) 245 6309
Toll Free: (800) 758 9160
Website: http://www.kpdisabilitylaw.com/

Firm focuses exclusively in Social Security Disability law.

Living Earth Investments
2307 NE 132nd Ave.
Portland, OR 97230
Tel: (503) 807 2062 or (503) 488 5845
Contact Name: Aaron Rivers, Down Syndrome Parent, Portfolio Manager
Email: aaron@livingearthinvestments.com
Website: http://www.LivingEarthInvestments.com

Offers financial counseling and guidance to families with special needs children.

Oregon FIRST
5825 N Greeley Avenue
Portland, OR 9717
Tel: (503) 232 0302
Email: info@orfirst.org
Website: http://www.orfirst.org

Non-profit Community Parent Resource Center serving special education families located in Portland, Oregon with children birth to age 26.

Oregon Office of Vocational Rehabilitation Services
500 Summer Street NE
Salem, OR 97301
(503) 945 5880
Email: vr.info@state.or.us
Website: http://www.oregon.gov/DHS/vr/

Oregon Supported Employment Center for Excellence
1215 SW G St.
Grants Pass, OR 97526
Tel: (541) 476 2373
Contact Name: Jeff Krolick
Email: jkrolick@optionsonline.org
Website: http://osece.org/

Community and Recreation Services

Abilitree
2680 NE Twin Knolls Dr. Suite 150
Bend, OR 97701
Tel: (541) 388 8103
Website: http://www.abilitree.org

Abilitree provides jobs, training, community service and independent living opportunities for people with disabilities.

Adult Learning Systems of Oregon (ALSO)
345 E Columbia River Hwy
Troutdale, OR 97060
Tel: (503) 489 6565
Contact Name: Alison Burt
Email: aburt@adultlearningsystems.org
Website: http://adultlearningsystems.org

Offers a variety of residential and vocational supports to cater to each person's needs.

Autism Society of Oregon
PO Box 69635
Portland, OR 97239
Toll Free: (888) 288 4761
Website: http://autismsocietyoregon.org/

Arc of Multnomah Clackamas
619 S.W. 11th Avenue, Suite 106
Portland, OR 97205-2692
Tel: (503) 223 7279
Website: http://www.thearcmult.org

Columbia Care Services, Inc.
1175 E Main St. Suite 1B
Medford, OR 97504
Tel: (541) 858 8170
Email: info@columbiacare.org
Website: http://www.columbiacare.org

Creative Housing Solutions, LLC
910 Coburg Rd
Eugene, OR 97401
Tel: (541) 685 1406
Email: info@gbcchs.com
Website: http://gbcchs.com/

Family And Community Together (FACT)
13455 SE 97th Avenue
Clackamas, OR 97015
Toll Free: (888) 988 3228
Email: info@factoregon.org
Website: http://www.factoregon.org

Oregon Family to Family Health Information Center
OR
Tel: (855) 323 6744
Email: contact@oregonfamilytofamily.com
Website: http://www.oregonfamilytofamily.com

KindTree - Autism Rocks
2096 1/2 Arthur St
Eugene, OR 97405
Tel: (541) 521 7208
Email: autism@kindtree.org
Website: http://www.kindtree.org

LIFT Paratransit Program
Oregon
Tel: (503)-962-8000
Website: http://www.trimet.org/lift/index.htm

LTD EZ Access
Oregon
Tel: (541)-682-6100
Email: ltd@ltd.org
Website: http://www.ltd.org/ridingltd/
accessibleservices.html?SESSIONID=b579304f74ca1fc
c21c9f0c9509a6de1

The LTD EZ Access Program offers services and products to assist older adults and people with disabilities with transportation.

Mount Hood Kiwanis Camp for Children and Adults with Disabilities
9320 SW Barbur Boulevard Suite 165
Portland, OR 97219
Tel: (503) 452 7416
Email: info@mhkc.org
Website: http://www.mhkc.org

Six-day residential camp. Horseback riding, canoeing, swimming, arts and crafts, hiking, camping, outdoor cooking, skits, challenge course.

Upward Bound Camp
Stayton, OR 97383
Tel: (503) 897 2447
Contact Name: Evan Pierce
Email: upward.bound.camp@gmail.com
Website: http://www.upwardboundcamp.org

Provides recreational camp experiences for people with special needs, ages 12 and up.

PENNSYLVANIA

Doctors, Clinics, Hospitals, and Other Health Services

Autism Diagnostic Evaluations Resources & Services (ADERS)
Lewisburg, PA 17837
Tel: (570) 490 3017
Contact Name: Steve McAnnaney
Email: mcannaney@gmail.com
Provides ADOS-certified diagnostics and PA Adult Autism Waiver services.

Barry Gillespie, DMD MSD LMT
Gillespie Approach Craniosacral Facial Therapy
860 First Avenue
Suite 1B
King of Prussia, PA 19406
Tel: (610) 265 2522
Website: www.gillespieapproach.com

Center for Patients with Special Needs (CPSN)
University of Pittsburgh School of Dental Medicine
3501 Terrace St., Salk Hall
Pittsburgh, PA 15261
Tel: (412) 648 3039
Website: http://www.dental.pitt.edu/special_needs

Children's Hospital of Pittsburgh of UPMC
One Children's Hospital Drive 4401 Penn Ave.
Pittsburgh, PA 15224
Tel: (412) 692 5325
Website: http://www.chp.edu

Division of Neurology
The Children's Hospital Of Philadelphia, 3401 Civic Center Blvd. Wood Building, 6th Floor
Philadelphia, PA 19104
Tel: (215) 590 1719
Website: http://www.chop.edu/service/neurology

Franne Berez, MD ND
Squirrel Hill Family Wellness Center
5801 Beacon Street
Pittsburgh, PA 15217

Tel: (412) 422 5433
Website: www.drberez.com

Treatment for the entire family combining conventional medical care with natural modalities.

Geisinger Health System's ADMI
120 Hamm Drive Suite 2
Lewisburg, PA 17837
Tel: (570) 522 9430
Email: info@geisingeradmi.org
Website: http://www.geisingeradmi.org

Focuses on clinical care and cutting edge research on neurodevelopmental disorders, including ASD.

Geshay Pediatric Dentistry, P.C.
634 Pittsburgh Road
Uniontown, PA 15401
Tel: (724) 439 1576
Website: http://geshaypediatricdentistry.com

Good Shepherd Rehabilitation Hospital
Department of Pediatrics 850 S. 5th St.
Allentown, PA 18103
Tel: (610) 776 3578
Contact Name: Karen Johns
Email: kjohns@gsrh.org
Website: http://www.goodshepherdrehab.org

Family Care Chiropractic Center
1121 11th St 1st Floor
Conway, PA 15042
Tel: (724) 869 2167
Contact Name: Suzanne Fleeson-DaSilva
Email: familycarechiro@verizon.net
Website: http://www.fcchiropracticcenter.com

Iannessa Pediatric Dentistry, PC
Iannessa Pediatric Dentistry, PC
980 Beaver Grade Road Suite 101
Moon Township, PA 15108
Tel: (412) 329 7267
Contact Name:
Ryan Conover
Email: ryan@driannessa.com
Website:http://www.iannessapediatricdentistry.com

Jefferson Hospital
3905 Ford Road
Philadelphia, PA 19131
Tel: (215) 578 3400
Website: http://www.jeffersonhospital.org

Jefferson Regional Medical Center
Pittsburgh, PA 15236
Tel: (412) 469 5000
Website: http://www.jeffersonregional.com

Julie Lachman, ND LLC
196 W Ashland St.
Doylestown, PA 18901
Tel: (267) 915 6072
Contact Name: Julie Lachman, ND
Email: info@drlachman.com
Website: http://www.drlachman.com

Noah Erickson, D.C., Med. Ac.
Dr. Noah's ARC
12300 Perry Highway
Wexford, PA 15090
Tel: (877) 533 9993
Website: www.Drnoahsarc.com

Providing biomedical treatments for children with ASD and other conditions, using epigenetics and nutrigenomics to individualize treatment.

Pediatric Dental Associates, Ltd.
6404 Roosevelt Blvd.
Philadelphia, PA 19149
Tel: (215) 743 3700
Contact Name: Joyce Zuccarini
Email: zucc2000@aol.com
Website: http://www.teethforkids.com

Penn Foundation
Behavioral Health Services
807 Lawn Avenue P.O. Box 32
Sellersville, PA 18960
Tel: (215) 453 5178 x256
Contact Name: Debra Springer
Email: dspringer@pennfoundation.org
Website: http://www.pennfoundation.org

Saint Clair Memorial Hospital
1000 Bower Hill Road
Pittsburgh, PA 15243
Tel: (412) 561 4900
Website: http://www.stclair.org

Special Touch Dentistry
Special Touch Dentistry
240 Geiger Rd.
Philadelphia, PA 19115
Tel: (215) 508 4200

Provides dental services to patients over age 12.

St. Christopher's Hospital for Children
St. Christopher's Hospital for Children
E. Erie Ave. & N. Front St.
Philadelphia, PA 19134
Tel: (215) 427 5531
Website: http://www.stchristophershospital.com

Steven L. Kugler, MD
Specialty Care & Surgery Center, The Children's Hospital Of Philadelphia
500 W Butler Ave.
Chalfont, PA 18914
Tel: (215) 997 5730
Website: http://www.chop.edu/doctors/kugler-steven-l.html
Pediatric neurologist.

Turtle Creek Valley Mental Health Clinic
Steel Valley Therapeutic Activities Center
1705 Maple Ave
Homestead, PA 15120
Tel: (412) 464 1522
Website: http://www.tcv.net

Vision Development Institute
Vision Development Institute
1789 S Braddock Ave
Pittsburgh, PA 15218
Tel: (412) 731 5007
Contact Name: Dr. Hans Lessmann
Email: visiondevelopment1992@yahoo.com
Website: http://www.optometrists.org/lessmann

VDI offers vision therapy and rehabilitation to both children and adults.

Therapy Services

A Broader Spectrum Counseling Center and Parenting Education Center
196 Ashland St Suite 316
Doylestown, PA 18901
Tel: (267) 241 1424
Contact Name: Pam Hill
Email: pamhill@abscounseling.com
Website: http://www.abscounseling.com

Autism Education and Research Institute (AERI)
P.O. Box 1786
Greensburg, PA 15601
Toll free: (866) 727 AERI
Contact Name: Catherine Hughes, Director of Family Support Services
Email: support@aerionline.com
Website: http://www.aerionline.com

AERI provides psychological testing, training and consultation, autism services (throughout the lifespan), family-based mental health services, parent-child interaction therapy, trauma services, and transition services.

Community Counseling Center of Mercer County
2201 East State St.
Hermitage, PA 16148

Tel: (724) 981 7141
Toll Free: (866) 853 7758
Contact Name: Maggie Caesar-Myers, LCSW, BCBA
Email: Mcaesar@cccmer.org
Website: http://www.cccmer.org

Offers many of services covering the lifespan and for individual needs of those diagnosed with ASD.

Erik Young, M.Ed., LPC
828 Paoli Pike West Chester Wellness Center
West Chester, PA 19380
Tel: (484) 693 0582
Email: erikyounglpc@verizon.net
Website: http://www.erikyoungtherapy.com

Provides counseling and support to families and individuals struggling with the challenges of ASD.

Family Psychological Associates Ltd
1900 Murray Avenue Suite 301
Pittsburgh, PA 15217
Tel: (724) 543 1888
Website: http://www.kcifpa.com/

Horses 4 Hope Equestrian Center
927 Laurel Hill Road
Mt Bethel, PA 18343
Tel: (610) 674 0159
Contact Name: Aiyana Callaway
Email: horsesaremylife21@yahoo.com
Website: http://www.horses-4-hope.com

Equine-assisted therapy.

Marley's Dog Days
Erie, PA 16508
Tel: (814) 853 9208
Contact Name: Marley Winningham
Email: marleysdogdays@gmail.com
Website: http://www.marleysdogdays.weebly.com

Offers animal-assisted therapeutic techniques to help children attain therapy goals, such as improved communication, focus, sensory.

Music Works
2050 West Chester Pike Suite 115
Havertown, PA 19083-2742
Tel: (610) 449 9669
Contact Name: Lori O'Leary, Executive Director
Email: lori.oleary@musicworkswonders.org
Website: http://www.MusicWorksWonders.org

Provides music therapy services to children and young adults with ASD and other special needs.

Philadelphia Autism Center for Excellence (PACE)
NorthEast Treatment (NET) Centers, 499 N 5th St.
Suites D & E
Philadelphia, PA 19123

Tel: (215) 408 4937
Contact Name: Dr. Jayme Banks
Email: jhaynes@net-centers.org

Provides a comprehensive array of services for children and families with ASD.

Special Equestrians
2800 Street Rd
Warrington, PA 18976
Tel: (215) 918 1001
Contact Name: Tracey Dripps
Email: traceydripps@verizon.net
Website: http://www.specialequestrians.org

Therapeutic horseback riding serving Bucks, Montgomery, Philadelphia and surrounding PA counties.

Vision Development Institute
1789 S Braddock Ave
Pittsburgh, PA 15218
Tel: (412) 731 5007
Contact Name: Dr. Hans Lessmann
Email: visiondevelopment1992@yahoo.com
Website: http://www.optometrists.org/lessmann

VDI offers vision therapy and rehabilitation to both children and adults.

Schools and Educational Services

Achieving in Higher Education with Autism and Developmental Disabilities (AHEADD)
3945 Forbes Avenue Suite 470
Pittsburgh, PA 15213
Toll Free: (877) AHEADD1
Contact Name: Carolyn Komich Hare
Email: admin@aheadd.org
Website: http://www.aheadd.org

AHEADD provides coaching, mentoring, and personal advocacy for college students with ASD and other challenges.

ACLD Tillotson School
4900 Girard Road
Pittsburgh, PA 15227
Tel: (412) 881 2253
Contact Name: Bernice Martin
Email: bmartin@acldonline.org
Website: http://www.acldonline.org

Allegheny Valley School
1996 Ewings Mill Road
Coraopolis, PA 15108
Tel: (412) 299 7777
Contact Name: Regis G. Champ, President
Website: http://www.avs.net

Asperger Initiative at Mercyhurst (AIM)
501 East 38th Street Old Main, Room 314
Erie, PA 16546
Tel: (814) 824 2451
Contact Name: Bradley McGarry, Director
Email: bmcgarry@mercyhurst.edu
Website: http://www.mercyhurst.edu

Supports students in all areas of the college experience, including campus life and class work.

Barber National Institute
136 East Ave
Erie, PA 16507
Tel: (814) 453 7661
Email: BNIerie@barberinstitute.org
Website: http://www.barberinstitute.org/index.php

Camphill Special School
1784 Fairview Road
Glenmoore, PA 19343
Tel: (610) 469 9236
Contact Name: Bernard Wolf
Email: information@beaverrun.org
Website: http://www.camphillspecialschool.org

A state-approved Waldorf school that offers day and residential programs for children and youth with intellectual and developmental disabilities.

Eastern University - The College Success Program for Students Living with Autism Spectrum Disorder
1300 Eagle Road
St. Davids, PA 19087
Tel: (484) 654 2378 or (610) 341 5837
Contact Name: Douglas Cornman
Email: dcornman@eastern.edu
Website: http://www.eastern.edu/csp

Provides comprehensive academic, social, life skills, and cultural supports to undergraduate students living with ASD.

Familylinks: Therapeutic Learning Center
2644 Banksville Road
Pittsburgh, PA 15216
Tel: (412) 942 0417
Contact Name: Michele Hanzel
Email: mhanzel@familylinks.org
Website: http://www.familylinks.org

The Therapeutic Learning Center is a licensed School Based Partial Hospitalization Program for children grades pre k-5th grade.

Green Tree School & Services (GTSS)
1196 East Washington Lane
Philadelphia, PA 19138-1044
Tel: (215) 866 0200

Contact Name: Courtney Ridley
Email: cridley@gmail.com
Website: http://www.gts-s.org

Green Tree School & Services was established in 1957 in the Germantown section of Philadelphia to provide education and therapeutic services to children with learning, developmental and emotional needs, including Autism Spectrum Disorder and Emotional and Behavioral Disorders. Key programs currently include an Approved Private School, Behavioral Health Services, and On-Site Outpatient Clinic, Integrated Services - Innovation and Training, and Green Tree Partnerships.

The Graham Academy
469 Miller Street
Luzerne, PA 18709
Tel: (570) 283 0641
Email: info@thegrahamacademy.com
Website: http://www.thegrahamacademy.com

A special education school for children living with ASD or behavioral challenges in grades 1–8.

Kinney Center for Autism Education and Support
SJU 376 N Latchs Ln.
Lower Merion, PA 19066
Tel: (610) 660 2170
Email: kinneyautism@sju.edu
Website: http://kinneyautism.sju.edu

The Nexus School
1333 Old Wels Rd
Huntington Valley, PA 19006
Tel: (215) 947 2775
Contact Name: Vicki West
Email: vicki.west@thenexusschool.org
Website: http://www.TheNexusSchool.org

The Nexus School is a private school dedicated to children from kindergarten through age 21 with ASD.

Preparing Adolescents for Adult Life (PAAL)
115 Washington Avenue
Downingtown, PA 19335
Tel: (610) 873 6291
Email: louisc@cciu.org
Website: http://www.mecaautism.org

A community-based, specialty secondary educational program for students with ASD between the ages of 14 and 21.

Special Education at New Horizon School: Beaver Valley Intermediate Unit
128 Friendship Circle
Beaver, PA 15009
(724) 728 3730

Contact Name: Mrs. Docia Jacobs
Email: djj@bviu.org
Website: http://www.bviu.org/46384311014734/site/
default.asp

Valley Forge Educational Services
1777 North Valley Road
Malvern, PA 19355
Tel: (610) 296 6725
Website: http://www.vfes.net

Watson Institute: Autism College and Community Life Acclimation and Intervention Model
Pittsburgh, PA
Tel: (412) 749 2889
Website: http://www.thewatsoninstitute.org/

This program is specifically designed for college-bound teenagers with Asperger's disorder and high-functioning autistic disorder.

Legal, Government & Financial Services

Pennsylvania Bureau of Vocational Rehabilitation
1521 North Sixth Street
Harrisburg, PA 17102
Toll Free: (800) 442 6351
Website: http://www.portal.state.pa.us/portal/server.
pt?open=514&objID=552292&mode=2

PLAN of PA
P.O. Box 154
Wayne, PA 19087
Tel: (610) 687 4249
Contact Name: Kris Shaw
Email: kshaw@planofpa.org

PLAN of PA provides planning, care management, and Special Needs Trust services to families of adults with ASD and other challenges.

Community and Recreation Services

A B C 4 AUTISM SERVICES
307 Riverview RD
Swarthmore, PA 19081
Tel: (610) 543 8973 or (484) 844 9665
Contact Name: Mercedes Palma, Clinical Coordinator
Email: abc4autismservices@gmail.com

APS Autism Program
100 Louise Drive
Ivyland, PA 18974
Tel: (215) 672 9505, X232
Contact Name: Lindsay Goldberg
Email: lgoldberg@apspackage.com

Autism GUARDS
Lafayette Hill, PA 19444
Tel: (267) 250 9612
Contact Name: Tara Thompson-Horwitz
Email: tara@autismguards.org
Website: http://www.autismguards.org/
FB: https://www.facebook.com/AutismGuards
Resource/networking group providing educational information and recreational resources for adolescents with ASD.

Autism Living and Working: ALAW
1528 Walnut Street Suite 815
Philadelphia, PA 19102
Tel: (267) 322 5800
Email: alaw@autismlivingworking.org
Website: http://www.autismlivingworking.org

Boyertown Area YMCA - Special Needs Swim Instruction
144 Holly Rd
Gilbertsville, PA 19512
Tel: (610) 367 9622, X237
Contact Name: Kathy Undercuffler, Aquatic Director
Email: kundercuffler@boyertownymca.org
Website: https://philaymca.org/

Carousel Connections
Philadelphia, PA 19107
Tel: (215) 948 2527
Website: http://www.carouselconnections.com

Community Care Connections
114 Skyline Ln
Butler, PA 16001
Tel: (724) 283 3198
Website: http://www.communitycareconnect.org

Community Guidance Center
793 Old Route 19 Highway North
Indiana, PA 15701
Tel: (724) 465 5576
Website: http://www.thecgc.com

Community Integrated Services
441 N. 5th St. Suite 210
Philadelphia, PA 19123
Tel: (215) 238 7411
Email: info@cisworks.org
Website: http://www.cisworks.org
Provides individualized employment opportunities.

Emmaus Community of Pittsburgh
2821 Sarah Street
Pittsburgh, PA 15203
Tel: (412) 381 0277

Contact Name: Karen D. Jacobsen, Executive Director
Email: kdjacobsen@emmauspgh.org
Website: http://www.emmauspgh.org

Provides residential homes for persons with intellectual and developmental disabilities.

Exceptional Adventures
250 Clever Road
McKees Rocks, PA 15108
Tel: (412) 446 0713
Contact Name: Sarah Blonski
Email: sblonski@pfq.org
Website: http://www.exceptionaladventures.com

Provides vacation planning and arrangements for vacationers with disabilities.

Family Service Assn of Bucks County Asperger's Awareness, Community-Education, and Support Program
2300 Old Lincoln Highway Suite 102 at the Oxford Valley Mall
Langhorne, PA 19047
Tel: (215) 757 6916, x 351 or (215) 757 3300
Contact Name: Amy Conte
Email: aconte@fsabc.org
Website: http://www.fsabc.org

Family Services of Western Pennsylvania
Family Services of Western Pennsylvania
868 Fourth Avenue
New Kensington, PA 15086
Tel: (724) 334 2386
Website: http://www.fswp.org

Kaleidoscope Family Solutions, Inc.
1084 Lancaster Avenue 2nd Floor
Bryn Mawr, PA 19010
Tel: (267) 295 2222
Toll Free: (877) 384 1729
Contact Name: Dr. TaraColleen Macatee
Email: tcmacatee@kfamilysolutions.org
Website: http://www.kfamilysolutions.org

Keystone Human Services
124 Pine St.
Harrisburg, PA 17101
Tel: (717) 232 7509
Toll Free: (888) 377 6504
Contact Name: Madeleine DeHart, Corporate Secretary
Email: mdehart@keystonehumanservices.org
Website: http://www.keystonehumanservices.org

Kindermusik for Special Needs
3881 Skippack Pike
Skippack, PA 19474

Tel: (610) 584 0430
Contact Name: Joy Huff
Email: joy@skippackmusicschool.com
Website: http://www.skippackmusicschool.com

Lehigh Valley Center for Independent Living
435 Allentown Dr
Allentown, PA 18109
Tel: (610) 770 9781
Contact Name: Kristy Gehman-Brown, Director of Core & Housing Services
Email: kristygehman-brown@lvcil.org
Website: http://www.lvcil.org

Offers independent living skills education, peer support, advocacy and housing search and support services for people with disabilities.

Lisa Rae Music Studios, LLC
P.O. Box 142
Crescent, PA 15046-0142
Tel: (412) 638 7598
Contact Name: Lisa Rae Vaughan, Executive Director
Email: LisaRaeVaughan@yahoo.com
Tel: http://www.lisaraemusic.com

Medina Kenpo Karate
151 S. State Rd
Springfield, PA 19064
Tel: (610) 543 0544
Email: medinakenpokids@gmail.com
Website: http://www.medinakenpo.com

Pittsburgh's Joey Travolta Film Camp
Pittsburgh, PA 15213
Tel: (412) 848 9355
Contact Name: Carolyn Hare
Email: carolynkhare@gmail.com
Website: http://www.joeytravoltafilmcamp-pittsburgh.com
FB: http://www.facebook.com/JoeyTravoltaFilmCampPittsburgh

An inclusive program for students and young adults age 13-25; it also provides essential transition and career training experiences for adolescents and young adults with ASD.

Providing Autism Support Services to Achieve Gainful Employment (PASSAGES)
118 52nd St
Pittsburgh, PA 15201
Tel: (412) 632 1905
Contact Name: Jamia Cinelli
Email: Jamia.Cinelli@goodwillswpa.org
Website: http://www.goodwillswpa.org

SharpVisions
1425 Forbes Ave.
Pittsburgh, PA 15219
Tel: (412) 456 2144
Email: referrals@sharpvisions.org
Website: http://www.sharpvisions.org

Skills of Central Pennsylvania, Inc.
Blair Regional Office
805 Chestnut Ave
Altoona, PA 16601
Tel: (814) 949 4800
Website: http://www.skillsofcentralpa.org/public/
services/adult_autism_services.php

Committed to creating opportunities and providing support for people who need specialized services to enhance all aspects of their lives.

Synergy Recreation
43 Hetzel Road
Ridley Park, PA 19078
Tel: (610) 324 8307
Contact Name: Heather Johnson
Email: heather@synergyrecreation.com
Website: http://www.synergyrecreation.com

Theatre Horizon
401 DeKalb St.
Norristown, PA 19401
Tel: (610) 283 2230
Contact Name: Leigh Mallonee
Email: leigh@theatrehorizon.org
Website: http://www.theatrehorizon.org/education/
autism.html

Offering youth drama for ages 10–16, and adult playwriting.

Tindall Resource Group, Incorporated
2824 Cottman Avenue Suite 13
Philadelphia, PA 19149
Tel: (215) 273 6704
Contact Name: Wanda Tindall
Email: wtindall@tindallmail.com
Website: http://www.tindallresourcegroup.com

Verland Foundation
Adult Day Care Center
212 Iris Road
Sewickley, PA 15143
Tel: (412) 741 2375
Website: http://www.verland.org/

Person-centered, community homes and services supporting over 200 individuals with intellectual disabilities.

RHODE ISLAND

Doctors, Clinics, Hospitals, and Other Health Services

Bradley Hospital
1011 Veterans Memorial Parkway
East Providence, RI 02915
Tel: (401) 432 1000
Contact Name: Rowland P. Barrett, PhD
Email: RBarrett@Lifespan.Org
Website: http://www.bradleyhospital.org/

Catherine Labiak-Maher, MD FAAP
19 Friendship Street Suite 340
Newport, RI 2840
Tel: (401) 848 0008
Contact Name: Catherine Labiak-Maher

Specializes in children with disabilities and developmental and behavioral pediatrics.

Neurodevelopmental Center
Memorial Hospital of Rhode Island
555 Prospect Street
Pawtucket, RI 2860
Tel: (401) 729 2582 or (401) 729 6200
Contact Name: Joseph J Hallett, MD FAAP

Northstar Pediatrics Hasbro Children's Hospital
593 Eddy Street
Providence, RI 2903
Tel: (401) 444 6769 or (401) 444 4471
Contact Name: Robert Thomas Burke
Website: http://www.hasbrochildrenshospital.org/

R.I. CART
100 Shirley Blvd.
Cranston, RI 2910
Tel: (401) 461 6383
Contact Name: Glynis Forcht
Email: thenews@riautism.org
Website: http://www.riautism.org

Therapy Services

Center for Children and Families
50 Holden St. First Floor
Providence, RI 02908
Tel: (401) 274 1122, X48935
Website: http://www.womenandinfants.org/
centerforchildrenandfamilies/index.cfm

The Center offers services to children of a broad age range with ASD, including diagnostic and behavioral assessments, psychiatric consultation, and outpatient child and family therapies.

Early Intervention and the Livingston Center
30 Livingston Street
Providence, RI 2904
Tel: (401) 274 6310
Contact Name: June Groden, Ph.D
Email: jgroden@grodencenter.org
Website: http://www.grodencenter.org/early-childhood

Hands in Harmony, LLC
Wakefield, RI 02880
Tel: (401) 783 4810
Contact Name: Nicole O'Malley
Email: nicolemtbc@yahoo.com
Website: http://www.handsinharmonyri.com

Provides music therapy services across Rhode Island.

Lend A Hand Therapeutic Riding Foundation
151 Laten Knight Road
Cranston, RI 02921-3216
Tel: (401) 826 9278
Contact Name: Jessica Moses
Email: info@lendahandri.org
Website: http://www.lendahandri.org

Provides therapeutic riding and hippotherapy to children with disabilities.

Looking Upwards Early Intervention Services
2974 East Main Road PO Box 838
Portsmouth, RI 2871
Tel: (401) 293 5790
Contact Name: Carolyn Souza
Email: csouza@lookingupwards.org
Website: http://www.lookingupwards.org/early-intervention.html

Provides evaluations, therapeutic services including OT, ST, and PT, and support in families' homes or other convenient locations.

Perspectives Corporation
1130 Ten Rod Road Building C Suite 201
North Kingstown, RI 2852
Tel: (401) 294 8181
Contact Name: Brenda Verdi
Email: bverdi@perspectivescorporation.com
Website: http://www.perspectivescorporation.com

Early Intensive Behavioral Intervention (EIBI) program uses ABA principles of to provide language, social, cognitive, and daily living skill acquisition. Their Behavioral Health division addresses daily living skills, social skills, and behavior reduction.

Schools and Educational Services

Bradley School-East Providence
Bradley Hospital
1011 Veteran's Memorial Parkway
East Providence, RI 2915
Tel: (401) 432 1411
Website: http://www.lifespan.org/bradley/services/school

Cornerstone School
665 Dyer Avenue
Cranston, RI 2920
Tel: (401) 942 2388 or (401) 941 1112
Contact Name: Pat Krakowsky
Email: pkrakowsky@cranstonarc.org
Website: http://www.cranstonarc.org

Cornerstone School is a small, year round, private special education school serving students 18 months through 21 years in both Rhode Island and Massachusetts.

The Groden Center
86 Mount Hope Ave.
Providence, RI 2906
Tel: (401) 274 6310 or (401) 751 0459
Contact Name: Peggy Stocker
Email: pstocker@grodencenter.org
Website: http://www.grodencenter.org

The Groden Center, Inc. is a school and residential treatment center in Rhode Island for children and youth with ASD and developmental disabilities providing early intervention services, an early childhood education program and functional and social development instruction to school-age children.

Kingston Hill Academy
The Groden Network
850 Stony Fort Road
Saunderstown, RI 2874
Tel: (401) 783 8282
Contact Name: Steve Panikoff
Email: spanikoff@kingstonhill.org
Website: http://www.kingstonhill.org

Meeting Street
1000 Eddy Street
Providence, RI 2905
Tel: (401) 533 9100
Contact Name: Laurie Kiely
Email: info@meetingstreet.org
Website: http://www.meetingstreet.org

Pathways Strategic Training Center
3445 Post Road
Warwick, RI 2886
Tel: (401) 739 2700

Email: info@trudeaucenter.org
Website: http://www.trudeaucenter.org/pathways.asp

Pathways Strategic Teaching Center is a comprehensive education and treatment program servicing children with ASD and related disorders.

Legal, Government & Financial Services

Department of Behavioral Healthcare, Developmental Disabilities and Hospitals (BHDDH)
Department of Developmental Disabilities 14
Harrington Rd.
Cranston, RI 2920
Tel: (401) 462 3234
Website: http://www.mhrh.state.ri.us/ddd

Family Service of Rhode Island
55 Hope Street
Providence, RI 2906
Tel: (401) 331 1350
Website: http://www.familyserviceri.org

Rhode Island Disability Law Center
275 Westminster Street Suite 401
Providence, RI 2903
Tel: (401) 831 3150
Toll Free: (800) 733 5332

Rhode Island Office of Rehabilitation Services
40 Fountain Street
Providence, RI 02903
Tel: (401) 421 7005
Website: http://www.ors.state.ri.us/

Community and Recreation Services

The Autism Project
1516 Atwood Ave
Johnston, RI 02919
Tel: (401) 785 2666
Contact Name: Susan Baylis, Parent Consultant, RIPIN
Email: susan@theautismproject.org
Website: http://www.theautismproject.org

The Cove Center
610 Manton Ave
Providence, RI 02909
Tel: (401) 851 0459
Contact Name: Patricia Fiske
Email: pfiske@covecenter.org
Website: http://www.grodennetwork.org/adults/cove-center.asp

Offers a range of instructional, vocational, and residential programs for adults.

The Fogarty Center
220 Woonasquatucket Ave.
North Providence, RI 2911
Tel: (401) 353 7000
Email: csalerno@fogartycenter.org
Website: http://www.fogartycenter.org

Provides services to adults with developmental disabilities.

James L. Maher Center
120 Hillside Ave.
Newport, RI 2840
Tel: (401) 846 0340
Email: jackm@mahercenter.org
Website: http://www.mahercenter.org

Magic and Miracles
Equine Interactive Programs
27 Arthur Richmond Road
West Greenwich, RI 2817
Tel: (401) 524 7117
Contact Name: Gina Morro
Email: gmorro@cox.net
Tel: http://www.quarterturns.org

Pairs equine facilitated learning and social skills lessons.

Sensational Child
650 Ten Rod Road Box 1
North Kingstown, RI 2852
Tel: (401) 667 2797
Contact Name: Sean Delong
Email: sean@sensationalchild.com
Website: http://sensationalchild.com

SOUTH CAROLINA

Doctors, Clinics, Hospitals, and Other Health Services

Coastal Pediatric Associates
1952 Long Grove Dr Suite 202
Mt. Pleasant, SC 29464
Tel: (843) 971 2992
Contact Name: Kim Covington
Email: covington@coastalpediatricassociates.com
Website: http://www.coastalpediatricassociates.com

Crockett Pediatric Dentistry P.A.
102 S. Venture Drive
Greenville, SC 29615
Tel: (864) 234 9800
Email: jerry@crockettpediatricdentistry.com
Website: http://www.crockettpediatricdentistry.com

EcoHealth Wellness Center
1051 Johnnie Dodds Blvd. Suite B
Mount Pleasant, SC 29464
Tel: (843) 884 4466
Email: info@ecohealthwellness.com
Website: http://www.ecohealthwellness.com

Greenville Hospital System University Medical Center
Department of Developmental Behavioral Pediatrics
200 Patewood Drive
Suite A200
Greenville, SC 29615
Tel: (864) 454 5115 or (864) 560 1471
Website: http://www.ghs.org

MUSC Children's Hospital
The Carolina Autism Resource and Evaluation (CARE) Clinic
171 Ashley Ave.
Charleston, SC 29425
Tel: (843) 876 0444
Website: http://www.musckids.com

Palmetto Pediatrics
1970 Augusta Hwy.
Lexington, SC 29072
Tel: (803) 358 2370
Contact Name: Kim Conant, Special Needs Care Coordinator
Email: specialneeds@palmettopeds.net
Website: http://www.palmettopediatric.com

SpringBrook Behavioral Health System
1 Havenwood Ln.
Travelers Rest, SC 29690
Tel: (864) 843 8013
Contact Name: Mary Ann Bennett
Email: maryann.bennett@springbrookbhs.com
Website: http://www.springbrookbehavioral.com

Therapy Services

ASPIRE
222 Redbank Road
Goose Creek, SC 29445
Tel: (843) 628 2935
Email: info@aspire-clinic.com
Website: http://www.aspire-clinic.com

Aspire provides ABA programming, Speech/Language Therapy, and Occupational therapy in a multi-disciplinary team approach to maximize each child's learning, while minimizing challenging behavior.

Bayada Habilitation
Greenville, SC 29607
Tel: (864) 242 1211

Contact Name: Kimberly Phillips
Email: kphillips@bayada.com
Website: http://www.bayada.com

Bayada Habilitation offers in-home behavioral consultation through insurance companies to families of children with ASD. Treatment plans include educational, social, communicative, and behavioral goals and objectives.

Beacon, Inc.
4501 Old Spartanburg Road, Suite 7
Eastside Professional Court
Taylors, SC 29687
Tel: (864) 292 5154
Contact Name: Jeannie C. Turley, MSP, CCC-LSLP
Email: jeannie@BEACONSLPS.com
Website: http://www.BEACONSLPS.com

Provides a variety of traditional and innovative treatment programs.

Blooming Kids Learning Center, LLC
1105 Mt Gallant Rd
Rock Hill, SC 29732
Tel: (704) 345 7168 or (704) 737 7542
Contact Name: Christy Knecht
Email: bloomingkidslearningcenter@yahoo.com
Facebook: https://www.facebook.com/pages/Blooming-Kids-Learning-Center-LLC/414174262027326?sk=info&tab=overview

ABA-based program that focuses on academic, social, and language excellence.

The Building Futures Autism Clinic
PO Box 7136
Myrtle Beach, SC 29572
Tel: (843) 449 0554
Contact Name: Sarah Pope
Email: sosed@sc.rr.com
Website: http://www.sos-healthcare.com

Provides individualized ABA therapy in a clinic setting and in home.

Carolina Center for ABA
Various locations
Tel: (919) 402 7051
Contact Name: Leigh Mahan
Email: leigh@carolinacenterforaba.com
Website: http://www.creativeconsultantsnc.com

Carolina Speech & Language Center Inc.
221 Stallsville Road
Summerville, SC 29485
Tel: (843) 832 1795
Contact Name: Mary Balderson
Email: m.balderson@mycsal.com
Website: http://carolinaspeechandlanguage.com

Center for Developmental Services
29 North Academy Street
Greenville, SC 29601
Tel: (864) 331 1445
Email: CDS@CDServices.org
Website: http://www.cdservices.org

Chrysalis Autism Center
410 Oakland Avenue
Suite 101
Rock Hill, SC 29730
Tel: (803) 792 0771
Website: Http://www.chrysalisautismctr.com/default_
v3.aspx

Provides ABA-based Early Intensive Behavior Intervention to children with ASD.

Crescent Child Development Services, LLC
966 Governor's Court
Mount Pleasant, SC 29464
Tel: (843) 813 1538
Contact Name: Tara Gregori, MSP, CCC-SLP, NBCT, BCBA
Email: info@crescentchilddevelopmentservices.com
Website: http://www.
crescentchilddevelopmentservices.com

Provides assessment, speech-language therapy, behavioral consulting, and ABA therapy and educational resources for children with ASD.

The Dakota Center
4011-B Belle Terre Blvd.
Myrtle Beach, SC 29579
Contact Name: Tracy or Donald Terrell
Email: thedakotacenter@msn.com
Website: http://www.thedakotacenter.com

Evaluates children with ASD and offers multiple treatment interventions including floortime model, relationship development research based group therapy programs, summer camps, a listening program, movement therapy, and primitive reflex programs.

Early Autism Project
2630-B Hardee Cove
Sumter, SC 29150
Tel: (803) 905 4427
Website: http://www.sceap.com

Develops customized ABA therapy programs.

EdSolutions, LLC
Florence, SC 29501
Tel: (843) 460 4777 or (843) 230 3039
Contact Name: Spears Beckham
Email: spearsatedsolutions@gmail.com
Website: http://www.EdSolutionsABA.com

Provides ABA therapy.

Navigation Behavioral Consulting (NBC), LLC
Goose Creek, SC 29445
Tel: (719) 459 8374 or (850) 348 5724
Contact Name: Megan Miller, M.S., BCBA, LBA, Managing Supervisor
Email: mmillernbc@gmail.com
Website: http://www.navigateaba.com

In home 1:1 ABA services, school consultations, verbal behavior approach, toilet training, parent training, and consultations provided.

Encouraging Steps
7900 Park Place Road PO Box 30
Rock Hill, SC 29731
Tel: (803) 628 5800
Contact Name: Sonya Lopes - Early Interventionist Supervisor
Email: slopes@yorkdsnb.org
Website: http://www.yorkdsnb.org/services/
encouraging-steps/

Early Intervention services for children from birth through 5 years of age.

Happy Hooves
4700 Dacusville Highway
Marietta, SC 29661
Tel: (864) 898 0043
Contact Name: Becky Sweeney
Email: edenfarms@nuvox.net
Website: http://www.edenfarms.net/happy-hooves-
therapeutic-riding.html

Therapeutic riding lessons for children and adults.

One Piece At A Time (OPAT), LLC
Blythewood, SC 29016
Tel: (925) 236 0494
Email: opat.llc@gmail.com
Website: http://www.opatllc.com

Provides ABA services for children with ASD in home and community settings.

Outlaw's Vision Quest Farm, Inc.
2919 Jeffords Rd N.
Lamar, South Carolina 29069
Tel: (843) 256 2277
Contact Name: Tina C. Outlaw-Kennett
Email: ovqf@bellsouth.net
Facebook: https://www.facebook.com/OutlawsVision.
QuestFarm
Website: http://www.outlawsvisionquestfarm.net/

Provides support groups and therapeutic riding.

Red House Behavior Resources, Inc.
Columbia, SC 29205
Tel: (888) 362 3970
Email: contact@redhousebehavior.com
Website: http://www.redhousebehavior.com

Red House provides in-home ABA treatment with Board Certified Behavior Analysts.

Sprout Pediatrics, LLC
Irmo, SC 29063
Tel: (803) 629 1981
Email: sproutpeds@gmail.com
Website: http://www.sproutpeds.com

Offers adaptive wellness, physical therapy, occupational therapy, feeding therapy and speech and language therapy.

Star, LLC
474 Wando Park Blvd. Suite 104
Mt. Pleasant, SC 29492
Tel: (843) 324 1464
Contact Name: Maria Averill
Email: maria@starcarolina.com
Website: http://www.starcarolina.com

Applied Behavior Analysis (ABA) services, community outreach and education, diagnostic testing, educational consultation, individual and group consultation, parent training, psychiatric services, social skills groups & summer camps.

Young Talkers
8703 Highway 17 Byp. South Suite I
Myrtle Beach, SC 29575
Tel: (843) 457 1053
Contact Name: Nicole Young-Cline
Email: Nicole@YoungTalkers.com
Website: http://www.YoungTalkers.com

A pediatric speech therapy clinic serving ages birth to 18 specializing in feeding disorders and working with children with ASD.

Schools and Educational Services

Autism Academy of South Carolina
2243 Percival Road
Columbia, SC 29223
Tel: (803) 790 7997
Contact Name: Matt Wood
Email: matt@autismacademyofsc.com
Website: http://www.autismacademyofsc.com

A year-round day program addressing the therapeutic and educational needs of children with ASD, providing individualized ABA-based programs.

CarolinaLIFE Program at University of South Carolina
240 Wardlaw – College of Education 820 Main Street
Columbia, SC 29208
Tel: (803) 576 5590
Contact Name: Laura C. Chezan, M.Ed., BCBA
Email: sclife@mailbox.sc.edu
Website: http://www.sa.sc.edu/carolinalife/

ClemsonLIFE Program at Clemson University
201E Godfrey Hall
Clemson, SC 29634
Tel: (864) 656 0501
Contact Name: James Collins, Ed.S., NCSP, BCBA
Email: clemsonlife@clemson.edu
Website: http://www.clemson.edu/culife/index.html

Coastal Carolina University LIFE Program
Biddle Center for Teaching, Learning, & Community Engagement
Baxley Hall 205
Conway, SC 29528
Tel: (843) 349 2387
Contact Name: Sandra Saunders
Email: ssaunders@coastal.edu
Website: http://www.coastal.edu/education/LIFE/index.html

Hidden Treasure Christian School
500 West Lee Road
Taylors, SC 29687
Tel: (864) 235 6848
Email: info@hiddentreasure.org
Website: http://www.hiddentreasure.org

Provides K-12 special education instruction to children with mental, physical, emotional, and developmental disabilities.

Pine Grove, Inc.
1500 Chestnut Road P.O. Box 100
Elgin, SC 29045
Tel: (803) 438 3011
Contact Name: David S. Perhach
Email: davep@pinegroveinc.com
Website: http://www.pinegroveinc.com

A comprehensive residential facility and school serving children and adolescents with ASD. Also offers educational day services.

REACH Program at the College of Charleston
175 Calhoun St. 234 Robert Scott Small Building, Room 233
Charleston, SC 29424
Tel: (843) 953 4849
Email: REACHProgram@cofc.edu
Website: http://reach.cofc.edu

The REACH (Realizing Educational and Career Hopes) Program is a 4-year inclusive non-degree program for students with mild intellectual disabilities.

St. John Catholic School
3921 St. John Avenue
North Charleston, SC 29405
Tel: (404) 966 1626
Contact Name: Crissie McCormack
Email: crissiemccormack@yahoo.com
Website: http://www.saintjohncatholicsc.org

Trident Academy
1455 Wakendaw Road
Mt. Pleasant, SC 29464
Tel: (843)8847046 or 8438843494
Contact Name: Niki Leiva
Email: nleiva@tridentacademy.com
Website: http://www.tridentacademy.com

A program designed to assist cognitively capable students to transition to conventional learning environments.

Legal, Government & Financial Services

Burton Center – Various locations
2605 Hwy 72/221 E.
Greenwood, SC 29649
Email: jfeltonburton@burtoncenter.org
Website: http://www.burtoncenter.org/

Clingman Law Firm
1201 Main Street, Suite 1980
PO Box 7096
Columbia, SC 29202
Tel: (803) 787 0557
Contact Name: Sarah Clingman, CELA*
Email: Sarah@Clingmanlaw.com
Website: Http://clingmanlaw.net/

Cutchin Law Firm
1473 Stuart Engals Blvd.
Mt. Pleasant, SC 29464
Tel: (843) 216 0809
Contact Name: Bill Cutchin
Email: bill@cutchinlaw.com
Website: http://www.cutchinlaw.com

Law practice primarily focused on trusts and estates, including special needs trusts.

Evan Guthrie Law Firm
164 Market Street Suite 362
Charleston, SC 29401
Tel: (843) 926 3813
Contact Name: Evan Guthrie

Email: contact@ekglaw.com
Website: http://www.ekglaw.com

Evan Guthrie Law Firm is a special need and estate planning attorney.

South Carolina Health and Human Services
P.O. Box 8206
Columbia, SC 29202
Tel: (888) 549 0820
Contact Name: info@scdhhs.gov
Website: http://www.scdhhs.gov/

South Carolina Vocational Rehabilitation Department
1410 Boston Avenue
West Columbia, SC 29171
Tel: (800) 832 7526
Email: info@scvrd.state.sc.us
Website: http://www.scvrd.net/

Community and Recreation Services

Active Day Center
Various locations
Find your location: Website: http://www.seniorcarectrs.com/adult-day-centers-location/?loc=SC
Tel: (877) 435 3372
E-Mail: info@seniorcarectrs.com
Website: http://www.seniorcarectrs.com/

Autism Advocate Foundation
P.O. Box 7061
Myrtle Beach, SC 29572
Tel: (843) 213 0217
Contact Name: Amy Gary, Executive Director
Website: http://www.autismadvocatefoundation.com

The Autism Advocate Foundation offers Project Lifesaver, Richards summer program, Life Lessons, high-functioning kids respite care and social skills programs.

Babcock Center
P.O. Box 4389
West Columbia, SC 29170
Tel: (803) 799 1970
Email: info@babcockcenter.org
Website: http://www.babcockcenter.org/

Believe
Aiken, SC 29801
Tel: (803) 474 1154
Contact Name: Jaime Hansen
Email: jnhhansen@gmail.com

A Parent-led Autism Support and Advocacy Group

Berkeley Citizens, Inc.
PO Drawer 429
Moncks Corner, SC 29461
Tel: (843) 761 0300
Email: bciadmin@bciservices.org
Website: http://www.berkeleycitizens.org/

Boyd Hill Recreation Center 1165 Constitution Blvd.
Rock Hill, SC 29732
Tel: (803) 329 5659
Contact Name: Wendy Waddle
Website: Http://www.cityofrockhill.com/departments/
parks-recreation-tourism/more/parks-recreation-
tourism/therapeutic-recreation

Therapeutic recreation programs.

Camp Good Times of Charleston
P.O. Box 81114
Charleston, SC 29416
Tel: (843) 817 2221
Email: bethweiner@cgtkids.com
Website: http://www.campgoodtimesofcharleston.org

Camp Spearhead
4806 Old Spartanburg Rd
Taylors, SC 29687
Tel: (864) 288 6470
Contact Name: Randy Murr
Email: randy@gcrd.org
Website: http://www.campspearhead.org

Offers residential camp programs in the summer and
weekend programs throughout the school year. Serves
children 8 and older and adults with special needs.

CCTA ParaTransit Services
Tel: (803) 864 0211
Email: info@cctaride.org
Website: http://www.cctaride.org/bus-information/ada-
paratransit.html

Chittenden County Transportation Authority (CCTA) provides ADA paratransit services for persons unable to
use CCTA fixed route bus system because of a disability.

Charles Lea Center
195 Burdette Street
Spartanburg, SC 29307
Tel: (864) 585 0322
Email: dkiely@charleslea.org
Website: http://www.charlesleacenter.org

Charleston Young Adult AS's
Charleston, SC 29407
Tel: (843) 364 3696
Contact Name: Danielle Gilbert
Email: dkgilbert2008@yahoo.com

Website: http://www.meetup.com/Charleston-Young-
Adult-ASDs

A group for young adults (17-32) with ASD.

Darlington County Autism Support Group
2300 East Home Avenue
Hartsville, SC 29550
Tel: (843) 307 3386 or (843) 307 4179
Contact Name: Coretta Bailey or Wendy Stokes
Email: coretta.bailey@yahoo.com

Family Connections of South Carolina
2712 Middleburg Drive Suite 103-B
Columbia, SC 29204
Tel: (800) 578 8750
Contact Name: Andy Pope
Email: andypope@familyconnectionSC.org
Website: http://www.familyconnectionsc.org

Links families of children with special healthcare needs
and disabilities with resources, support and education.

**Family Resource Center For Disabilities and Special
Needs**
1575 Savannah Highway Suite 6
Charleston, SC 29407
Tel: (843) 266 1318
Email: frc@frcdsn.org
Website: http://www.frcdsn.org

Healing Farms
P.O. Box 2002
Mt. Pleasant, SC 29465
Tel: (843) 971 9300
Contact Name: Mary Tutterow
Website: http://www.healingfarms.com

Creating sustainable community-based programming
for adults with developmental disabilities.

Lowcountry Autism Consortium (LAC)
Charleston, SC 29492
Tel: (843) 225 5835
Contact Name: Dr. Robert Scharstein
Email: rob@lowcountryautismconsortium.org
Website: http://www.lowcountryautismconsortium.org

Merry Pranksers Theatrical Troupe
Boyd Hill Recreation Center 1165 Constitution Blvd.
Rock Hill, SC
Tel: (803) 329 5659
Contact Name: Wendy Waddle
Website: Http://www.unctv.org/content/laughatus

Provides individuals with disabilities the opportunity to
perform on stage in an original production.

Project HOPE Foundation - Hope Link
2258 Woodruff Road, Suite 2100-358
Simpsonville, SC 29681
Tel: (864) 676 0028
Contact Name: Executive Directors, Lisa Lane & Susan Sachs
Email: administration@projecthopesc.org
Website: http://www.projecthopesc.org/hope-link

Hope Link, a nonprofit program of Project HOPE Foundation, provides community outreach to assist families newly diagnosed with ASD in navigating the systems.

Rockin' & Ridin' for Autism
3043 Old Powderhouse Road E - 4
Aiken, SC 29803
Tel: (803) 292 9847 or (321) 576 4819
Contact Name: Lisanne Harrell-Walke
Email: lisanne_walke@yahoo.com
Facebook: Website: http://www.facebook.com/RockinRidinForAutism

South Carolina Autism Society
5 Century Dr. Suite 130
Greenville, SC 29607 1578
Tel: (864) 241 8669
Email: scas@autism.org
Website: http://www.scautism.org

SOUTH DAKOTA

Doctors, Clinics, Hospitals, and Other Health Services

Dr. Jerome M. Blake
Developmental Pediatrics
1305 W. 18th St.
Sioux Falls, SD 57117
Tel: (605) 312 1000

Sanford Children's Hospital
1305 W 18th St.
Sioux Falls, SD 57117
Tel: (605) 333 7188
Website: http://www.sanfordhealth.org/sioux-falls

Speech & Hearing Center & USD Scottish Rite Children's Clinic
University of South Dakota-Communication Sciences & Disorders
414 E. Clark St.
Vermillion, SD
Tel: (605) 677 5474
Email: csd@usd.edu
Website: Http://www.usd.edu/arts-and-sciences/communication-sciences-and-disorders/clinics.cfm

Therapy Services

Accelerate Center for Intensive Early Intervention
1908 W. 42nd St., Suite B
Sioux Falls, SD 57105
Tel: (605) 351 7976
Contact Name: Paul Graumann
Email: pgraumann@sfearlyintervention.org
Website: http://www.sfearlyintervention.org

Provides center-based occupational and speech therapy services to children ages 2-5 in small groups of 4 children for 3 hours per day, 5 days per week. The Early Start Denver Model is used, incorporating ABA and developmental components.

Adaptivation Inc.
2225 W 50th Suite 100
Sioux Falls, SD 57105
Tel: (800) 723 2783
Contact Name: Lori Dahlquist
Email: lori@adaptivation.com
Website: http://www.adaptivation.com

Provides augmentative communication devices and services.

Autism Behavioral Consulting, LLC
25792 Packard Lane
Renner, SD 57055
Tel: (605) 351 1002
Contact Name: Brittany Schmidt
Email: brittanyabc@gmail.com
Website: http://www.abc-autism.com

Behavior Care Specialists
6009 W. 41st St. Suite 4
Sioux Falls, SD 57106
Tel: (605) 271 2690
Contact Name: Vannapha Halseide
Email: vannaphah@behaviorcarespecialists.com
Website: http://www.behaviorcarespecialists.com

Offers early intervention services for children diagnosed with autism, pervasive development disorders and related developmental disabilities.

Music Therapy Services of South Dakota
3304 S. Florence Ave.
Sioux Falls, SD 57103
Tel: (605) 371 1529
Contact Name: Lora Barthelman
Email: musictherapyservices@sio.midco.net
Website: http://www.musictherapyservicessd.com

Theratime, Inc.
2115 Pendar Lane
Sioux Falls, SD 57105

Tel: (605) 359 3842
Contact Name: Cory Faber
Email: coryfab@msn.com
Website: http://www.theratime.com

Provides a wide array of early intervention services including speech therapy, occupational and physical therapies, and ABA therapy.

Legal, Government & Financial Services

Department of Housing and Urban Development
4301 West 57th St Suite 101
Sioux Falls, SD 57108
Tel: (605) 330 4223
Contact Name: Roger Jacobs
Email: SD_webmanager@hud.gov
Website: http://www.hud.gov/local/index.
cfm?state=sd&topic=offices

Office of Special Education
Kneip Building 700 Governors Drive
Pierre, SD 57501-2291
Tel: (605) 773 4698
Contact Name: Elizabeth Gordon, 619 Coordinator
Email: elizabeth.gordon@state.sd.us
Website: http://doe.sd.gov/oess/sped.asp

Respite Care Program
Department of Human Services
Hillsview Plaza
E. Hwy. 34, c/o 500 East Capital
Pierre, SD 57501-5070
Website: http://dhs.sd.gov/dd/respite/index.aspx

South Dakota Advocacy Services
221 South Central Avenue
Pierre, SD 57501
Tel: (605) 224 8294
Toll Free: (800) 658 4782
Contact Name: Robert J. Kean
Website: http://www.sdadvocacy.com

South Dakota Department of Social Services
700 Governors Drive
Pierre, SD 57501
Tel: (605) 773 3495
Website: http://dss.sd.gov/medicalservices/

South Dakota Division of Rehabilitation Services
3800 E. Highway 34 500 East Capitol
Pierre, SD 57501
Tel: (605) 773 3195
Email: infodhs@state.sd.us
Website: http://dhs.sd.gov/drs/vocrehab/vr.aspx

Community and Recreation Services

Aberdeen Transit Services
123 S. Lincoln St.
Aberdeen, SD 57401
Tel: (605) 626 3333
Website: http://www.aberdeen.sd.us/index.
aspx?NID=182

Autism Awareness Aberdeen
37902 127th Street
Aberdeen, SD 57401
Tel: (605) 262 1055
Contact Name: Beth Schmitz-Biegler
Email: schaatz@hotmail.com
Facebook: https://www.facebook.com/
AutismAwarenessAberdeen

Autism Spectrum Disorders Program
Department of Pediatrics Sanford School of Medicine
of The University of South Dakota
1400 W 22nd St.
Sioux Falls, SD 57105
Tel: (605) 357 1439
Email: cd@usd.edu
Website: http://www.usd.edu/cd

DakotAbilities
3600 S. Duluth Ave
Sioux Falls, SD 57105
Tel: (605) 334 4220
Website: http://www.dakotabilities.org/

Dial - A - Ride
300 6th St.
Rapid City, SD 57701
Tel: (394) 6631
Website: http://www.rapidride.org/dial-a-ride.php

Lifescape
Various locations
Tel: (605) 444 9500
Website: Http://www.cchs.org/

Provides a wide range of services to children and adults.

OAHE
125 W. Pleasant Dr. Suite #1
Pierre, SD 57501
Tel: (605) 224 4501
Website: http://www.oaheinc.com

South Dakota Parent Connection (SDPC)
Sioux Falls, SD 57106
Tel: (605) 361 3171
Email: sdpc@sdparent.org
Website: http://www.sdparent.org

TENNESSEE

Doctors, Clinics, Hospitals, and Other Health Services

Center For Proactive Medicine
1916 Patterson Street Suite 203
Nashville, TN 37203
Tel: (615) 331 1973
Email: info@proactivemed.org
Website: http://www.proactivemed.org

Chattanooga Autism Center
1400 McCallie Avenue Suite 100
Chattanooga, TN 37404
Tel: (423) 531 6961
Email: ChattanoogaAutismCenter@gmail.com
Website: http://ChattanoogaAutismCenter.org

Specializing in serving people of all ages with ASD providing comprehensive services.

Children's Primary Care Center
611 22nd Street
Knoxville, TN 37916
Tel: (865) 522 4153

Cool Springs Family Medicine
4091 Mallory Lane Suite 118
Franklin, TN 37067
Tel: (615) 791 9784
Contact Name: Daniel Kalb, M.D.

Cumberland Pediatric Dentistry and Orthodontics
739 President Place #200
Smyrna, TN 37167
Tel: (615) 220 6161
Contact Name: Jack Stalker
Email: jackstalker@gmail.com
Website: http://www.cumberlandpediatricdentistry.com

Dr. Edward Perdue DDS
8120 Sawyer Brown Rd Suite 103
Nashville, TN 37221
Tel: (615) 662 2191
Contact Name: Chelcy Morrison
Email: drperduemarketing@comcast.net
Website: http://healthyteeth4kids.com

Dr. James Deberry
10261 Kingston Pike
Knoxville, TN 37922
Tel: (865) 691 1404

Dr. Jason Clopton
Center of Vision Development
1080 Neal Street Suite 300

Cookeville, TN 38501
Toll Free: (877) 372 2567
Email: DrClopton@covd.biz
Website: http://www.covd.biz

Dr. Mike D. Mysinger, D.D.S.
Dentistry for Children 120 Capitol Drive
Knoxville, TN 37922
Tel: (865) 693 7070

East Tennessee Children's Hospital
2018 Clinch Ave.
Knoxville, TN 37916
Tel: (865) 541 8805
Contact Name: Janis Neece, PhD
Email: JGNeece@etch.com
Website: http://www.etch.com

Monroe Carell Jr. Children's Hospital at Vanderbilt
2200 Children's Way
Nashville, TN 37232
Tel:(615) 936 1000
Website: http://www.vanderbiltchildrens.com

Natural Family Dentistry
216 3rd Avenue North
Franklin, TN 37064
Tel: (615) 595 6111
Contact Name: Graham B. Burcham D.D.S.

Pellissippi Pediatrics
1921 Topside Road
Louisville, TN 37777
Tel: (865) 681 8662

Rochester Pediatrics
224 S. Peters Road
Knoxville, TN 37923
Tel: (865) 693 5016

Snodgrass King Pediatric Dentistry
4761 Andrew Jackson Pkwy
Hermitage, TN 37076
Tel: (615) 885 3525
Website: http://www.snodgrassking.com

UT Medical Group
880 Madison Ave. 5th floor
Memphis, TN 38103
Tel: (866) 278 4966 or (901) 448 6610
Website: http://www.utmedicalgroup.com

Vaibhav Patel, DC
900 Conference Dr Suite 15A
Goodlettsville, TN 37072
Tel: (615) 448 6845

Website: http://www.vitalitychirotn.com

Provides chiropractic care along with nutritional counseling/workshops and focuses on exercise as well to achieve the state of true health.

Vanderbilt Bill Wilkerson Center
1215 21st Avenue South MCE Suite 6209
Nashville, TN 37221
Tel: (615) 936 5000
Contact Name: Jennifer Pilkington, MS, CCC-SLP
Email: jennifer.pilkington@vanderbilt.edu
Website: http://www.vanderbilthealth.com/billwilkerson/

Therapy Services

Bolton Music Therapy
P.O. Box 330434
Murfreesboro, TN 37129
Tel: (615) 715 1232
Contact Name: Kevin Bolton
Email: boltonmusictherapy@gmail.com
Website: http://www.boltonmusictherapy.com

Center of Development
1080 Neal St. Ste 300
Cookeville, TN 38501
Tel: (931) 372 2567
Contact Name: Heidi Clopton, OTR/L
Email: covd@covd.biz
Website: http://www.developmentaldelay.net

Communication Connection, Inc.
111 Suplhur Springs Rd
Murfreesboro, TN 37129
Tel: (615) 896 8046
Contact Name: Tammy Harvey, MS, CCC-SLP, Owner
Email: Tammy@CommunicationConnectionInc.Com
Website: http://www.CommunicationConnectionInc.Com

Elite Behavior Analysis
2115 Chapman Road STE 125
Chattanooga, TN 37421
Tel: (423) 531 7497 or (615) 483 3887
Contact Name: Kris Yi
Email: kyi@elitebehavior.com
Website: http://www.elitebehavior.com

Elite Behavior Analysis provides Behavior Analysis Services and training to a number of school districts, community agencies and private families across Middle and East Tennessee.

Health, Healing, Hope Outreach (H3O) Aquatics
236 Robert Rose Dr.

Murfreesboro, TN 37129
Tel: (615) 995 8027 or (615) 962 9500
Contact Name: Michael Burrows
Email: michael@h3oaquatics.com
Website: http://www.h3oaquatics.com

H3O Aquatics is a medical rehabilitation facility.

Internal Balance
1608 Westgate Center Ste. 2000
Brentwood, TN 37027
Contact Name: Tamara Mariea, Biomedical Nutritionist
Website: http://www.internalbalance.com

Music Therapy Network of Tennessee
Music Therapy Network of Tennessee Chattanooga, TN 37363
Tel: (931) 808 2838
Contact Name: Megan Taylor, MT-BC
Email: megantaylor@musictherapynetworkoftn.com
Website: http://www.musictherapynetworkoftn.com

Musical Bridges
Brentwood, TN 37024
Toll Free: (888) 687 2734
Contact Name: Melissa House Humphries, MT-BC
Email: mail@musicalbridges.com
Website: http://www.musicalbridges.com

Small Miracles Therapeutic Horseback Riding Center, Inc.
1026 Rock Springs Drive
Kingsport, TN 37663
Tel: (423) 349 1111
Email: smiracles@chartertn.net
Website: http://www.small-miracles.org

Waves ASD Program
435 Main Street
Franklin, TN 37064
Tel: (615) 794 9602
Contact Name: Terri Little
Email: tlittle@wavesinc.com
Website: http://www.wavesinc.com

Schools and Educational Services

Autism & Behavior Consulting Services, LLC
4721 Trousdale Drive Suite 129
Nashville, TN 37220
Tel: (615) 331 1141
Contact Name: Jane Barnes
Email: jane@abcservicesllc.net
Website: http://www.abcservicesllc.net

Learning in Focused Environment (L.I.F.E.) school program ages 3-11, ABA, speech therapy.

Camelot of Kingston
183 Fiddlers Lane
Kingston, TN 37763
Tel: (865) 376 1190
Website: http://www.camelotforkids.org

Faith Christian Academy
9114 Davies Plantation Road
Bartlett, TN 38133
Tel: (901) 382 2099
Contact Name: Tammy Mullins
Email: faith_christian_academy@yahoo.com

First Steps, Inc.
McWhorter Family Children's Center 1900 Graybar Ln.
Nashville, TN 37215
Tel: (615) 690 3091
Contact Name: Suzanne Satterfield
Email: ssatterfield@firststepsnashville.org
Website: http://www.firststepsnashville.org

First Steps provides education, outreach and therapy services to children with special needs.

Genesis Learning Centers/Genesis Academy
430 Allied Drive
Nashville, TN 37211
Tel: (615) 832 4222
Contact Name: Terry Adams or Chuck Goon
Email: cgoon@genesislearn.org
Website: http://www.genesislearn.org

Harwood Center
711 Jefferson Avenue
Memphis, TN 38105
Tel: (901) 448 6580
Contact Name: Claire Moss
Email: cmoss1@uthsc.edu
Website: http://www.harwoodcenter.org

Specialized education and therapeutic services for children age 18 months to 5 who are experiencing delays in their development or have a specific developmental disability.

The Phoenix School for Creative Learning
2404 Arthur Road
Germantown, TN 38138
Tel: (901) 757 4360
Website: http://www.thephoenixschool.net

Scenic Land School and Tutoring Center
1200 Mountain Creek Road Suite 300
Chattanooga, TN 37405
Tel: (423) 877 9711
Email: info@sceniclandschool.org
Website: http://www.sceniclandschool.org

University of Tennessee–Office of Disability Services
University of Tennessee Knoxville, TN 37996
Tel: (865) 974 9176
Contact Name: Elizabeth Fussell
Email: lizfuss@utk.edu
Website: http://ods.utk.edu

University of Tennessee FUTURE Program
431 Claxton Complex
Knoxville, TN 37996
Tel: (865) 974 9176
Contact Name: Liz Fussell
Email: lizfuss@utk.edu
Website: http://futureut.utk.edu

Vanderbilt University Next Step Program
Vanderbilt Kennedy Center 230 Appleton Place
Nashville, TN 37203
Tel: (615) 343 0822
Email: NextStep@Vanderbilt.edu
http://kc.vanderbilt.edu/site/nextstep

Next Step is a 2-year certification program for students with intellectual disabilities, providing individualized Programs of Study in the areas of education, social skills, and vocational training.

Legal, Government & Financial Services

Behavioral Health Services
Lentz Public Health Center 311 23rd Ave. North
Nashville, TN 37203
Tel: (615) 340 5616
Website: www.nashville.gov/Health-Department/Clinical-Health-Services/Behavioral-Health-Services.aspx

Tennessee Vocational Rehabilitation Services
400 Deaderick Street 2nd Floor
Nashville, TN 37243
Tel: (615) 313 4891
Website: http://www.tennessee.gov/humanserv/rehab/vrs.html

Community and Recreation Services

ASD Athletes
PO Box 24432
Knoxville, TN 37933-2432
Tel: (865) 604 8511
Contact Name: Terry or Jennifer Higgins
Email: info@asdathletes.org
Website: http://asdathletes.org

Autism Solution Center
9282 Cordova Park Road
Cordova, TN 38018

Tel: (901) 758 8288
Email: info@autismsolutioncenter.com
Website: http://www.autismsolutioncenter.com

Breakthrough Corporation
1805 Maryville Pike
Knoxville, TN 37920
Tel: (865) 247 0065
Contact Name: Tom Beeson
Email: info@breakthroughknoxville.com
Website: http://www.breakthroughknoxville.com

Empower Me Day Camp
2215 Callis Road
Lebanon, TN 37099
Tel: (615) 453 0005Contact Name:
Michelle Harnsberger
Email: EmpowerMeDayCamp@aol.com

Green's Karate
Green's Karate
4121 Hixson Pike
Chatanooga, TN 37415
Tel: (423) 432 5280
Contact Name: Sensei Corey Green
Email: cg@greenskarate.com
Website: http://www.greenskarate.com

Kerri Ruschival Piano Studio
204 Elberta St
Nashville, TN 37210
(615) 310 2377
Contact Name: Kerri Ruschival
Email: kerri@kerriruschivalpiano.com
Website: http://www.kerriruschivalpiano.com

Offers adaptive private lessons to students with special needs 7 and older to suit each student's needs.

The Michael Dunn Center
629 Gallaher Road
Kingston, TN 37763
Tel: (865) 376 3416
Website: http://www.michaeldunncenter.org

Mosaic
2170 Business Center Drive Suite 6
Memphis, TN 38134
Tel: (901) 372 6100
Contact Name: Sherry Taylor
Website: http://www.mosaicinfo.org

Nashville Children's Theatre Drama Class for ASD
25 Middleton St
Nashville, TN 37210
United States
(615) 254 9103

Contact Name: Alicia Fuss
Email: afuss@nashvillect.org
Website: http://nashvillechildrenstheatre.org/camp_asd.htm

New Beginnings Youth Ranch
204 Green Acres
Clarkrange, TN 38553
Tel: (931) 260 1650 or (931) 863 4664
Contact Name: Mike Archambault
Email: ccfarmag@yahoo.com
Website: http://www.newbeginningsyouthranch.com

Orange Grove Center
Orange Grove Center
615 Derby Street
Chattanooga, TN 37404
Tel: (423) 629 1451 or (423) 493 2954
Contact Name: Kyle Hauth or Dianne Aytes
Email: khauth@orangegrove.org
Website: http://www.orangegrovecenter.com

Progress Inc.
319 Ezell Pike
Nashville, TN 37217
Tel: (615) 399 3000
Contact Name: Meika McClendon
Email: m.mccleandon@progress-inc.org
Website: http://www.progress-inc.org/supportedemplyoment.html

Progress is a not-for-profit organization, dedicated to supporting adults with intellectual disabilities.

VSA Arts Tennessee
1210 Lake Rise Place
Gallatin, TN 37066
Tel: (615) 826 5252
Contact Name: Lori Kissinger PhD
Email: userk7706@aol.com
Website: http://www.vsaartstennessee.org

Provides opportunities for people with disabilities to participate in and express themselves through the arts and arts education.

TEXAS

Doctors, Clinics, Hospitals, and Other Health Services

Child Study Center
1300 W Lancaster Ave.
Fort Worth, TX 76102
Tel: (817) 336 8611
Email: info@cscfw.org
Website: http://www.cscfw.org

The Child Study Center (CSC) provides diagnosis and treatment services to children who have, or are at risk for, developmental disabilities and related behavioral and emotional problems.

Clear Lake Children's Center
16815 Royal Crest Drive Suite 160
Houston, TX 77058
Tel: (281) 407 5658
Contact Name: Dr. Becky Siekierski, PhD, LSSP, NCSP
Email: info@clearlakechildrenscenter.com
Website: http://www.clearlakechildrenscenter.com

Cook Children's Rehabilitation Services
750 Mid-Cities Blvd. #110
Hurst, TX 76054
Tel: (682) 885 4063
Website: http://www.cookchildrens.org

The Dental Anesthesia Group
San Antonio, TX 78258
Tel: (210) 460 0271
Contact Name: Dr. Albert Kang
Email: thedentalanesthesiagroup@gmail.com
Website: http://www.thedentalanesthesiagroup.com

DePelchin Children's Center
4950 Memorial Dr
Houston, TX 77007
Tel: (713) 730 2335
Contact Name: Rachel Halpern
Email: rhalpern@depelchin.org
Website: http://www.depelchin.org

Driscoll Children's Hospital
3533 S. Alameda Street
Corpus Christi, TX 788411
Tel: (361) 694 5678
Website: http://www.driscollchildrens.org

Evaluations/Assessments for Autism Spectrum Disorders
1203 Chandler Circle
Prosper, TX 75078
Tel: (214) 682 9164
Contact Name: Athena Bivens
Email: atbivens75078@gmail.com

Faye Elahi
6101 Windcom Court, Suite 100
Plano, TX 75093
Tel: (972) 743 1425
Contact Name: Faye Elahi
Email: specialneedsnutrition@gmail.com
Website: http://www.specialneedsnutrition.com
Offers nutritional services.

The Johnson Center for Child Health and Development
1700 Rio Grande, Suite 200
Austin, TX 78701
Tel: (512) 732 8400
Email: info@johnson-center.org
Website: http://www.johnson-center.org

Pediatric Gastroenterology Resources of Texas
Arthur Krigsman, MD
7901 Cameron Road
Building 3, Suite 110
Austin, TX 78754
Tel: (718) 327 2200, ext. 202
Fax: (512) 233 2397
Website: www.autismgi.com

Treatment for gastrointestinal disorders in children with ASD and others.

Therapy Services

ABA Center for Excellence
Various locations
Main office: 3201 Cherry Ridge Dr., Suite B 205
San Antonio, Texas 78230
Tel: (210) 685 2266
info@abacenter4excellence.com

ABA Center 4 Excellence provides behavioral services to individuals with autism, developmental disabilities, & other special needs.

Achieve Pediatric Therapy and Rehab
715 Discovery Blvd., Ste 115
Cedar Park, TX 78613
Tel: (512) 260 6990
Contact Name: Karen Hoover
Email: office@achievepediatrics.com
Website: http://www.achievepediatrics.com

Provides occupational, physical, and speech therapy services.

Andy's Voice, Inc.
Plano, TX 75075
Tel: (817) 715 9794
Contact Name: Lexi Furlong, M.Ed., BCBA
Email: lexifurlong@andys-voice.com
Website: http://andys-voice.com

Services include ABA, the verbal behavior approach, cognitive behavior therapy, social skills training, and academic tutoring.

A Therapy Connection (ATC)
1112 N Floyd Rd. #9
Richardson, TX 75080
Tel: (972) 470 5855

Contact Name: Anne Howard
Email: info@atherapyconnection.com
Website: http://www.atherapyconnection.com

A Therapy Connection is a speech, occupational, physical and feeding therapy clinic.

Autism Therapies, LLC
594 Garden Ct.
Southlake, TX 76092
Tel: (817) 925 2979
Contact Name: Lloyd Summy
Email: lloyd@autism-therapies.com
Website: http://www.autism-therapies.com

Provides ABA services to families of children with Autism and other developmental disorder.

Autism Treatment Center
Various locations
Website: http://www.atcoftexas.org/index.html

Behavior Exchange
6105 Windcom Court Suite 400
Plano, TX 75093
Tel: (972) 312 8733
Contact Name: Leanne Brown
Email: info@behaviorexchange.com
Website: http://www.behaviorexchange.com

Provides ABA therapy, parent training, school readiness programming, ARD advocacy, school consultations, and other services.

Brazoria County Association for Citizens with Handicaps Early Childhood Intervention Program
120 E. Hospital Dr
Angleton, TX 77515
Tel: (877) 714 1766
Email: contactus@bacheci.org
Website: http://www.bacheci.org

Brent Woodall Foundation
3021 Gateway Drive Suite 295
Irving, TX 75063
Tel: (972) 756 9170
Contact Name: Carley Waltenburg
Email: info@woodallkids.org
Website: http://www.woodallkids.org

Provides ABA therapy for children ages 2-12, social skills groups, parent trainings, free evaluations.

Castell Therapy
3724 Jefferson St. #221
Austin, TX 78731
Tel: (512) 298 2174
Contact Name: Amanda Dishner

Email: amanda@castelltherapy.com
Website: http://www.castelltherapy.com

Collaborative Autism Resources & Education (CARE), LLC
San Antonio, TX
Tel: (877) 712 2735 or 7132942952
Contact Name: Lauren Lanier
Email: llanier@educatorscare.com
Website: http://www.educatorscare.com

Analysis (ABA) trained tutors provide exclusively in-home and community-based one-on-one ABA services for children of active duty military families. Also offers in-home and community-based private pay services for children with developmental disabilities and/ or behavioral disorders in Houston and San Antonio.

Community REC Therapies, LLC
Various locations
Tel: (512) 897 1914
Contact Name: Christine Everitt
Email: ctrs@communityrectherapies.com
Website: http://www.communityrectherapies.com

Dallas Brain Changers
10000 N Central Expwy, Suite 400
Dallas, TX 75231
Tel: (214) 642 3976
Contact Name: Dr. Stephanie Golder, ThD
Email: BrainChangers@gmail.com
Website: http://www.DallasBrainChangers.com

Utilizes neurofeedback to address the symptoms associated with ASD.

ECI of Tarrant County
3840 Hulen Tower N #308
Fort Worth, TX 76107
Tel: (888) 754 0524
Contact Name: Grace White
Email: grace.white@mhmrtc.org
Website: http://www.mhmrtc.org/ECI

Early Childhood Intervention (ECI) provides services to families with children (birth to 36 months) who have developmental delays and disabilities in the following counties: Denton, Ellis, Erath, Hood, Johnson, Navarro, Palo Pinto, Parker, Somervell, Tarrant and Wise.

Epic Health Services
6800 Park Ten Boulevard Suite 246-E
San Antonio, TX 78213
Tel: (210) 377 3742
Contact Name: Ryan Henson
Email: Ryan.Henson@epichealthservices.com
Website: http://www.epichealthservices.com

Provides autism/ABA services.

First Leap
9901 North Capital Of Texas #250
Austin, TX 78759
Tel: (512) 887 2126
Contact Name: Laura Peroutka M.Ed BCBA
Email: Contact@first-leap.com
Website: http://First-Leap.com

First Leap offers in home & clinic based Applied Behavior Analysis (ABA) therapy for children with Autism Spectrum Disorders or other Developmental Disabilities.

Focus Behavioral Associates
635 N Robinson Dr. Suite K
Robinson, TX 76706
Tel: (254) 732 2262
Contact Name: Lisa Fuentes
Email: lisa@focusbehavioral.com
Website: http://www.focusbehavioral.com/

Provides clinical-based Applied Behavior Analysis (ABA) techniques.

FUSION Wellness
1527 Big Horn Dr.
Houston, TX 77090
Tel: (281) 723 2187
Contact Name: Sue Ellen Burch
Email: SueEllenBurch@me.com
Website: http://www.fusionwellnessgroup.com

FUSION utilizes a multiple modality program that integrates many different western and eastern alternative therapies.

Heartwood Children's Behavior Center of Texas
25432 Loop 494, Suite A
Porter, TX 77365
Tel: (281) 354 5424
Contact Name: Joanne Winkler, M.Ed.
Email: jkwinkler7@gmail.com
Website: http://www.heartwoodtx.org

Provides early intervention for children with developmental disabilities using components of ABA and Play Therapy.

Houston Autism Center
5246 Dow Road
Houston, TX 77040
Tel: (713).939.1229
Contact Name: Yvonne Habet, Ph.D.
Email: dryvonnehabet@sbcglobal.net
Website: http://www.houstonautismcenter.com

Identification, assessment, and treatment of children, teens, and adults with ASD. Therapies include ABA, Son Rise, Floor time, and biomedical approaches.

Kids Developmental Clinic (KDC)
Various locations
Email: info@kidsdevelopmentalclinic.com
Website: http://www.kidsdevelopmentalclinic.com/index.php

Pediatric Outpatient Clinic providing Speech, Occupational and Physical Therapy services to children from newborn to 18 years of age.

Line Leader Pediatric Therapy
3303 Northland Drive Suite 214
Austin, TX 78731
Tel: (512) 619 0303
Contact Name: Sharon Wisnieski
Email: walksharon@yahoo.com
Website: http://www.lineleadertherapy.com

Provides occupational, physical, and speech therapy services for children.

Little Behavior Consulting, LLC
Austin, TX 78701
Tel: (512) 200 4948
Contact Name: Lindsey Hamm
Email: info@littlebehaviorconsulting.com
Website: http://www.littlebehaviorconsulting.com

Provides individualized ABA therapy, parent training, toilet training, positive behavior supports, and IEP/ARD advocacy among others.

Dr. Michelle Kandalaft
4100 West 15th Street Suite 204
Plano, TX 75093
Tel: (972) 985 1100
Contact Name: Dr. Michelle Kandalaft
Email: drmkandalaft@gmail.com
Website: http://www.spectrumandbeyond.com

Offers therapies and evaluations for individuals with Asperger's Syndrome and other conditions related to social deficits.

Morning Glory Ranch
31500 Charter Lane
Waller, TX 77484
Tel: (936) 372 2207
Contact Name: Mira Schiff
Email: mira@morninggloryranch.org
Website: http://www.morninggloryranch.org

Experiential outdoor education & equine therapeutic riding wellness.

Pastoral Counseling Center
4525 Lemmon Avenue Suite 200
Dallas, TX 75219
Tel: (214) 526 4525

Toll Free: (800) 340 7557
Website: http://www.pccdallas.org

PediaPlex
2425 E. Southlake Blvd. Suite 100
Southlake, TX 76092
Tel: (817) 442 0222
Email: info@pediaplex.net
Website: http://www.pediaplex.net

Positive Enlightenment, Inc.
Austin, TX 78769
Tel: (512) 377 1118
Website: http://www.positiveenlightenment.com/
Provides ABA-based services.

Seek East
908 Town & Country Blvd Ste 130-D
Houston, TX 77024
Tel: (713) 984 7513
Contact Name: Gabrielle Seekely, M.Ed, LPC-S, BCPC
& Penelope Eastham, MA. CCC SLP
Email: SeekEast@SeekEast.com
Website: http://www.SeekEast.com

SLP and psychotherapist providing services working to address many challenges faced by those with social, cognitive, and communication differences.

The Shape of Behavior
Multiple locations
Corporate office: 12941 North Freeway, Suite #750
Houston TX 77060
Tel: (832).358.2655
Website: Http://www.shapeofbehavior.com/
Provides ABA, HBI, behavior medicine, EEG biofeedback, behavioral services and autism therapy.

Southeast Texas Behavioral Solutions
80 Interstate 10 North, Suite 205
Beaumont, TX 77702
Tel: (409) 225 5796
Contact Name: Julie Sherman, Ph.D.
Email: Drsherman4@gmail.com
Website: http://www.southeasttexasbehavioralsolutions.com
Provides ABA-based behavioral services and biofeedback and neurofeedback to children and adolescents.

Texana Children's Center for Autism
4910 Airport Avenue Building F
Rosenberg, TX 77471
Tel: (281).239.1497
Contact Name: Ellen Catoe
Email: ellen.catoe@texanacenter.com
Website: http://www.texanacenter.com

Center using ABA-based strategies to teach children with ASD.

Texas Young Autism Project
3730 Kirby Drive Suite 540
Houston, TX 77098
Tel: (713) 353 0254
Toll Free: (800) 673 2110
Email: info@drharris.org
Website: http://www.texasyoungautismproject.com

Provides individualized ABA services to children on the spectrum as well as other children with neurological or developmental difficulties.

Schools and Educational Services

Austin Community College VoCAT Program
5930 Middle Fiskville Road
Austin, TX 78752
Contact name: Mariah Bukowski
Tel: (512) 223 7515
Email: vocat@austincc.edu
https://sites.google.com/site/vocatprogram/

A Continuing Education college experience for special needs adults whose disabilities may prevent them from participation in traditional adult education programs.

College Living Experience (CLE)
11801 Stonehollow Drive Suite 100
Austin, TX 78758
Tel: (512) 339 7878
Contact Name: Bronwyn Towart, Program Director
Email: Btowart@experiencecle.com
Website: http://www.experiencecle.com

Disability Support Services
Midwestern State University, 3410 Taft Blvd. Clark Student Center, Room 168
Wichita Falls, TX 76308
Tel: (940) 397 4140
Contact Name: Debra Higginbotham, Director
Email: debra.higginbotham@mwsu.edu
Website: http://students.mwsu.edu/disability/

Edge Transition Academy
2007 N Collins Blvd. Suite 301
Richardson, TX 75080
Tel: (214) 808 0370
Contact Name: Rosalind Funderburgh
Email: administration@edgetransitionacademy.org
Website: http://www.edgetransitionacademy.org

Edge Transition Academy is a post high school transition program.

The Helping House
919 Jack Lock
Nacogdoches, TX 75964
Tel: (936) 371 1536
Contact Name: Amanda Johnson
Email: ajohnson@the-helping-house.org
Website: http://www.the-helping-house.org

Offers private school, after school care, summer clinics, behavioral consulting, feeding therapy, toilet training, teacher training, as well as a Spanish Language support group.

Houston Community College VAST Academy
VAST Department/Occupational Life Skills HCC
Central 1301 Alabama, 101G
Houston, TX 77004
Tel: (713) 718 6297
Contact Name: Ana Calvo, MSW
Email: ana.calvo@hccs.edu
Website: http://vast.hccs.edu

VAST Academy provides post-secondary transition programs and comprehensive support services.

Lake Pointe Resource Center & Lake Pointe Academy
1921 Acton Hwy
Granbury, TX 76049
Tel: (682) 936 4112 or (817) 937 4332
Contact Name: Madalyn Cano, MSSW, LMSW or
Susan Miller, MS, CCC-SLP
Email: admin@lakepointegranbury.com
Website: http://www.lakepointegranbury.com

LoneStar Solutions
1981 Stadium Oaks
Arlington, TX 76011
Tel: (817) 522 5061
Contact Name: Ashley Fogle
Email: ashleyfogle@rvbh.com
Website: http://www.lonestarsolutions.org

The Monarch School
2815 Rosefield
Dr. Houston, Texas 77080
Tel: (713) 479 0800
Fax: (713) 933 0567
Website: www.monarchschool.org

St. Mary's Center for Exceptional Children
2300 Highland Village Rd.
Building 8, Suite 810
Highland Village TX 75077
Tel: (214) 998 8262
Website: http://www.autismtherapyonline.com/index.php

Teach-Me-In-Autism
Houston, TX
Tel: (713) 849 5993
Contact Name: Gina Mouser
Email: ginaam@sbcglobal.net
Website: http://www.teach-me-in-autism.com

Legal, Government & Financial Services

101 Advocacy
2141 Encino Cliff
San Antonio, TX 78259
Tel: (210) 722 9974
Contact Name: Sylvia Farber
Email: SFarber@101advocacy.com
Website: http://www.101advocacy.com

Helping families of greater San Antonio navigate through the special education process.

Advocacy, Inc.
6800 Park Ten Blvd #208-N
San Antonio, TX 78213
Tel: (210) 737 0499
Website: http://www.advocacyinc.org

Statewide legal rights advocacy system that provides services to people with developmental disabilities and mental illness.

ArcherConsulting
1717 St. James Place Suite 205
Houston, TX 77056
Tel: (713) 572 1717
Contact Name: Joe Rivera
Email: joe@archerconsulting.com
Website: http://www.archerconsulting.com

Special needs financial planning.

Christiansen Law Firm, PC
315 S Jupiter Rd, Suite 115
Allen, TX 75002
Tel: (214) 924 9215
Contact Name: Scott Christiansen
Email: scott@scottclawfirm.com
Website: http://www.scottclawfirm.com

Estate planning, including special needs trusts.

Department of Housing and Urban Development
Locations in Fort Worth, Houston, and San Antonio
Tel: (817) 978 5965
Contact Name: Mark J. Brezina
Email: TX_webmanager@hud.gov
Website: http://portal.hud.gov/hudportal/HUD?src=/states/texas/offices

Hayes & Wilson (HW), PLLC
1235 North Loop West Suite 907
Houston, TX 77008
Tel: (713) 880 3939
Website: Http://www.hayeswilsonlaw.com

Estate planning, probate, special needs planning and other asset protection matters.

The Forsberg Law Firm, PC
15899 Hwy 105 W
Montgomery, TX 77356
Tel: (936)5886226
Contact Name: Kevin Forsberg
Email: kevin@forsberglaw.net
Website: http://www.forsberglaw.net

Special education law.

The Franklin Law Firm, LLP
400 S. Zang Boulevard Suite 1400
Dallas, TX 75208
Tel: (214) 948 6464
Contact Name: Jason Franklin
Email: franklinlawdallas@yahoo.com
Website: http://www.franklin-lawfirm.com

The Franklin Law Firm is an injury, accident, and disability law firm located in Dallas, TX.

GrayStar Investments, LLC
PO BOX 30373
Austin, TX 78755
Tel: (512) 809 9024
Contact Name: Yolanda Baker
Email: mail@graystarinvestments.com
Website: http://www.graystarinvestments.com

Special needs tax and financial planning.

Jennifer Fitzhugh Advocacy
4014 Angel Trumpet
San Antonio, TX 78259
Tel: (210) 497 8685
Contact Name: Jennifer Fitzhugh
Email: jenniferlayne@sbcglobal.net

Special education advocacy.

Law Office of Kathryn Craven
1130 South Henderson St. Suite 106
Ft Worth, TX 76104
Tel: (817) 923 5557 or (817) 946 2805
Contact Name: Kathryn Craven, Attorney
Email: kcraven@kcravenlaw.com
Website: http://www.kcravenlaw.com

Comprehensive legal services for families with special needs.

The Livens Law Firm
2516 Harwood Rd 4213 Wiley Post
Dallas, TX 76021
Tel: (817) 545 3425
Contact Name: Lina Martinez
Email: lmartinez@livenslaw.com
Website: http://www.livenslaw.com

Special needs planning and special needs trusts.

National ARD/IEP Advocates
Sugarland, TX 77496
Tel: (281) 265 1506
Contact Name: Louis Geigerman
Email: louis@narda.org
Website: http://www.narda.org

Special education advocacy.

Nickerson Law Group PC
3801 North Capital Of Texas Hwy, Suite J-220
Austin, TX 78746
Tel: (512) 461 1383
Contact Name: Julia Nickerson
Email: ccd@julianickerson.com
Website: http://www.julianickerson.com

Special needs legal planning.

Noteboom The Law Firm
669 Airport Freeway
Hurst, TX 76053
Tel: (817) 282 9700
Contact Name: Chuck Noteboom, Founder
Email: noteboomlawfirm@yahoo.com
Website: http://www.noteboom.com

Disability law and other practice areas.

Philpot Law Office, P.C.
7314 Offats Pointe
Galveston, TX 77551
Tel: (281)9892010
Contact Name: Dorene Philpot
Email: fape4kids@gmail.com
Website: http://www.dphilpotlaw.com

Special education law.

Texas Council on Autism & Pervasive Development Disorders
4800 North Lamar Blvd.
MC 1423
Austin, Texas 78756
Tel: (1-(800) 628 5115 (DARS Inquiries Line)
Email: AutismServices@dars.state.tx.us
Website: http://www.dars.state.tx.us/councils/autism/autism.shtml

Texas Department of Assistive and Rehabilitative Services
4900 N. Lamar Blvd.
Austin, TX 78751
Tel: (800) 628 5115
Email: DARS.Inquiries@dars.state.tx.us
Website: http://www.dars.state.tx.us/drs/index.shtml

Texas Health and Human Services Commission

Brown-Heatly Building
4900 N. Lamar Blvd.
Austin, TX 78751-2316
Tel: (512) 424 6500

Email: webmaster@hhsc.state.tx.us.
Website: http://www.hhsc.state.tx.us/index.shtml

Weeks Law Firm
2201 N. Central Expressway Suite 225
Richardson, TX 75080
Tel: (214) 269 4290
Contact Name: Tresi Weeks
Email: tresi@weekslawtexas.com
Website: http://www.weekslawtexas.com

Special needs planning, special needs trusts and estate planning.

Community and Recreation Services

Adventurers Academy of Life Long Learning
7106 Shadywood Dr
Austin, TX 78745
Tel: (512) 443 4514
Contact Name: Diane Mackey
Email: dimacktx@gmail.com
Website: http://www.austinadventurers.org

Any Baby Can
Various locations
Tel: (210) 227 0170
Contact Name: Hugo Hernandez
Email: hhernandez@anybabycansa.org
Website: http://www.anybabycansa.org

Association For Neurologically Impaired Children (AFNIC)
1412 West 9th Street
Austin, TX 78703
Tel: (972) 264 7983
Contact Name: Phil Ferrara, Executive Director
Email: ferrara54@tx.rr.com
Website: http://www.afniconline.org/

Autism Spectrum Resource Center
3440 Alameda
Corpus Christi, TX 78411
Tel: (361) 851 5111
Contact Name: Bill Butler
Email: bill@spectrumcounseling.us
Website: http://www.asrc-cc.org

Autumn's Dawn Transitional Center
7702 FM 1960 E sat Suite 212
Humble, TX 77346
Tel: (281)9134990 or 2816361342
Contact Name: Jenise Cronan
Email: jenisec@autumnsdawn.org
Website: http://www.autumnsdawn.org

A transitional center for young adults with Autism/Aspergers 18-30 years of age.

Avondale House
3737 O'Meara Dr.
Houston, TX 77025
Tel: (713) 993 9544
Contact Name: Kelly Adams, LMSW
Email: kellya@avondalehouse.org
Website: http://www.avondalehouse.org

Avondale House provides services to children and young adults with autism.

Betty Hardwick Center
2626 S. Clack
Abilene, TX 79606
Tel: (325) 691 2033
Contact Name: Jenifer Farrar
Email: jfarrar@bhcmhmr.org
Website: http://www.bhcmhmr.org

Blessed Be Hope for Three, Inc.
10200 W Airport Blvd. Suite 100
Stafford, TX 77477
Tel: (800) 317 0787
Contact Name: Darla Farmer
Email: darla@hopeforthree.org
Website: http://www.hopeforthree.org

Primary goal is to provide financial assistance to families in Fort Bend County who have children with autism and are in need of help to pay for therapies and treatments.

Breckenridge Village of Tyler (BVT)
15062 County Road 1145
Tyler, TX 75704
Tel: (903) 596 8100
Contact Name: Jim Anderson
Website: http://www.breckenridgevillage.com

BVT is a faith-based residential community, offering a variety of services for adults with mild to moderate cognitive/developmental disorders.

The Bridge: Social Learning Center
1516 E Palm Valley Blvd Building A-4
Round Rock, TX 78664
Tel: (512) 238 5858
Contact Name: Carolyn Peterson
Email: carolyn@thebridgesocial.com
Website: http://www.thebridgesocial.com

Offers LEGO-based social skills groups and camps, executive function coaching, parent and school training, in-home and school support, and individualized tutoring services for all ages of children to young adults with ASD and related challenges.

Brighton: The Center for Inclusive Communities
14207 Higgins Rd.
San Antonio, TX 78217
Tel: (210) 826 4492
Email: info@brightonsa.org
Website: http://brightonsa.org

Brighton provides family & community education and developmental services to children (birth to age 22) with disabilities or delays.

Brookwood Community
1752 FM 1489 –
Brookshire, TX 77423
Tel: (281) 375 2100
Website: http://www.brookwoodcommunity.org/

A God-centered educational, residential, and entrepreneurial community for adults with disabilities.

The Clubhouse
PO Box 1196
Euless, TX 76039
Tel: (817) 835 0446
Email: director@theclubhouse.org
Website: http://theclubhouse.org

Coastal Bend Autism Advocacy
3124 South Alameda Street
Corpus Christi, TX 78404
Tel: (361) 537 0503
Email: cbaa4u@sbcglobal.net
Website: http://www.coastalbendautismadvocacy.org

Down Home Ranch
20250 FM 619
Elgin, TX 78621
Tel: (888) 926 2253
Email: info@downhomeranch.org
Website: http://downhomeranch.org/

Easter Seals Greater Houston
4500 Bissonnet, #340
Bellaire, TX 77401
Tel: (713) 838 9050
Contact Name: Elise Hough
Email: ehough@eastersealshouston.org
Website: http://www.eastersealshouston.org

Ethiopian and Eritrean Families Raising Kids with Special Needs
100 Bald Cypress circle
Irving, TX 75063
Tel: (972)4329711

A support group for families in the DFW area raising kids with all disabilities.

Eva's Heroes
11107 Wurzbach Road, Suite 203
San Antonio, TX 78230
Tel: (210) 694 9090
Contact Name: Christiane Perkins-Garcia
Email: cgarcia@evasheroes.org
Website: http://www.evasheroes.org

ExcellentCare Management
9516 North Freeway
Houston, TX 77037
Tel: (713) 697 9235
Website: http://www.excellentcaremanagement.com

Provides services to children of all ages, from birth to 21 that have developmental disabilities and/or special needs.

Families for Effective Autism Treatment (FEAT) - Houston
3946 Glade Valley Drive
Kingwood, TX 77339
Tel: (281) 361 3328
Email: feathouston@yahoo.com
Website: http://www.feathouston.org

Heart of Texas Autism Network
PO 2484
Waco, TX 76703
Tel: (254) 733 8965
Contact Name: Betsy Klesse
Email: hotanwaco@gmail.com
Website: http://www.hotautismnetwork.org

Independent Living Experience
11801 Stonehollow Dr. Suite 100
Austin, TX 78758
Tel: (832) 452 3155
Contact Name: James Williams, Regional Coordinator
Email: JWilliams@independentlivingexperience.com
Website: http://www.independentlivingexperience.com

It's a Sensory World (ISW)!
13617 Neutron Road
Farmers Branch, TX 75244
Tel: (972) 239 8100
Contact Name: Rekha Suryanarayana
Email: rekha@itsasensoryworld.com
Website: http://www.itsasensoryworld.com

Multi-sensory, educational, recreational, and therapeutic services for children with special needs.

LaunchAbility
4350 Sigma Road Suite 100
Farmers Branch, TX 75244
Tel: (972) 991 6777
Email: info@LaunchAbility.org
Website: http://www.LaunchAbility.org

Life Point
580 Pleasant Ridge Drive
Mansfield, TX 76063
Tel: (817) 473 7125
Contact Name: Nancy Ryals, Director
Email: nancy@lifepointinc.org
Website: http://www.lifepointinc.org

A day program for all young adults, ages 18-29, with special needs.

Life/Run Center for Independent Living
4902 34th St. Suite #5
Lubbock, TX 79410
Tel: (806) 795 5433
Website: http://www.liferun.org

Marbridge Foundation
P.O. Box 2250
Manchaca, TX 78652
Tel: (512) 282 1144 x 1204
Contact Name: Sandra Lantz
Email: slantz@marbridge.org
Website: http://www.marbridge.org

Morgan's Wonderland: A Special Place for Special Friends
5223 David Edwards Drive
San Antonio, Texas 78233
Tel: (210) 495 5888 or (877) 495 5888
Website: http://morganswonderland.com

A 25 acre park is specifically designed for children and adults with special needs, providing outdoor recreational opportunities for individuals with special needs, their families, friends and the entire community.

Mosaic
Various locations
National Supports Office
4980 S. 118th St.

Omaha, NE 68137
Tel: (877)3MOSAIC
Website: http://www.mosaicinfo.org
Contact form: Website: http://www.mosaicinfo.org/contact-mosaic

My Possibilities
1631 Dorchester Dr.
Plano, TX 75075
Tel: (469) 241 9100
Contact Name: Lena Carrera, Program Manager
Email: lcarrera@mptx.org
Website: http://www.mypossibilities.org

nonPareil Institute
5240 Tennyson Parkway, Suite 105
Plano, TX 75024
Tel: (972) 900 9476
Contact Name: Gary W. Moore
Email: gary@npitx.org
Website: http://npitx.org

Provides technical training, employment and housing to individuals with ASD.

North Texas SNAP
P.O. Box 3294
Grapevine, TX 76099
Tel: (817) 481 6522
Contact Name: Rita Goodner
Email: rita.goodner@tx.rr.com
Website: http://www.ntxsnap.org

Partners Resource Network
1090 Longfellow
Beaumont, TX 77706
Tel: (409) 898 4684
Contact Name: Alexis Smith
Email: asmith_prnpath@sbcglobal.net
Website: http://www.partnerstx.org

Operates Texas parent training and information centers, which provide training, education, information, referral, emotional support, and individual assistance in obtaining appropriate services.

Ratcliff Youth and Family Services
P.O. Box 380391
Duncanville, TX 75138
Tel: (972) 298 0200
Contact Name: Tammi Abney
Email: ryfs1@aol.com
Website: http://www.ratcliffyouthandfamilyservices.com

The Sean Ashley House
5606 Parkersburg Drive
Houston, TX 77036

Tel: (713) 667 6460
Website: http://www.seanashleyhouse.org/

Tee Time for Autism
Pearland, TX 77588
Tel: (281) 851 5431 or (832) 314 5010
Contact Name: Brittany Jewell
Email: teetimeforautism@gmail.com
Website: http://www.teetimeforautism.com

United Through Hope, Inc.
503 Bolivar
Denton, TX 76201
Tel: (1-(866) 857 7751
Contact Name: Dr. Laurie Harrier
Email: info@unitedthroughhope.org
Website: http://www.unitedthroughhope.org

Social skills group in the naturalistic setting for pre-K through Adults, vocational training, support groups, parent nights out, advocacy, summer camp.

VIA Transportation Services
800 W. Myrtle
San Antonio, TX 78212
Tel: (210) 362 2000
Website: http://www.viainfo.net

Public transportation for those with disabilities.

Village Learning & Achievement Center at Stoney Glen
2225 Stoney Glen
Kingwood, TX 77339
Tel: (281) 358 6172
Contact Name: Sandy Parks
Email: sparks@villagelac.org
Website: http://www.villagelac.org

Village at Stoney Glen provides independent living opportunities in a residential setting for adults with disabilities.

Work Ready
Various locations
Tel: (214) 763 1500
Email: contact@workreadytexas.com
Website: http://workreadytexas.com

UTAH

Doctors, Clinics, Hospitals, and Other Health Services

Autism Assessment and Treatment Center
4505 Wasatch Blvd Suite 190
Salt Lake City, UT 84124

Tel: (801) 386 8069
Contact Name: Leanne Beale
Website: http://www.autismutah.com

Autism and Psychological Services for Children and Families
2290 E. 4500 S. Ste. 210
Holladay, UT 84117
Tel: (801) 200 2760 or (801) 719 7036
Contact Name: Dr. Brill
Email: autismslc@gmail.com

Provides comprehensive assessments for all ages. Free screenings are provided for children under the age of three, to determine if testing is necessary. Individualized treatment may include developmental and behavioral therapies, social skills groups, sibling support groups, mentoring, school support, individual and family therapy.

Autism Spectrum Disorder Clinic (ASDC)
University of Utah, 650 Komas Dr. Suite 206
Salt Lake City, UT 84108
Tel: (801) 587 8020
Contact Name: Hailey Hodel
Email: hailey.hodel@hsc.utah.edu
Website: http://healthcare.utah.edu/uni/asdc/

Focuses on diagnostic assessments of autism spectrum disorders. Also provides therapy (individual and family) to help with associated psychiatric and behavior issues, as well as groups, including social skills groups, groups to help reduce rigidity, art/music/recreational therapy, and parent training for children, adolescents, and adults.

Bodin: An Educational Consulting Group
2274 South 1300 East #G15-114
Salt Lake City, UT 84106
Tel: (801) 364 1680
Toll Free: (800) 874 2124
Email: info@thebodingroup.com
Website: http://www.thebodingroup.com

BYU Comprehensive Clinic
1190 North 900 East
Provo, UT 84602
Tel: (801) 422 7759
Website: http://cc.byu.edu

The BYU Comprehensive Clinic offers affordable mental health services to children, adults, couples, and families. These services include counseling, psychological and neuropsychological assessments, and groups.

The Children's Center
1855 East Medical Drive
Salt Lake City, UT 84112

Tel: (801) 582 5534
Website: http://www.tccslc.org

Provides comprehensive mental health care to enhance the emotional well being of infants, toddlers, preschoolers and their families.

The NeuroAssessment and Development Center (NADC)
1486 South 1100 East Suite 100
Salt Lake City, UT 84105
Tel: (801) 649 5300
Email: info@neurodevelop.com
Website: http://www.neurodevelop.com

Offers an integrated, neuro-specialty approach towards Assessment and Treatment of ASD and other conditions, serving children, adolescents, and adults.

Timpanogos Assessment and Psychological Services
Clear Horizons Academy
1875 S. Geneva Rd.
Orem, UT 84097
Tel: (801) 810 8378
Contact Name: Mikle South, PhD
Email: timp.testing@gmail.com
Website: http://www.timptesting.com

Provides comprehensive diagnostic ASD evaluations from toddlers through adults and evaluates for other concerns, including anxiety, depression, ADHD, and learning disabilities. Provides social skills groups for children and adolescents diagnosed with ASD.

Utah Center for Psychological Health (UCPH)
124 S 400 East, Suite 300
Salt Lake City, UT 84111
Tel: (801) 355 0188
Contact Name: Dr. Heidi Block
Email: info@utahpsychhealth.com
Website: http://www.utahpsychhealth.com

Provides comprehensive and individualized diagnostic evaluations for people across the lifespan, as well as skill groups, individual and family therapy, and consultation services.

Wasatch Pediatrics
Various locations
Tel: (801) 947 0830
Website: http://www.wasatchpeds.net/

Therapy Services

Amy Peters Therapy Services, LLC
3986 W. Lilac Ln.
Mountain Green, UT 84050
Tel: (801)784-8074
Contact Name: Amy Peters
Email: peters1015@yahoo.com
Website: http://www.amypeterstherapy.com

Providing in-home ABA services to children with ASD.

Apex Behavior Consulting
243 E 400 South, Suite 300
Salt Lake City, UT 84111
Tel: (801) 674 5352
Contact Name: Jennifer Call, M.Ed, BCBA, Clinical Director
Email: Jennifer@apexbehavior.com
Website: http://www.apexbehavior.com

Uses Positive Behavior Support practices and ABA to provide individualized treatment programs.

Autism Links, LLC
3134 Broadway Street
Magna, UT 84044
Tel: (801) 560 5742
Contact Name: Robyn Anderson, Owner
Email: asdconnections@hotmail.com
Website: http://www.infoonautism.blogspot.com

Services Offered: ABA Therapy, Social Groups, Academic Tutoring, Consultation, IEP Meetings, and others.

Browning Speech Therapy, LLC
11634 Summer Stone Dr
South Jordan, UT 84095
Tel: (801) 493 9690
Contact Name: Beth Browning MS CCC SLP
Email: bethbrowning@me.com
Website: http://Browningspeech.com

Specializes in working with children (birth–18 years old) in their home environment using an eclectic therapy style.

Chrysalis
West Jordan, UT 84084
Tel: (801) 404 6023
Contact Name: Jesse Yarger
Email: jesse.yarger@gochrysalis.com
Website: http://gochrysalis.com/services/autism

Chrysalis provides intensive in-home ABA services to children between the ages of two and six.

Courage Reins
5879 W 10400 N
Highland, UT 84003
Tel: (801) 756 8900
Contact Name: Vicki Armstrong, Director
Email: vrarm@mstarmetro.net
Website: http://www.couragereins.org

Therapeutic horseback riding and other equine based activities.

Hoofbeats To Healing
1006 West 5000 South
Palmyra (Spanish Fork), UT 84660
Tel: (801) 836 4325
Contact Name: Tamera Tanner
Email: tamtrot@gmail.com
Website: http://www.hoofbeatstohealing.org

Provides therapeutic horseback riding.

iBehave Therapy Group, LLC
2985 N 935 East Suite 7
Layton, UT 84040
Tel: (801) 564 2794
Contact Name: Nicole Nordello, B.S., Co-Owner
Email: nicole@ibehavetg.com
Website: http://www.ibehavetg.com

Kids On The Move (KOTM)
475 West 260 North
Orem, UT 84057
Tel: (801) 221 9930
Contact Name: Courtney Smith, Autism Specialist Lead
Email: csmith@kotm.org
Website: http://www.kotm.org

Provides services through three main programs: Early Intervention; Early Head Start and Autism Bridges.

Kids Who Count
345 N. SR 198
Salem, UT 84653
Tel: (801) 423 3000
Website: http://www.kidswhocount.org

Early intervention program for children under the age of 3 with a disability or a delay in development.

The Learning Center for Families
1192 West Sunset Blvd.
St. George, UT 84770
Tel: (435) 673 5353 x25
Contact Name: Anita Gardner
Email: anitag@infowest.com
Website: http://www.tlc4families.org

A private, non profit health, social service and school readiness agency.

P.L.A.Y. Along
6754 S Oquirrh Ridge Rd
West Jordan, UT 84081
Tel: (801) 955 2688
Email: playalongdir@yahoo.com
Website: http://www.playproject.org

The P.L.A.Y. Project is a community based/regional autism training and early intervention program.

Pryor Consulting
265 West 1250 North
American Fork, UT 84003
Tel: (801) 492 4874
Website: http://www.pryorconsulting.net

Pryor Consulting provides quality consultative services for families of children with ASD.

Pure Progression Music Therapy
Sandy, UT 84092
Tel: (801) 618 3323
Contact Name: Mary Whyte, MT-BC
Email: info@pureprogression.com
Website: http://www.pureprogression.com

Turning Leaf Wellness Center
1240 W 100 S Bldg 22 Suite 121
St. George, UT 84790
Tel: (435) 652 1202
Contact Name: Mary Ellen Crase MFT-I
Email: MaryEllencrase@hotmail.com
Website: http://www.turningleafwellnesscenter.com/index.html

Utah Behavior Services
6013 Redwood Rd.
Salt Lake City, UT 84123
Tel: (801) 255 5131 X101
Contact Name: Sarah Sanders, M.Ed., BCBA, Co-CEO
Email: info@utbs.com
Website: http://www.utahbehaviorservices.com

Private, in-home, one-on-one ABA therapy and Behavior Consultation services.

Schools and Educational Services

Carmen B. Pingree Center for Children with Autism
780 Guardsman Way
Salt Lake City, UT 84108
Tel: (801) 581 0194
Contact Name: Pete Nicholas, Ph.D., Director
Email: petern@vmh.com
Website: http://www.carmenbpingree.com

Clear Horizons Academy
1875 S. Geneva Road
Orem, UT 84058
Tel: (801) 437 0490
Website: http://www.clearhorizonsacademy.org

GIANT Steps
Foothill Elementary School 921 North 1240 East
Orem, UT 84097
Tel: (801) 226 5437
Website: http://www.wasatch.org/GiantSteps/GiantSteps.html

GIANT Steps is a treatment program for children ages three years through five years who have been diagnosed with ASD using discrete trial, TEACCH, and Greenspan's Floortime, along with preschool activities. Also provides to qualifying students speech therapy, occupational therapy, and/or adaptive physical education.

Redwood Learning Center
P.O. Box 902277
Sandy, UT 84090-2277
Tel: (801) 523 0715
Contact Name: Dara and Steve Michalski
Email: redwoodlc@comcast.net
Website: http://www.redwoodlc.com

Scenic View Academy
5455 Heritage School Drive
Provo, UT 84604
Tel: (801) 226 2550
Website: http://www.svacademy.org/

A school for adults with learning disabilities providing case management, clinical services, education, employment, health/fitness, and recreational therapy.

Southwest Educational Development Center (SEDC)
520 West 800 South
Cedar City, UT 84720
Tel: (435) 586 2865
Contact Name: Bob Wasden
Email: bob.wasden@m.sedc.k12.ut.us
Website: http://www.sedc.k12.ut.us

Legal, Government & Financial Services

Alder & Robb, P.C.
623 East 2100 South
Salt Lake City, UT 84106
Tel: (801) 463 2600
Contact Name: James P. Alder
Website: http://www.alder-robb.com

Salt Lake City estate planning law firm focused on special needs planning.

Bodin: An Educational Consulting Group
2274 South 1300 East #G15-114
Salt Lake City, UT 84106
Tel: (801) 364 1680
Toll Free: (800) 874 2124
Email: info@thebodingroup.com
Website: http://www.thebodingroup.com

Brandon D. Ross, Certified Special Needs Advisor
60 E. South Temple Suite 200-61
Salt Lake City, UT 84110

Tel: (801) 535 1376 / (888) 869 5682
Contact Name: Brandon Ross
Email: brandon_ross@ml.com
Special needs financial planning.

Department of Housing and Urban Development
125 S. State Street, Suite 3001
Salt Lake City, UT 84138
Tel: (801) 524 6070
Contact Name: Kelly Jorgensen
Email: UT_webmanager@hud.gov
Website: http://www.hud.gov/local/index.cfm?state=ut&topic=offices

Disability Law Center
205 North 400 West
Salt Lake City, UT 84103
Tel: (801) 363 1347
Toll Free: (800) 662 9080
Website: http://www.disabilitylawcenter.org

Guardian & Conservator Services
716 East 4500 South Suite N160
Salt Lake City, UT 84107
Tel: (801) 281 1100
Email: kelly_saunders@xmission.com
Website: http://www.guardianconservatorservices.com

Legal Aid Society of Salt Lake
205 North 400 West
Salt Lake City, UT 84103
Tel: (801) 328 8849
Website: Http://legalaidsocietyofsaltlake.org/welcome/

Spectrum Advocates, L.L.C.
6153 Vinecrest Dr United States
Salt Lake City, UT 84121
Tel: (801)9539149
Contact Name: Heather Cannon
Email: spectrumadvocates@gmail.com

Utah State Office of Rehabilitation
P.O. Box 144200
Salt Lake City, UT 84114
Tel: (801) 538 7530
Website: http://www.usor.utah.gov/

Community and Recreation Services

Bear River Activity and Skill Center
Center for Persons with Disabilities
6800 Old Main Hill
Logan, UT 84322
Tel: (435) 797 1981

Cache Valley Call-A-Ride
150 E. 500 N
Logan, UT 84321
Tel: (435) 753 0993
Website: Http://www.cvtdbus.org/index.php

Easy to Love
Layton, UT 84040
Tel: (801) 532 4331
Contact Name: Lindsay Bartholomew
Email: Utaheasy2love@gmail.com
Website: http://www.utaheasytolove.org

Support group in Davis and Salt Lake Counties providing monthly support, special needs friendly family activities, social activities for parents and parent training and workshops.

Fairmont Aquatic Center
1044 East Sugarmont Drive
Salt Lake City, UT 84106
Tel: (801) 486 5867
Website: http://www.recreation.slco.org/fairmont

Families of Autism and Asperger's Standing Together (F.A.A.S.T.)
P.O. Box 645
Roy, UT 84067
Tel: (801) 917 4014
Contact Name: James S. Vaughan
Email: faastutah@gmail.com
Website: http://faastutah.weebly.com/
Facebook: https://www.facebook.com/pages/
Families-of-Autism-and-Aspergers-Standing-Together-
FAAST/193999220626397?ref=hl

Kostopulos Dream Foundation
2500 Emigration Canyon
Salt Lake City, UT 84108
Tel: (801) 582 0700
Email: information@campk.org
Website: http://www.campk.org

Offering recreational opportunities for individuals of all ages and abilities.

National Ability Center
1000 Ability Way
Park City, UT 84068
Tel: (435) 649 3991
Email: DaleS@discoverNAC.org
Website: http://discovernac.org

Offers alpine and Nordic skiing, snowboarding, sled hockey, horseback riding, rock climbing, cycling, canoeing, river rafting, water skiing, archery, and bobsled for people with disabilities of all ages. Also have summer camps specifically for children with ASD.

Parents for Choice in Education
8 E Broadway # 730
Salt Lake City, UT 84111
Tel: (801) 532 1448
Email: info@choiceineducation.org
Website: http://www.choiceineducation.org

Resolution Horse Company
15467 S. Rose Canyon Road
Herriman, UT 84096
Tel: (385) 232 6273
Contact Name: Bruce Cavender
Email: bruce@resolutionhorse.org
Website: http://www.resolutionhorsecompany.org

Provides free horse riding lessons for special-needs and at-risk children.

Rise Services
40 West Cache Valley BLVD Building 8 Suite D
Logan, UT 84341
Tel: (801) 995 2357
Contact Name: Kasey Peterson
Email: kaseyp@riseservicesinc.org
Website: http://www.riseservicesinc.org

Offers day programs, supported living, supported employment, residential, and after school programs.

Snowbird Ski and Summer Resort
Snowbird, UT 84092
Tel: (801) 933 2188
Website: http://www.snowbird.com

Programs offered include; ski lessons, snow shoe tours and sledge hockey throughout the winter, and numerous outdoor recreational activities such as hiking on barrier free trails, fishing, biking, tram rides and environmental awareness programs in the summer.

Splore | Accessible Outdoor Recreation
774 East 3300 South, Suite 105
Salt Lake City, UT 84106
Tel: (801) 484 4128
Email: info@splore.org
Website: http://www.splore.org

Splore is a Utah based non-profit organization that specializes in promoting empowering experiences in an active friendly world through affordable, customized, inclusive recreation and education programs for people of all abilities.

United Angels Foundation
2335 South State Street
Provo, UT 84606
Email: info@unitedangelsfoundation.org
Website: http://www.unitedangelsfoundation.org

US Autism & Asperger Association
P.O. Box 532
Draper, UT 84020-0532
Tel: (801) 816 1234
Website: http://www.usautism.org

Utah Family Voices
University of Utah 44 North Medical Drive
P.O. Box 144650
Salt Lake City, UT 84111
Tel: (801) 584 8236
Toll Free: (800) 829 8200
Website: http://www.utahfamilyvoices.org

Utah Parent Center
2290 East 4500 South, Suite 110
Salt Lake City, UT 84117-4428
Tel: (801) 272 1051
Toll Free: (800) 468 1160 in UT
Email: autisminfo@utahparentcenter.org
Website: http://www.utahparentcenter.org

Work Activity Center
1275 West 2320 South
West Valley City, UT 84119
Tel: (801) 977 9779
Contact Name: Debbie Rooks
Email: debbie.rooks@workactivitycenter.org
Website: http://www.workactivitycenter.org

Provides day, residential, employment, and health services.

VERMONT

Doctors, Clinics, Hospitals, and Other Health Services

The Healer Within You
528 Essex Road Suite 205
Williston, VT 5495
Tel: (802) 318 5329
Contact Name: Dr. Pam Halton
Email: healerwithinu@gmail.com
Website: http://www.thehealerwithinyou.com

Mousetrap Pediatrics
44 Center Street
Enosburg Falls, VT 5450
Tel: (802) 527 8189
Contact Name: Daniel Larrow, MD

The University of Vermont Medical Center
111 Colchester Avenue
Burlington, Vermont 05401
Tel: (802) 847 0000

https://www.uvmhealth.org/medcenter/Pages/default.aspx

Therapy Services

High Horses Therapeutic Riding Program
Norwich, VT 05055
Tel: (802) 356 3386
Contact Name: Liz Claud, Director
Email: Liz.Claud@HighHorses.org
Website: http://www.HighHorses.org

A therapeutic equine experience.

Howard Center
208 Flynn Ave. Suite 3J
Burlington, VT 5401
Tel: (802) 488 6000
Website: http://www.howardcenter.org

Inger Dybfest, M.Ed., RMT
41 John Street
Shelburne, Vermont 05482
Tel: (802).985.3883
Contact Name: Inger Dybfest, M.Ed., RMT
Email: idybfest1@gmail.com

Registered Music Therapist providing evaluation and sessions for children with special needs.

Rhythm of the Rein
386 US Route 2 P.O. Box 67
Marshfield, VT 5658
Tel: (802) 426 3781
Contact Name: Dianne Lashoones
Email: RhythmOfTheRein@aol.com
Website: http://www.rhythmoftherein.org

Therapeutic riding center.

Sd Associates LLC
PO Box 6308
Rutland, VT 05702-6308
Tel: (802) 236 0121 or (802) 235 9533
Contact Name: David Powsner
Email: powsnerd@me.com

Vt Hippotherapy: Hearts, Hands and Horses
Destiny Morgan Farm
Creek Farm Road
Colchester, Vermont
Tel: (802) 860 6072
Contact Name: Kelly Fitzpatrick
Email: ftzptrk2@gmail.com
Website: http://vthippotherapy.com

Medical treatment provided by a licensed occupational, physical therapist where the therapist uses the multidemensional movement of the horse to facilitate the achievement of therapeutic goals.

Schools and Educational Services

Augmentive Learning and Movement Center
122 Park Street
Morrisville, VT 5661
Tel: (802) 879 3011
Email: info@almc-vermont.com
Website: http://www.almc-vermont.com

Center on Disability and Community Inclusion
University of Vermont and State Agricultural College
Burlington, VT 5405
Tel: (802) 656 1143
Contact Name: Susan Ryan
Email: Susan.Ryan@uvm.edu
Website: http://www.uvm.edu/cdci

Hinesburg Community School
10888 Route 116
Hinesburg, VT 5461
Tel: (802) 482 2106
Contact Name: Laura Smith
Email: lsmith@hcsvt.org
Website: http://www2.cssu.org/hcsvt

I.N.S.P.I.R.E. for Autism, Inc.
77 Dylan Road
Brattleboro, VT 05301
Tel: (802) 251 7301
Contact Name: Brenda L. Seitz
Email: bseitz@theinspireschool.org
Website: http://www.theinspireschool.org

Serving individuals 7 through 22 years, whose primary diagnosis is ASD.

Kidpower Vermont
P.O. Box 94
North Ferrisburgh, VT 5473
Tel: (802) 425-KIDS
Contact Name: Laura Slesar
Email: Kidpowervermont@gmail.com
Website: http://www.kidpowervermont.org

Mansfield Hall
371 Pearl St.
Burlington, VT 05401
Tel: (802) 870 0862
Website: http://www.mansfieldhall.org

A post-secondary program for young adults who have the academic potential to be successful in college, but need additional individualized supports to realize their possibilities.

Shelburne Community School
345 Harbor Road
Shelburne, VT 05482
Tel: (802) 985 3331
Contact Name: Toni Dunn
Email: tdunn@cssu.org
Website: Http://www.scsvt.org/Page/291

Stern Center for Language and Learning
183 Talcott Road Suite 101
Williston, VT 05495
Tel: (802) 878 2332
Website: http://www.sterncenter.org

Sunglow Literacy Consulting
Essex Junction, VT 05452
Tel: (802) 879 0898
Contact Name: Jan Ellis-Clements
Email: janellisclem@comcast.net
Facebook: https://www.facebook.com/pages/Sunglow-Literacy-Consulting/149044351797790

Literacy Tutoring and Consulting.

The University of Vermont SUCCEED Program
102 S. Winooski Avenue
Burlington, VT 05401
Tel: (802).488.6542
Contact Name: Jen Mitchell
Email: jenm@howardcenter.org
Website: http://www.howardcenter.org/succeed/

William Center Deaf Autism Program
209 Austine Drive
Brattleboro, VT 05301
Tel: (802) 258 9500
Contact Name: Bert Carter
Email: bcarter@vcdhh.org
Website: http://www.vcdhh.org

Residential school program for students ages 8-22 who are deaf and on the Autism Spectrum.

Legal, Government & Financial Services

Baystate Financial Services
302 Mountain View Drive
Colchester, VT 5446
Tel: (802) 863 280
Website: http://www.baystatefinancial.com

Special needs financial planning.

Caffry Law, PLLC
55 South Main Street Suite 1
Waterbury, VT 05676
Tel: (802) 882 8163
Contact Name: Maria Davies
Email: info@caffrylaw.com

Website: http://www.caffrylaw.com

Provides special needs planning for individuals with disabilities and their families.

Daniel S. Allen Financial Planning Services
441 West River Rd 2nd Floor North
Brattleboro, VT 05301
Tel: (802) 254 7756
Contact Name: Scott Gordon-Macey
Email: sgordonmacey@metlife.com
Website: http://www.dsallen.metlife.com

Special needs financial planning.

Department of Housing and Urban Development
95 St. Paul street Suite 440
Burlington, VT 05401
Tel: ((802) 951 6320
Contact Name: Michael McNamara
Email: VT_webmanager@hud.gov
Website: http://www.hud.gov/local/index.
cfm?state=vt&topic=offices

Department of Vermont Health Access
312 Hurricane Lane
Williston, VT 05495
Tel: (1-(800) 250 8427 or 1-(802) 879 5900
Email: gmcmemberservices@ahs.state.vt.us
Website: http://www.hcr.vermont.gov

Family, Infant and Toddler Program
Department for Children and Families
103 S Main Street
Waterbury, VT 5671
Tel: (802) 241 3622
Contact Name: Helen Keith, Part C Coordinator
Email: helen.keith@ahs.state.vt.us
Website: http://dcf.vermont.gov/cdd/reports/IDEA_Part_C

Law Office of Claudia I. Pringles
32 Main St. #370
Montpelier, VT 05602
Tel: (802) 778 0306
Website: http://www.specialneedslawattorney.com

Special Education Unit
120 State Street
Montpelier, VT 05620-2501
Tel: (802) 828 5114
Contact Name: Kate Rogers, 619 Coordinator
Email: kate.rogers@state.vt.us
Website: http://education.vermont.gov/new/html/
pgm_sped.html

Vermont Division of Vocational Rehabilitation
103 S. Main Street Weeks 1A
Waterbury, VT 05671

Tel: (866) 879 6757
Website: http://vocrehab.vermont.gov/

Community and Recreation Services

Advance Transit Access
P.O. Box 1027
Wilder, VT 05088
Tel: (802) 295 1824
Website: http://www.advancetransit.com/accessAT.htm

APTO LLC
905 Roosevelt Hwy Suite 115
Colchester, VT 05446
Contact Name: Thomas Moore
Email: info@aptollc.com
Website: http://www.aptollc.com
Facebook: Website: http://www.facebook.com/pages/
APTO-LLC/487274924653271

APTO™ is a sports class developed and led by Thomas Moore, MSS, BCBA.

Autism Support Daily
PO Box 4556
Burlington, VT 5482
Tel: (802) 985 8773
Contact Name: Laurie
Email: mjustlaurie@aol.com
Website: http://www.AutismSupportDaily.com

Camp Akeela
One Thoreau Way
Thetford Center, VT 5075
Tel: (866) 680 4744
Contact Name: Debbie & Eric Sasson, Directors
Email: eric@campakeela.com
Website: http://www.campakeela.com

Camp Kaleidoscope
473 Tatro Road
Starksboro, VT 5487
Tel: (800) 430 2667
Email: peg@cgcvt.org
Website: http://www.cgcvt.org

Champlain Community Services, Inc.
512 Troy Ave. Suite #1
Colchester, VT 5446
Tel: (802) 655 0511
Website: http://www.ccs-vt.org

Easter Seals of Vermont
641 Comstock Road Suite 1
Berlin, VT 5602
Tel: (802) 223 4744
Website: http://www.vt.easterseals.com

Going All Out For Autism, Inc.
1182 Route 4A West
Castleton, VT 05735
Tel: (802) 236 9360
Contact Name: Sara Hathaway Stark
Email: info@autismvt.org
Website: http://autismvt.org/

Marble Valley Paratransit Services
Tel: (802) 747 3502
Toll Free: (800) 339 3191
Website: http://www.thebus.com/routes/special.htm

Transition II, Inc.
346 Shelburne Road
Burlington, VT 05401
Tel: (866) 572 7127
Contact Name: Kara Artus
Website: http://www.transitionii.com/

Vermont Autism Network
2993 Chester Arthur Road
Enosburg Falls, VT 05450
Tel: (802) 782 5301
Contact Name: Jess Poirier
Email: jesslpoirier@gmail.com
Facebook: https://www.facebook.com/
VermontAutismNetwork

Vermont Autism Task Force VT
Email: info@autismtaskforce.com
Website: http://www.autismtaskforce.com

Vermont Parent Information Center
600 Blair Park Road Suite 301
Williston, VT 5495
Tel: (802) 876 5315
Toll Free: (800) 639 7170
Email: vpic@vtpic.com

The Vermont Parent Information Center (VPIC) is a statewide network of support and information for families who have a child with special needs or disabilities, and the professionals who work with them.

VIRGINIA

Doctors, Clinics, Hospitals, and Other Health Services

Commonwealth Autism Service
2201 W. Broad St. Suite 107
Richmond, VA 23220
Tel: (800) 649 8481 or (804) 355 0300
Website: http://www.autismva.org

CAS offers resources across the state of VA as well as a Diagnostic & Assessment Clinic. Serves children 18 months to 7 years old.

Continuum Autism Spectrum Alliance (CASA)
1651 Old Meadow Road Suite 600
McLean, VA 22102
Tel: (800) 828 5659
Contact Name: Marc Rose
Email: mrose@continuumgroup.net
Website: http://www.autismspectrumalliance.com

Provides a continuum of care that includes diagnosis, assessment, and treatment.

Highlands Community Services (HCS)
610 Campus Drive
Abingdon, VA 24210
Tel: (276) 525 1550
Website: http://www.highlandscsb.org

Reston Sunrise Dentistry
12359 Sunrise Valley Drive Suite #330
Reston, VA 20191
Tel: (703) 860 4148
Contact Name: Dr. Hanah Pham
Email: restonsunrise@yahoo.com
Website: http://www.sedationdentistreston.com

The Rimland Center for Integrative Medicine—Advocates for Families
Elizabeth Mumper, MD, FAAP
2919 Confederate Ave.
Lynchburg, VA 24501
Tel: (434) 528 9075
Website: www.rimlandcenter.com

A medical practice specializing in integrative treatment of children with ASD and similar challenges.

UVA Children's Hospital
PO Box 800386
Charlottesville, VA 22903
Tel: (434) 924 0000
Website: http://www.healthsystem.virginia.edu/internet/
pediatrics

Therapy Services

Blue Ridge Autism and Achievement Center
312 Whitwell Dr
Roanoke, VA 24019
Tel: (540) 366 7399 or (540) 777 1218
Contact Name: Angie Leonard
Email: BRAAC.Roanoke@gmail.com
Website: http://www.braacroanoke.org

Provides education and services for children and families affected by autism and unique learning challenges, such as learning disabilities.

Dare to Care Charities Life Enrichment Center
P.O. Box 688 2494 Camp Jaycee Rd
Blue Ridge, VA 24064
Tel: (540) 947 5697
Contact Name: Jan Keister
Email: jan.dtcc@yahoo.com

Providing comprehensive therapeutic services and programming to individuals with developmental and intellectual disabilities through farm programs, respite, day and residential programs.

DKB Therapy Services & More, PLLC
800 Westwood Office Park
Fredericksburg, VA 22401
Tel: (540) 693 6997
Contact Name: Deniece M. Payne
Email: deniece_p@yahoo.com
Website: http://www.dkbtherapyservices.com

Provides speech, OT, PT, autism & assistive technology services assessments, music, dance therapy, bilingual speech therapy, psycho-educational services & assessments, IM, bio feedback, ABA/AVB, independent assessments, and advocacy assistance.

Dower and Associates
9845 Business Way
Manassas, VA 20110
Tel: (703) 330 0554
Contact Name: Nikia Dower, MS, CCC-SLP/L, BCBA/L
Email: information@dowerandassociates.com
Website: http://www.dowerandassociates.com

A multi-disciplinary private practice with a focus in speech/language, education and behavior analysis.

FAITH Autism Services
Richmond, VA 23235
Tel: (615) 294 1221
Contact Name: Doemiko Flores
Email: hr@faithisallyouneed.net
Website: http://www.faithisallyouneed.net

Furtherance of Autism with Intervention, Treatment, and Health (FAITH) Autism Services is a Tricare Network Provider. Offering comprehensive ABA therapy services to include direct services, advocacy, consultation and training.

Golden Dreams Therapeutic Horseback Riding
21197 St. Louis Rd.
Middleburg, VA 20117
Tel: (540).687.5800
Email: info@goldendreamsriding.org

Website: http://www.goldendreamsriding.org
Therapeutic riding and other equine activities.

Grafton
Locations in Leesburg, Richmond, Berryville, Winchester
P.O. Box 2500
Winchester, VA 22604
Toll Free: (888) 955 5205
Admissions: admissions@grafton.org
Human Resources: humres@grafton.org
Website: http://www.grafton.org

Provides a continuum of services to children, youth and adults including ABA, early intervention, psychiatric residential treatment facilities, a short-term stabilization program, special education programs, community-based group homes, intensive outpatient program and outpatient services.

Learn Behavior Consultation Services
3414 Flint Hill Place
Woodbridge, VA 22192
Tel: (724) 448 9653
Contact Name: Kerry Dillman, MA, BCBA, President, Lead Behavior Analyst
Email: kdillman.learn@gmail.com
Website: http://www.learnbehaviorconsult.com

Service options include direct 1:1 therapy sessions; paraprofessional supervision; functional assessments; treatment plan development; social skills groups; IEP support.

Metropolitan Pediatric Therapy, LLC
Woodbridge, VA 22192
Tel: (703) 919 7974
Contact Name: Sascha Rogers, MS, OTR/L
Email: InfoMetroPeds@gmail.com

Occupational therapy with a focus on sensory integration.

Northern Virginia Therapeutic Riding Program
6429 Clifton Rd.
Clifton, VA 20124
Tel: (703).764.0269
Contact Name: Maryrose Bornhorst
Email: info@nvtrp.org
Website: http://www.nvtrp.org

Provides therapeutic horseback riding and equine therapy for children age 6 and up and adults with disabilities, youth-at-risk, military service personnel, and their families.

Pediatric Feeding & Speech Solutions, PLLC
704 South King Street Suite #1
Leesburg, VA 20175

Tel: (703) 771 2200
Contact Name: Kelly Benson-Vogt, MA CCC/SLP
Email: kelly@pediatricfeedingandspeec.com
Website: http://pediatricfeedingandspeech.com

Pediatric Feeding & Speech Solutions offers individualized and specialized treatment options for pediatric feeding and speech and language disorders.

Rainbow Therapeutic Riding Center
5605 Antioch Road
Haymarket, VA 20169
Tel: (703) 754 6159
Email: rainbow@rainbowriding.org
Website: http://rainbowriding.org

Provides therapeutic equestrian activities to individuals with physical and mental challenges.

Reaching Potentials
1602 William Street Upper Floor
Fredericksburg, VA 22401
Tel: (540) 368 8087
Contact Name: Pamela Gorski
Email: RPforAutism@aol.com
Website: http://www.reachingpotentials.org

Recognizing Children's Gifts (RCG) Behavioral Health Network
Richmond Office (804) 897 1753 Williamsburg Office
(757) 561 0234 Email: info@rcghealthnetwork.com
Website: http://www.rcghealthnetwork.com/

Provides children with developmental delays and autism one-on-one ABA services in the child's natural environment or a clinical setting.

Spectrum Psychological Services
1020 Independence Blvd, Suite 204
Virginia Beach, VA 23455
Tel: (757) 640 1882
Website: www.spectrumpsychological.net

Provides psychological testing/evaluation, counseling and neurofeedback to children and adults, including those with ASD.

Spectrum Transformation Group
11311 Business Center Dr. Suite C
Richmond, VA 23236
Tel: (804) 378 6141
Contact Name: Cedric Moore
Email: cedric@spectrumtgrp.com
Website: http://www.spectrumtgrp.com

Offering intensive, one-on-one treatment services for children with autism and related neurodevelopmental disorders.

Sprout Therapeutic Riding and Education Center
40685 John Mosby Hwy
Aldie, VA 20105
Tel: (703) 965 8628
Contact Name: Brooke Waldron
Email: Brooke.Waldron@sproutcenter.org
Website: http://www.sproutcenter.org

Equine assisted activities and therapies.

Thrive ABA Consulting, LLC
120 Bowery St. #308
Virginia Beach, VA 23462
Tel: (843) 714 4266
Contact Name: Zack Migioia, BCBA,LBA
Email: zack.migioia@gmail.com

Wings to Fly Therapy and Play Center
4530 Walney Rd. Suite 203
Chantilly, VA 20151
Tel: (703) 608 8817 or (703) 466 5533
Contact Name: Donna Shank, MA, Director/Owner
Email: donna@wingsoflytherapy.com
Website: http://www.wingsoflytherapy.com

Schools and Educational Services

Charterhouse School
3900 West Broad Street
Richmond, VA 23230
(804) 254 9669
Contact Name: Brendan Folmar, Associate Director of Education
Website: http://www.charterhouseschool.org

Offers year-round comprehensive educational services for students 11 to 22 years of age from the Greater Richmond area and students in the Child & Family Healing Center. The school offers integrated programs designed for middle, high school, and college students with Asperger's Syndrome.

Dominion Academy
1002 Wilmer Avenue
Richmond, VA 23227
Tel: (804) 266 9014
Contact Name: Donnovan Miller, Executive Director
Website: http://dominionyouthservices.com/wp/services/academy/

East End Academy
2000 27th Street Newport News, VA 23607 OR
2607 Colonial Avenue Norfolk, VA 23517
Tel: (757) 247 0039 or (757) 275 7498
Contact: Ruby Eley – Principal, Newport News school
Email: reley@eastendacademy.com

Contact: Maxine Jarvis-Dancy – Principal, Norfolk school
Email: mjarvis-dancy@eastendacademy.com
Website: http://eastendacademy.com/

The Faison School for Autism
1701 Byrd Ave
Richmond, VA 23230
Tel: (804) 612 1947
Email: contact@thefaisonschool.org
Website: http://www.thefaisonschool.org

Services are based on the principles of ABA and the Comprehensive Application of Behavior Analysis to Schooling (CABAS®) philosophy. The school serves students ages 16 months to 22 years, and The Faison Centers of Excellence provides outpatient clinic services, an afterschool program, residential support, adult day support, and summer programs.

Mason LIFE Program at George Mason University
Helen A. Kellar Institute for Human Disabilities 4400 University Drive, MSN 1F2
Fairfax, VA 22030
Tel: (703)993-3905
Contact Name: Heidi J. Graff
Email: hgraff@gmu.edu
Website: http://masonlife.gmu.edu/

The Mason LIFE (Learning into Future Environments) Program is a supportive academic university experience offering a four year curriculum of study to post-secondary students, 18-23 years of age, with intellectual and developmental disabilities.

Partners in Learning
503 Faulconer Drive Suite 7A
Charlottesville, VA 22903
Tel: (434) 996 8161
Contact Name: Stacy P. Dean, PhD, NCED
Email: stacy@drstacydean.com
Website: http://www.drstacydean.com

Paxton Campus
601 Catoctin Cir. Northeast
Leesburg, VA 20176
Tel: (703) 777 1939 x 104
Contact Name: Jennifer Lassiter, Executive Director
Email: jlassiter@paxtoncampus.org
Website: http://www.paxtoncampus.org

Virginia Commonwealth University–Disability Support Services
Richmond, VA 23284
Tel: (804) 827 0748
Contact Name: Elizabeth E. Getzel
Email: lgetzel@vcu.edu
Website: http://www.students.vcu.edu/dss

Legal, Government & Financial Services

Belkowitz Law, PLLC
10427 North Street Suite 200
Fairfax, VA 22030
Tel: (703) 246 9272 or (703) 246 9270
Contact Name: Cheri Belkowitz, Attorney at Law
Email: CBelkowitz@belkowitzlaw.com
Website: http://www.belkowitzlaw.com

Special education law.

Department of Housing and Urban Development
600 East Broad Street, Third Floor
Richmond, VA 23219-4920
Tel: (804) 822 4805
Contact Name: Carrie S. Schmidt
Email: VA_webmanager@hud.gov
Website: http://www.hud.gov/local/index.cfm?state=va&topic=offices

Elder & Disability Law Center
1950 Old Gallows Road Suite 700, Tysons Corner
Vienna, VA 22182
Website: http://www.edlc.com

The Homeschool Legal Defense Association
P. O. Box 3000
Purcellville, VA 20134-9000
Tel: (540) 338 5600
Email: info@hslda.org
Website: http://www.hslda.org

Kelly A. Thompson, Attorney at Law
6045 Wilson Blvd, Suite 101
Arlington, VA 22205
Tel: (703) 237 0027
Email: kelly@kellythompsonlaw.com
Website: http://www.kellythompsonlaw.com

Focuses on special needs planning, including benefits planning, guardianship, special needs trusts and other estate planning services.

Law Office of Melissa K. Waugh, PC
1900 Memorial Ave.
Lynchburg, VA 24501
Tel: (434) 200 8287
Contact Name: Melissa K. Waugh, JD, MPH
Email: mwaugh@waughlaw.net
Website: http://www.waughlaw.net

Special education law.

Merrill Lynch Special Needs Group of DC, MD, and VA
8075 Leesburg Pike
Vienna, VA 22182
Tel: (202) 659 6138

Contact Name: Mark Friese
Email: Mark_Friese@ml.com
Website: http://www.fa.ml.com/menick_friese

Special needs financial planning.

Virginia Department of Rehabilitative Services
8004 Franklin Farms Drive
Richmond, VA 23299
Tel: (800) 552 5019
Email: DRS@drs.virginia.gov
Website: http://www.vadrs.org/

Virginia Guardianship Association
Post Office Box 9204
Falls Church, VA 22046
Tel: (703) 532 3214 x402 or (804) 261 4046
Email: Nmercer@TheArcofNoVa.org
Website: http://www.VGAvirginia.org

Virginia Medical Assistance Program
801 E. Main Street
Richmond, VA 23219
Tel: (1-(800) 552 3431
Email: citizen.services@dss.virginia.gov
Website: http://www.dmas.virginia.gov/

Waddell Group - Special Needs Planning
1952 Gallows Road Suite 102
Vienna, VA 22182
Tel: (703) 881 9173
Contact Name: Theresa Waddell
Email: Theresa.Waddell@raymondjames.com
Website: http://www.waddellgroup.net

Special needs financial planning.

Community and Recreation Services

A Better Understanding, LLC
Mechanicsville, VA 23116
Tel: (804) 572 3132
Contact Name: Tim W. Sutton
Email: info@a-betterunderstanding.com
Website: http://www.a-betterunderstanding.com

Law enforcement veteran teaching autism and Alzheimer's awareness.

Access Chesterfield
7321 Whitepine Road
Richmond, VA 23237
Tel: (804) 279 8489
Website: http://www.chesterfield.gov/content.aspx?id=2949

Chesterfield County's Coordinated Transportation Program.

Camp Easter Seals UCP
900 Camp Easter Seals Rd.
New Castle, VA 24127
Tel: (540) 777 7325
Contact Name: Alex Barge
Email: alex.barge@eastersealsucp.com
Website: http://www.campeastersealsucp.com

Chimes Virginia & Potomac Region
3957 Pender Dr. Suite 103
Fairfax, VA 22030
Tel: (703) 267 6558
Website: http://www.chimes.org/VA.aspx

Endependence Center
6300 E. Virginia Beach Blvd.
Norfolk, VA 23502
Tel: (757) 461 8007
Email: ecinorf@endependence.org
Website: http://www.endependence.org

Provides an array of independent living services to individuals with disabilities and to the community.

Hanover Adult Center
7225 Stonewall Parkway
Mechanicsville, VA 23111
Tel: (804) 746 2250
Contact Name: Terry Seward
Email: Terry@HanoverAdultCenter.com
Website: http://www.hanoveradultcenter.com

The Linking Lives program at the Hanover Adult Center is a community based day support program for adults with intellectual disabilities including ASD.

HEAART: Helping Expand Autism Awareness Resource Team
628 Lake Street
Wise, VA 24293
Tel: (276) 328 8017
Contact Name: Jerri Adams
Email: jadams@wise.k12.va.us

Linda S. Young, LPC
641 Lynnhaven Parkway Suite #204
Virginia Beach, VA 23452
Tel: (757) 306 4232

Nova Cool Cats Special Hockey Inc.
Various locations
Contact: Randy Brawley, Head Coach
Tel: (703) 395 6278
Email: madref@verizon.net
Website: http://www.novacoolcats.org/

Parent Educational Advocacy Training Center (PEATC)
100 N. Washington Street Suite 234
Falls Church, VA 22046
Tel: (703) 923 0010
Toll Free: (800) 869 6782
Email: partners@peatc.org
Website: http://www.peatc.org

Phillips Programs for Children and Families
7010 Braddock Road
Annandale, VA 22003
Tel: (703) 941 8810
Contact Name: Piper Phillips Caswell, President & CEO
Email: Piper.Phillips@phillipsprograms.org
Website: http://www.phillipsprograms.org

Richmond Autism Integration Network
North Chesterfield, VA 23225
Tel: (804) 908 7246
Contact Name: Robin Davis, Executive Director
Email: RobinDavis@RichmondAutism.org
Website: http://www.RichmondAutism.Org

Richmond House
5302 Fitzhugh Avenue
Richmond, VA 23226
Tel: (804) 288 3122
Contact Name: Leslie Hundley - Executive Director
Email: lesliehundley@richmondhouse.org
Website: http://richmondhouse.org

A group home for young adults with ASD who live independently with support; also offers SNAP Club for middle and high school students and young adults.

ServiceSource
11150 Fairfax Blvd., Suite 401
Fairfax, VA 22030
Tel: (571) 337 9076
Contact Name: Theresa Piccolo
Email: theresa.piccolo@servicesource.org
Website: http://www.servicesource.org

SkillQuest Services
400 Investors Place
Virginia Beach, VA 23452
Tel: (757) 385 4040
Website: http://www.vbgov.com/Pages/home.aspx
Contact Name: ask for program supervisor

Adult day support services, for person's diagnosed with ID and ASD, CP, behavioral challenges, medical issues, mental health diagnosis, and other disabilities.

Specialized Transit Arranged Rides
P.O. Box 13247
Roanoke, VA 24032

Tel: (540) 982 2703 or (540) 982 2222
Website: http://www.valleymetro.com/star.htm

St. Joseph's Villa for Children
8000 Brook Road
Richmond, VA 23227
Tel: (804) 553 3265 or (804) 553 3200
Contact Name: Susan Pokorski
Website: http://www.stjosephsvilla.net

Supported Employment of Virginia
4901 Fitzhugh Ave Suite 100
Richmond, VA 23230
Tel: (804) 353 7956
Email: info@supported-employment.com
Website: http://www.supported-employment.com/v8/

Offers group supported employment, situational assessment, job coach training services, follow alongs, individual supported and extended employment services.

VersAbility Resources
2520 58th St.
Hampton, VA 23661
Tel: (757) 896 6461
Website: http://www.versability.org

Wall Residences
PO Box 235
Floyd, Virginia 24091
Tel: (540) 745 4216
Email: info@wallresidences.com
Website: http://www.wallresidences.com

WASHINGTON

Doctors, Clinics, Hospitals, and Other Health Services

Adult Autism Clinic
4225 Roosevelt Way NE
Seattle, WA 98105
Tel: (206) 598 7792
Website: http://www.uwmedicine.org/locations/adult-autism

Alan P. Lloyd, Licensed Acupuncturist
5370 Wilson Ave. S.
Seattle, 98118
Tel: (206) 218 9527
Contact Name: Alan P Lloyd
Email: mulloyd@juno.com
Website: http://www.essentialbirthandfamily.com

Specializes in children with ASD.

Autism Evaluation Clinic
Valley Medical Center
400 S. 43 Street
Renton, WA, 98055
Tel: (425) 228 3450
Website: http://www.valleymed.org/

Children's Village Yakima
3801 Kern Road
Yakima, WA 98902
Tel: (509) 574 3200
Toll Free: (800) 745 1077
Website: http://www.yakimachildrensvillage.org

The Village provides over 30 different services to children with special health care needs and their families including medical specialty clinics, development evaluations, dental services, OT, ST, PT, mental health counseling, education services, and care resource coordinators.

Hirsch Holistic Family Medicine
1017 4th Ave East, #6
Olympia, WA 98506
Tel: (360) 326 6436
Contact Name: Dr. Evan Hirsch
Email: Drevan@Onebox.com
Website: http://www.doctorevan.com

Trained in a variety of modalities including Functional Medicine, Medical Acupuncture, Nutritional Therapy, ASD, Kripalu Yoga and Pranayama, Reiki, Clinical Hypnosis and Intravenous Vitamin and Mineral Therapies and board certified in family medicine and holistic medicine.

Janel Newman-Kovacev ND
27121 174th Place SE Suite 203
Covington, WA 98042
Tel: (253) 277 1308
Website: http://www.mygenerationsclinic.com

Naturopathic physician offering alternative therapies including diet modification.

Nutrition Counseling
3856 260th Avenue SE
Issaquah, WA 98029
(425) 312 3246
Contact Name: Yuchi Yang
Email: yuchinutrition@yahoo.com
Website: http://www.anutritioncounseling.com

Yuchi Yang is a registered dietitian specializing in pediatric nutrition, including children with ASD.

Northwest Healthcare & Wellness Center
1901 George Washington Way Suite E
Richland, WA 99354

Tel: (509) 943 2101
Email: info@NWhealthcare.net
Website: http://NWhealthcare.net

Treatment of ASD to improve detoxification, relieve oxidative stress, and remove the accumulated toxins.

Robust Life Center
155 NE 100th St Suite 205
Seattle, WA 98125
Tel: (206) 365 1030
Contact Name: Holly Guentz
Email: info@robustlifecenter.com
Website: http://www.robustlifecenter.com

Nutritional healing specifically designed for ASD.

Seattle Children's Autism Center
4909 25th Ave Northeast
Seattle, WA 98105
Tel: (206) 987 8080
Website: http://www.seattlechildrens.org/clinics-programs/autism-center/

Seattle Children's Autism Center provides assessment, diagnosis, treatment and support for autism spectrum disorders.

Sendan Center
1616 Cornwall Ave Suite 103
Bellingham, WA 98225
Tel: (360) 305 3275
Website: http://www.sendancenter.com

Provides assessment and diagnostic services as well as individualized ABA-based treatment.

Sophia Health Institute
Dietrich Klinghardt, MD, PhD, and others
18106 140th Ave NE
Suite 102
Woodinville, WA 98072
Tel: (425) 402 4401
Email: info@sophiahi.com
Website: www.sophiahi.com

The practitioners at Sophia Health Institute take a patient-centered approach in treating the underlying causes of complex chronic illnesses, including ASD.

Trios Health
900 S. Auburn St.
Kennewick, 99336
Tel: (509) 221 7000

Therapy Services

Autism Behavioral Consulting (ABC)
9901 NE 7th Ave. Suite C-116
Vancouver, WA 98685

Tel: (360) 571 2432
Contact Name: Audra Jensen, M.ED.,BCBA, Executive Director
Email: info@autismabc.org
Website: http://www.autismabc.org

AutismPathways
37933 278th Ave SE
Enumclaw, WA 98022
Tel: (253) 709 3250
Contact Name: Julie C. Schrag
Email: julie@autismpathways.com
Website: http://autismpathways.com

Providing parent consultation and coaching for challenging behaviors, direct social-emotional-behavioral instruction to children, and school interventions and advocacy.

Blue Water Behavioral Consulting
Various locations
Tel: (360) 333 5684
Contact Name: Rachel Wagner, M.S., BCBA
Email: rachel.wagner@bluewateraba.com
Website: http://www.bluewateraba.com

Blue Water Behavioral Consulting provides home-based and community-based ABA/VB therapy for children, adolescents, and young adults diagnosed with autism spectrum disorders and other developmental disabilities.

Carnett Counseling
2120 State avenue NE Suite 219-B
Olympia, 98506
(360) 870 2130
Contact Name: Deborah Carnett
Email: deborah@carnettcounseling.com
Website: http://www.carnettcounseling.com

Chris Rebholz, Psy.D.
10512 NE 68th St. Suite C-104
Kirkland, 98033
Contact Name: Chris Rebholz, Psy.D.
Email: chrisrebholzpsyd@gmail.com

Specializes in diagnosing and treating adults with high-functioning autism.

InnerWave Neurofeedback Center
125 E. Washington
PO Box 399
La Conner, WA 98257 and
Kincaid Landing Ste 224
Mount Vernon, WA 98273
Tel: (360).708.1516
Contact Name: Joan Cross
Email: joan@innerwavecenter.com
Website: http://www.innerwavecenter.com/

K. Hardy Counseling
2804 Grand Ave Suite 207
Everett, WA 98201
Tel: (425) 270 8590
Contact Name: Kimberly Hardy
Email: khardycounseling@gmail.com
Website: http://www.khardycounseling.com

Lakeside Center for Autism
1871 NW Gilman Blvd. Suite 2
Issaquah, WA 98027
Tel: (425) 657 0620
Contact Name: Amy Stachelski, Admissions Director
Email: amy@lakesideautism.com
Website: http://www.lakesideautism.com

MOSAIC Physical Therapy & Massage
21907 64th Ave W, #110
Mountlake Terrace, 98043
Tel: (425) 673 5220
Email: mltclinic@mosaicrehab.com
Website: http://www.mosaicrehab.com/mlt/

A private outpatient practice using a combination of functional neuromuscular reeducation, hands on manual therapy, movement awareness techniques, and therapeutic exercise.

Puget Sound Psychology and Counseling
5105 200th Street Southwest Suite 100
Lynnwood, 98036
Tel: (425) 314 7618 or (206) 883 6175
Contact Name: Patrick Gray
Email: patrickgraycounselor@gmail.com
Website: http://www.pugetsoundpsychology.com

Therapy and vocational counseling for teens and adults with ASD; services include cognitive behavioral therapy, video modeling, DBT, mindfulness, adventure based therapy, social skills groups, and job clubs.

Responding to Autism (RTA) Center
4206 W 24th Ave B101
Kennewick, 99338
Tel: (509) 396 9230
Email: info@respondingtoautism.net
Website: http://www.respondingtoautism.net/

Ryther Child Center
2400 NE 95th Street
Seattle, WA 98115
Tel: (206) 525 5050
Website: http://www.ryther.org

Social Bridge
Seattle or Bellevue
Contact Name: Lisa Iland, M.S.
Tel: (425) 533 9671

Email: lisa@socialbridgeseattle.com
Website: http://www.socialbridgeseattle.com

Social Bridge helps teens and young adults with Autism Spectrum Disorders develop independent living, communication, and job skills at their home, college, or workplace.

Sonia Story
Move Play Thrive
PO Box 676
Chimacum, WA 98325
Tel: (360) 732 4356
Website: www.moveplaythrive.com

Tavon Center
24017 SE Black Nugget Road
Issaquah, WA 98027
Tel: (425) 503 6481
Email: contactus@tavoncenter.org
Website: http://www.tavoncenter.org

Connects people with disabilities to the community and nature through horticultural therapy.

Schools and Educational Services

Academy Schools
14601 Interurban Ave. S.
Tukwila, WA 98168
Tel: (206) 588 0860
Contact Name: Janelle Neil
Email: principal@academyschools.org
Website: http://www.academyschools.org

Bellevue Community College Venture Program
10700 Northup Way
Bellevue, WA 98004
Tel: (425) 564 2844
Contact Name: Becky Boberg
Email: rboberg@bcc.ctc.edu

Kindering Center
Bellevue and Bothell locations
Tel: (425) 747 4004
Email: info@kindering.org
Website: http://www.kindering.org

Magnolia Autism Center
1570 Wilmington Dr. Suite 220
DuPont, WA 98327
Tel: (253) 507 7004or(206) 453 4882
Contact Name: McCullough Campbell
Email: info@magnoliabehaviortherapy.com
Website: http://www.magnoliabehaviortherapy.com/magnolia-autism-center.html

Northwest Center Kids
3201 E. Republican Street
Seattle, WA 98112
(206) 963 3025
Contact Name: Amy Bender
Email: abender@nwcenter.org
Website: http://www.nwcenterkids.org/teens.html

Provides individualized programs of education, advocacy, therapy and family support.

Sum of Learning
Bellevue, WA 98009
Tel; (425) 802 6655
Contact Name: Ivy Chung
Email: info@sumoflearning.com
Website: http://www.sumoflearning.com

Sum of Learning offers behavioral and educational services to families and children, aged 2 to 18 years, affected by ASD and other related developmental disorders.

Legal, Government & Financial Services

Carolee H. Densley
1201 Monster Rd. SW Suite 320
Renton, WA 98057
(425) 463 7734
Email: cdensley@mycstone.com
Website: http://www.mycstone.com

Special needs financial planning.

Department of Social and Health Services
Division of Developmental Disabilities
DSHS Customer Service Center
P.O. Box 11699
Tacoma, WA 98411-9905
Website: http://www1.dshs.wa.gov/ddd/

Division of Vocational Rehabilitation
Mailing address: PO Box 45340
Olympia, WA 98504-5340
Location: 4565 7th Avenue SE
Lacey, WA 98503
Tel: (360) 725 3636
Toll-free: (800) 637 5627
Website: http://www.dshs.wa.gov/dvr/

Freel Sparks Law Firm
1455 NW Leary Way Suite 400
Seattle, WA 98107
Tel: (206) 850 8624
Contact Name: Kara Freel-Sparks
Email: info@freelsparkslaw.com
Website: http://www.freelsparkslaw.com

Special education law.

Law Office of Jenny Cochrane
4122 Factoria Blvd. SE Suite 310
Bellevue, WA 98006
Email: jennycochrane@gmail.com
Website: http://estateplansanddisabilitylaw.
wordpress.com
Special education law.

Special Education Advocacy
432 Tracy Ave N
Port Orchard, WA 98366
Tel: (206) 914 0975
Contact Name: Larry Davis
Email: larrydavis@specialeducationadvocacy.org
Website: http://www.specialeducationadvocacy.org

Special Solutions
520 Kirkland Way, Suite 102
Kirkland, WA 98033
Tel: (425) 828 7540
Contact Name: John James
Email: john@specialsolutions.org
Website: http://www.specialsolutions.org
Special needs planning.

Community and Recreation Services

AAA Residential Services
9027 Pacific Ave Suite #4
Tacoma, WA 98444
Tel: (253) 536 5803
Contact Name: Chandra Jones Program Director
Email: chandihomecare@aol.com

Alyssa Burnett Adult Life Center
Seattle Children's Autism Center 19213 Bothell Way
Northeast
Bothell, WA 98011
Tel: (425) 488 6173
Website: http://www.seattlechildrens.org/contact/
alyssa-burnett-adult-life-center
Year-round classes for adults age 18 or older.

Blue Compass Camps: Trailhead Young Adult Program
Seattle, WA 98106
Toll Free: (866) 683 6262
Contact Name: Jordan Maki
Email: jmaki@bluecompasscamps.com
Website: http://www.bluecompasscamps.com

Everett Para Transit
2930 Wetmore Ave
Everett, WA 98201
Tel: (425) 257 8801
Email: etmail@ci.everett.wa.us

Website: http://www.everettwa.org/default.
aspx?ID=300

Families for Effective Autism Treatment (FEAT) of Washington
Lake Sammamish Foursquare Church 14434 NE 8th St.,
Second Floor
Bellevue, WA 98007
Tel: (425) 223 5126
Website: http://www.featwa.org

Heart of Sailing
Corinthian Yacht Club of Tacoma
5624 Marine View Drive
Tacoma, WA 98422
(949) 236 7245
Toll Free: (866) 368 5350
Contact Name: George Saidah/ Founder
Email: gsaidah@heartofsailing.org or info@
heartofsailing.org
Website: http://www.heartofsailing.org
Website: http://www.cyct.com
Introduces sailing to special needs children and adults as a form of education and recreational therapy.

Highland Community Center
14224 Bel-Red Rd.
Bellevue, WA 98007
Tel: (425) 452 6105or(425) 452 7686
Contact Name: Kim Indurkar, Community Services
Program Coordinator
Email: Kindurkar@bellevuewa.gov
Website: http://www.bellevuewa.gov/highland_center.
htm
The Highland Community Center provides summer camps and after school programs for youth and evening/weekend programs for adults.

Innovative Services NW
9414 NE Fourth Plain Rd.
Vancouver, WA 98662
Tel: (360) 892 5142
Website: http://www.innovativeservicesnw.org

Life Enrichment Options
P.O. Box 117
Issaquah, WA 98027
Email: finneganrm@aol.com

L'Arche Tahoma Hope
Tel: (253) 535 3178
Email: info@larchetahomahope.org
Website: http://larchethc.org

MindSource Center
27023 164th Ave SE
Covington, WA 98042

Tel: (253) 639 7146
Email: help@mindsourcecenter.com
Website: http://www.mindsourcecenter.com
Website: http://www.carriesheppard.com

Northwest Autism Center
127 W. Boone
Spokane, WA 99201
Tel: (509) 328 1582
Email: info@nwautism.org
Website: http://www.nwautism.org

Northwest Child's
1823 N. 85th Street
Seattle, 98103
Tel: (206) 526 2493
Email: nwc.ap.office@gmail.com
Website: http://www.northwestchild.org/

Provides care in home and community settings to children, teens and adults with moderate to severe disabilities.

Open Doors for Multicultural Families
24700 Military Rd. South #105
Kent, WA 98032
Tel: (206) 216 4479
Email: info@multiculturalfamilies.org
Website: http://www.multiculturalfamilies.org

Outdoors for All
2 Nickerson Street, Suite 101
Seattle, WA 98109-1652
Tel: (206) 838 6030 or (206) 838 4995
Email: edbronsdon@outdoorsforall.org
Website: http://www.outdoorsforall.org

Offers a variety of on-snow and off-snow recreational activities for children and adults with disabilities.

Partnerships for Action Voices for Empowerment
6316 S. 12th St.
Tacoma, WA 98465
Tel: (253) 565 2266 or (800) 572 7368
Email: pave@wapave.org
Website: http://www.wapave.org

Person First Adult Family Home
11116 East Ferret Drive
Spokane Valley, WA 99206
Tel: (509) 927 4466 or (509) 979 6500
Contact Name: Amy Finkel: President & Provider
Email: amysf56@yahoo.com
Website: http://www.personfirstafh.com

Puget Sound Autism Aspergers Support Associates WA
Tel: (206) 617 2131
Contact Name: Glenna Clouse

Email: info@psaasa.org
Website: http://www.psaasa.org

Seattle Special Education PTSA
Website: http://www.seattlespecialedptsa.org

Sunridge Ranch
Ellensburg, WA
Email: mail@thesunridgeranch.com
Website: http://www.thesunridgeranch.com/index.html

Thrive Housing
Seattle, WA 98036
(760) 408 9936 or (888) 613 5306
Contact Name: Christy Bateman
Email: christy@thrivehousing.com
Website: http://www.thrivehousing.org

Yakima Valley School
609 Speyers Road
Selah, WA 98942
Tel: (509) 698 1300
Website: http://www.dshs.wa.gov/ddd/YVS.shtml

Provides a comprehensive residential care program for people of all ages with severe developmental disabilities.

WEST VIRGINIA

Doctors, Clinics, Hospitals, and Other Health Services

Cranio Sacral Therapy
707 5th St
New Glarus, WI 53574
Tel: (608) 235 9002
Contact Name: Jeanne Ruegsegger
Email: jruegsegger@tds.net

Offers cranio sacral therapy as well as other massage therapy options.

James Marvin Lewis, MD FAAP
6007 U.S. 60
Barboursville, WV 25504
Tel: (304) 733 9087

Specializes in Children with Disabilities and Developmental and Behavioral Pediatrics.

WVU Children's Hospital
930 Chestnut Ridge Rd
Morgantown, WV 26506
Tel: (304) 598 4835 or (800) 842 3627
Website: http://www.wvukids.com

Therapy Services

AAC Devices provided by Dynavox Mayer Johnson WV
Tel: (304) 377 0392
Contact Name: Stacy Riegel
Email: Stacy.riegel@dynavoxtech.com
Website: http://www.dynavoxtech.com

ABA by Board Certified Behavior Analyst
Kenova, WV 25530
Tel: (304) 972 7628
Contact Name: Rebecca Hubbard
Email: bcbagirl@gmail.com

Autism Services Center
The Keith Albee Building 929 4th Avenue
Huntington, WV 25701
Tel: (304) 525 8014
Website: http://www.autismservicescenter.org

Best Life Therapy
141 State Street
Bridgeport, WV 26330
Tel: (304) 933 3073
Contact Name: Rhea Dyer
Email: rhea.dyer@bestlifewv.com
Website: http://www.bestlifewv.com

Provides speech and occupational therapy and specializes in children with ASD.

Circle of Friends
2440 US Rt. 60
Hurricane, WV 25526
Tel: (304) 406 6106
Contact Name: Jill McLaury
Email: info@circleoffriendsaba.com
Website: http://circleoffriendsaba.com

Provides ABA services to children with autism.

Cornerstone Pediatric Center
PO Box 1276
Bridgeport, WV 26330
Tel: (304) 842 0044
Contact Name: Kathy Citerone, MOT, OTR/L
Email: kciterone@cornerstonepediatriccenter.com
Website: http://www.cornerstonepediatriccenter.com

Cornerstone Pediatric Center specializes in children with special needs and implements a brain-based therapy approach to treat the nervous system dysfunction causing delays and/or difficulties.

Diversified Assessment & Therapy Services
1401 Chestnut Street
Kenova WV 25530

Tel: (304)-453-2800
Website: http://www.datswv.com/
For individuals who have developmental disorders.

Early Intervention Program
Department of Health and Human Resources 350 Capital Street
Charleston, WV 25301
Tel: (304) 558 6311
Contact Name: Pam Roush, Part C Coordinator
Email: pamroush@wvdhhr.org
Website: http://www.wvdhhr.org/birth23

The Mental and Social Health Center
667 Huyett Rd
Charles Town, WV 25414
Tel: (304) 997 4161
Contact Name: Michel Shor
Email: michael@thementalandsocialhealthcenter.com
Website: http://www.thementalandsocialhealthcenter.com

Schools and Educational Services

Applied Behavior Learning Center
1006 Sixth Street
Charleston, WV 25302
Tel: (304) 546 0897
Website: http://www.ablcharleston.org

Augusta Levy Learning Center, Inc.
P.O. Box 6711
99 N. Main Street
Wheeling, WV 26003
Tel: (304)-242-6722
ABA-based learning center.

Barnes Learning Center
100 Naomi Street
Fairmont, WV 26554
Tel: (304) 367 2127
Contact Name: Debbie Blankenship
Website: http://www.wvschools.com/barnes

Hands on Communication
P.O. Box 6147
Wheeling, WV, WV 26003
Tel: (304) 218 9634
Contact Name: Bree Blum
Email: bree@signingtimeacademy.com
Website: http://www.hands-on-communication.com

North Marion High School
1 North Marion Drive
Farmington, WV 26571
Tel: (304) 986 3063

Contact Name: Barbara High
Email: mhuffman@access.k12.wv.us
Website: http://www.nmhswv.com

Legal, Government & Financial Services

West Virginia Advocates
1207 Quarrier St. Litton Building
Charleston, WV 25301-1842
Tel: (304) 346 0847 or Tel: (800) 950 5250
Contact Name: Linda A. Leasure
Email: wvainfo@wvadvocates.org
Website: http://www.wvadvocates.org

West Virginia Bureau for Medical Services
350 Capitol street Room 251
Charleston, WV 25301
Tel: (304) 558 1700 or (888) 483 0797

West Virginia Division of Rehabilitation Services
P.O. Box 1004
Institute, WV 25112
Tel: (304)-766-4600
Website: http://www.wvdrs.org/

Community and Recreation Services

Autism Management Group, LLC
4552 Route 152
Lavalette, WV 25535
Contact: Torrey Baker
Tel: (304)-586-6501
E-mail: phillips@autismgroup.org
Website: http://www.autismmanagementgroup.org/

Autism Training Center
Old Main 316
1 John Marshall Drive
Huntington, West Virginia 25755
Toll Free: Tel: (800)-344-5115 All others: Tel: (304)-696-2332
Website: http://www.marshall.edu/atc/

Dial-A-Ride
P.O. Box 7965
Huntington, WV 25779
Website: http://www.tta-wv.com/dialAride.html

Kanawha Valley Regional Transportation Authority
Tel: (304) 343 7586

Mainstream Services
4757 C Route 152
Lavalette, WV 25535
Tel: (304)-522-1945

Contact Name: Deana Prince
Email: dprince@mainstreamservices.org
Website: http://www.mainstreamservices.org

Northwood Health Systems
2121 Eoff Street Wheeling, 26003
Tel: (304) 234 3500
Email: communications@northwoodhealth.com

Licensed 6 bed facility in a quiet residential area. Must be 18 years or older with an intellectual disability.

Russell Nesbitt Services
431 Fulton Street
Wheeling, WV 26003
Tel: (304)-232-0233
Website: http://www.rns-watch.org/index.html

West Virginia Parent Training and Information (WVPTI), Inc.
Various locations
Tel: (800)-281-1436 (in WV) or Tel: (304)-624-1436
Email: WVPTI@aol.com

WISCONSIN

Doctors, Clinics, Hospitals, and Other Health Services

Arch Medical Center
9612 South Franklin Drive
Franklin, WI53132
Tel: (414) 855 0240
Email: info@archmedicalcenter.com
Website: http://www.archmedicalcenter.com

Provides inclusive biomedical treatment for adults and children.

Children's Hospital of Wisconsin
9000 W. Wisconsin Avenue
Wauwatosa, WI 53226
Tel: (414) 266 2000 or Tel: (877) 266 8989
Website: http://www.chw.org

Gundersen Lutheran Medical Center
1900 South Ave
La Crosse, WI54601
Tel: (608) 782 7300
Toll Free: (800) 362 9567
Email: info@gundluth.org
Website: http://www.gundluth.org

Jeffrey Neale Seltz, MD FAAP
317 Knutson Drive
Madison, WI 53704

Tel: (608) 301 9201

Specializes in children with disabilities and developmental and behavioral pediatrics

Marquette Autism Clinic
604 N 16th ST.
Milwaukee, WI 53233
Tel: (414) 288 4438
Contact Name: Amy Van Hecke, Ph.D.
Email: amy.vanhecke@marquette.edu
Website: http://www.marquette.edu/psyc/cps_autism.shtml

Offers comprehensive diagnostic evaluations for ASD and serves individuals from age 2 up.

Norm Schwartz, MD
Integrative Medicine Specialists
10602 N Pt Washington Rd
Suite 101
Mequon, WI 53092
Tel: (262) 240 0133
Website: www.normschwartzmd.com

Racine Dental Group
1320 South GreenBay Road
Racine, WI 53406
Tel: (262)-637-2911
Contact Name: Pediatric Dentists: Dr Jay Oksiuta, D.D.S. Jerry Oksiuta, D.D.S. Jenny Quizon, D.D.S
Website: http://www.racinedentalgroup.com/

Rollefson Trochlell and Associates
16655 W. Bluemound Rd.
Brookfield, WI 53005
Tel: (262) 786 1270
Website: http://www.thefunkidsdentist.com
Dental care.

Scott Theirl DC DACNB FACFN
Functional Restoration
10408 N. Baehr Road
Mequon, WI 53092
Tel: (800) 385 1655
Website: www.yourbestbrain.com

Chiropractic neurologist providing integrative care to children with ASD and others.

Walk of Wellness Healing Center
N27W23953 Paul Road Suite 100
Pewaukee, WI53072
Tel: (262)-347-2850
Contact Name: Dr. Hundt
Email: wowhealingcenter@gmail.com
Website: http://www.wowhealingcenter.com/

Dr. Hundt is a natural healthcare practitioner, specializing in specific nutrition and neurological balancing protocols for individuals living with ASD.

Therapy Services

ABA of Wisconsin
Enrollment Information: Tel: (602)-471-6802
Email form: Website: http://www.abaofwisconsin.org/contact-us.html

Achieve Center Inc.
Achieve Center
2600 Stewart Avenue Suite 38
Wausau, WI 54401
Tel: (715) 845 4900
Contact Name: Carol Wesley, Director
Email: carolw@uachievecenter.com
Website: http://www.uachievecenter.com

Achieve Center provides assessment and treatment services to children and their families impacted by neuropsychological developmental disorders, chronic health issues, and physical disabilities.

Applied Therapies & Wellness Center
1233 N. Mayfair #206
Wauwatosa, WI 53226
Tel: (414) 302 1233
Contact Name: Lisa Hill
Email: lhill@appliedtherapiesandwellness.com
Website: http://appliedtherapiesandwellness.com

Autism Therapy Group
Milwaukee, WI 53211
Tel: (224) 554 9634
Contact Name: Patrica Ostrow
Email: patricia.ostrow@theautismtherapygroup.com
Website: http://www.theautismtherapygroup.com

Specializes in ABA therapy in home and community environments.

Behavior Analysis of Wisconsin, Inc.
301 E. Buffalo St. Suite 148
Milwaukee, WI 53202
Tel: (414) 847 5722
Contact Name: Danielle Deller
Email: WIInfo@Behavior-Analysis.org
Website: http://www.behavior-analysis.org

Providers of Early Intensive Behavioral Intervention to children with autism as well as behavioral intervention and education to older children, adolescents, and adults with autism and related disorders using ABA-based methods.

The Center for Autism Treatment, Inc.
388 Woodside Drive
Cedarburg, WI 53012
Office: Tel: (262)-365-9063
Fax: Tel: (262)-922-4444
Contact Name: Tamara S. Kasper, MS, CCC-SLP, BCBA
Email: contact@centerautismtreatment.org
Website: http://www.centerautismtreatment.org/home

Children's Behavioral Health Services
4039 80th Street Suite D
Kenosha, WI 53142
(262) 657 5026
Email: childbehavior@msn.com
Website: http://www.cbhs-kenosha.com

Children's Therapy Network, LLC
14 Ellis Potter Ct. Ste 200
Madison, WI 53711
Tel: (608)-234-5990
Contact Name: Jen Krull
Email: jen.krull@ctn-madison.com
Website: http://www.ctn-madison.com

A therapy clinic specializing in the treatment of children with sensory processing disorders, autism spectrum disorders, behavioral and social difficulties, developmental delay, and feeding and eating concerns.

Common Threads Family Resource Center
5979 Siggelkow Road
McFarland, WI 53558
(608) 838 8999

Communication Innovations (CI)
Locations in Fitchburg, Middleton, and Sun Prairie
Tel: (608) 819 6394
Email: info@communicationinnovations.com
Website: http://www.communicationinnovations.com

Communication Innovations (CI) provides pediatric therapy services to individuals from birth through young adulthood. Services include occupational therapy, speech/language therapy, physical therapy, feeding therapy, sensory integration therapy, educational support and tutoring, social skills groups, daily living skills, music therapy, and aquatic therapy.

Deb Berrang, M.Ed. Dynamic Connections, LLC
2995 S. Delaware Ave.
Milwaukee, WI 53207
Tel: (414)-510-7523
Contact Name: Deb Berrang
Email: deb@remediatingautism.com

Guides families in identifying their family's needs, concerns, and goals for intervention, and then designs a developmental, relationship-based intervention plan that specifically works toward those goals. RDI® Program Certified Consultant.

Early Intervention Program – KAC
1218-79th Street
Kenosha, WI 53143
Tel: (262)-658-9500
Website: http://thekac.com/content/early-intervention-program

Provides service coordination, special education, physical, occupational and speech therapies for children ages birth to three years, who exhibit developmental delays.

Educational Solutions, Inc.
Eau Claire, WI 54703
Tel: (715) 552 1620
Contact Name: Kristin Wegner
Email: kristin@edso.co
Website: http://www.edso.co

Educational Solutions Inc., provides in-home and out-patient ABA services for children and adolescents with autism.

Hurd Psychology
700 Rayovac Drive, Suite 103
Madison, WI 53711
Tel: (608) 228 0750
Contact Name: Dr. Heather D. Hurd
Email: drheather@hurdpsychology.com
Website: http://www.hurdpsychology.com

Imagine a Child's Capacity
2875 Fish Hatchery Road Fitchburg, WI 53713
Contact: (608) 204 6247
Website: http://www.icc-wi.org/index

Offers individualized therapy, education and community partnerships that foster inclusion, acceptance and independence.

Integrated Development Services, Inc.
815 Forward Dr.
Madison, WI 53711
Tel: (608) 441 0123 or Tel: (800) 218 3781
Contact Name: Samantha Garlock
Email: intake@ids-wi.com
Website: http://www.ids-wi.com

KGH Consultation & Treatment
2990 Cahill Main Suite 204
Fitchburg, WI 53711
Tel: (608)-819-6810
Contact Name: Megan Gilbert

Email: megangilbert@kghconsultation.org
Website: http://www.KGHconsultation.org

Provides comprehensive services to individuals from 0-18 with social, developmental, learning and behavioral difficulties.

Listen and Learn, LLC
P.O. Box 4
Waunakee, WI 53597
(608) 335 2043
Contact Name: Jane Kenyon, M.Ed
Email: Jane.Kenyon@listen-and-learn.com
Website: http://www.listen-and-learn.com

Licensed Solisten Practitioner offering Sound Training Therapy in the home, as well as variety of child-centered developmentally appropriate activities to support learning, increase language, improve behavior, and enhance social skills.

Nature's Edge Therapy Center, Inc.
2523 14 3/4 Ave.
Rice Lake, WI 54868
Tel: (715) 859 6670
Contact Name: Becky Payne, MATCCC/SLP/HPCS, Founder and Director
Email: naturesedge@citizens-tel.net
Website: http://www.naturesedgetherapycenter.org

Providing intensive speech, occupational and physical therapy. Specializing in nonverbal learning and sensory integrative dysfunction. Therapy provided on a ranch setting, incorporating hippotherapy, animal assisted therapy and horticulture therapy.

Phoenix Behavioral Health Services, LLC
115 E. Waldo Blvd.
Manitowoc, WI 54220
Tel: (920) 682 1131
Contact Name: Todd Eiden Ph.D.
Email: info@phoenixbhc.com
Website: http://www.phoenixbhc.com

Provides outpatient psychology, counseling, and autism services.

P.L.A.Y. Project
325 S. Main St.
Oconomowoc, WI 53066
Tel: (262) 424 8521
Contact Name: Terri Enters
Email: tenters@lsswis.org
Website: http://www.playproject.org

Sonnenberg Consultants
723 58th St. Suite 200
Kenosha, WI 53140

Tel: (414) 416 4427
Email: sonnenbergconsultants@live.com
Website: http://www.sonnenbergconsultants.com

Provides a variety of individualized therapy approaches.

Therapeutic Links, PC
RecPlex 9900 Terwall Ter.
Pleasant Praire, WI 53158
Tel: (847) 548 3458
Contact Name: Sharon Silverberg, Office Manager
Email: sharon@therapeuticlinks.com
Website: http://www.therapeuticlinks.com

Provides occupational therapy.

Wiebusch and Nicholson Center for Autism
N27 W23953 Paul Road Suite 206
Pewaukee, WI 53072
Tel: (262) 347 0701
Contact Name: Jennifer Nicholson & Dr. Christopher Wiebusch
Email: wnca@wi.rr.com

Wisconsin Early Autism Project
150 N. Sunnyslope Road Suite 100
Brookfield, WI 53005
Tel: (608) 288 9040
Email: weap.mil@wiautism.com
Website: http://www.wiautism.com

A program and clinic for the treatment of children with ASD using ABA-based therapies.

Schools and Educational Services

Giggly Hugs Child Care Center
W246 S3145 Industrial Lane
Waukesha, WI 53189
United States
Tel: (414)-422-1678
Contact Name: Sarah Kirschling
Email: gigglyhugs@aol.com
Website: http://www.gigglyhugs.com

Has a separate special needs program for autism, sensory disorders and down syndrome. Also offers speech and occupational therapy, and a music program.

Islands of Brilliance
415 E. Menomonee St.
Milwaukee, WI 53202
Tel: (646)-505-8904
Email: kiko@islandsofbrilliance.org
Website: http://www.islandsofbrilliance.org/

Shepherds College
1805 15th Avenue
Union Grove, WI 53182-1597
Tel: (262) 878 5620
Website: http://www.shepherdscollege.org

A three-year post-secondary educational program for individuals with intellectual disabilities.

Wisconsin Independent Life College
PO BOX 239
Waterford, WI 53185
Tel: (262)-488-2071
Tel: (414)-940-1658
Contact Name: Stephanie Mauck, Administrative Director
Email: info@wisconsinilc.org
Website: http://wisconsinilc.org/about/

Legal, Government & Financial Services

Angela E. Canellos, CELA
631 North Mayfair Road
Wauwatosa, WI 53226
(414) 257 9200 or (414) 774 4499
Email: canelloslaw@aol.com

Annen Roetter, LLC
211 S. Paterson Street, Suite 340
Madison, WI 53703
Tel: (608)-251-6700
Contact Name: Jennifer Annen
Email: jannen@annenroetter.com
Website: http://www.annenroetter.com

Special needs legal planning including special needs trusts, social security, Medicaid guardianship/conservatorship and powers of attorney (financial, health and education).

Attorney Timothy P. Crawford, S.C.
840 Lake Ave. Suite 200
Racine, WI 53403
Tel: (262) 634 6659
Contact Name: Tim Crawford
Email: tpc@execpc.com
Website: http://www.TpcLaw.com
Legal planning/disability benefits.

Barbara Hughes, Esq.
2010 Eastwood Drive Suite 201
Madison, WI 53704-5459
(608) 244 5459 or (608) 244 4018
Email: bhughes@hill-law-firm.com
Website: http://www.hill-law-firm.com/hughes2.htm

Practice focusing on estate planning (including disability trusts), probate and trust administration, marital property, and elder law.

Clemment Law Office, LLC
222 N. Midvale Blvd, Ste.14
Madison, WI 53705
Tel: (608) 442 0506
Contact Name: Sarah C. Clemment, J.D.
Email: sarah@clemment.com
Website: http://www.clemment.com

Disability Rights Wisconsin
16 North Carroll Street Suite 400
Madison, WI 53703
Tel: (608) 267 0214 or Tel: (800) 928 8778
Contact Name: Lynn Breedlove
Email: yochupa@wp.dhss.state.wi.us
Website: http://www.disabilityrightswi.org

Division for Learning Support: Equity and Advocacy
125 S Webster Street
Madison, WI 53707
Tel: (608) 267 9172
Contact Name: Mary Peters, Early Childhood Consultant
Email: mary.peters@dpi.state.wi.us
Website: http://dpi.wi.gov/dlsea

Orchard Financial LLC
2201 East Enterprise Avenue Ste. 101
Appleton, WI 54911
Tel: (920) 205 8322
Contact Name: Jason K.Henderson
Email: jason@orchard-financial.com
Website: http://www.orchard-financial.com
Special needs financial planning.

Private Wealth Management at Robert W. Baird & Co.
777 E. Wisconsin Ave. Floor 29
Milwaukee, WI 53202
(414)298-5106
Contact Name: Brian Walsh, CFP®, CLU
Email: bwalsh@rwbaird.com
Special needs financial planning.

Schott, Bublitz & Engel, s.c.
16655 West Bluemound Road Suite 270
Brookfield, WI 53005
Tel: (262) 827 1700
Contact Name: Kristin P. Fredrick
Email: kfredrick@sbe-law.com
Website: http://www.sbe-law.com

Special Needs Planning, LLC
10200 Innovation Drive, Suite 800
Milwaukee WI, 53226
Tel: (414) 203 1932
Email: johnston.robert@principal.com
Special needs financial planning.

Wisconsin Division of Vocational Rehabilitation
201 East Washington Avenue
Madison, WI53707
(800) 442 3477
Email: dwddvr@dwd.wisconsin.gov
Website: http://dwd.wisconsin.gov/dvr/

Community and Recreation Services

Alianza Latina Aplicando Soluciones (ALAS)
1615 S. 22nd Street Suite 109
Milwaukee, WI 53204
Tel: (414) 643 0022 or Tel: (866) 249 5055
Email: Alasinc@Alianzalatinawi.org
Website: http://www.alianzalatinawi.org

ASPIRO
1673 Dousman St.
Green Bay, WI 54303
Tel: (920)-498-2599
Email: aspiro@aspiroinc.org
Website: http://www.aspiroinc.org
Website: http://www.facebook.com/ASPIROinc

Athletes for Autism Foundation
1850 N. MLK Drive #210
Milwaukee, WI 53212
Tel: (414) 562 9480
Contact Name: Ronny Thompson
Email: ronny.thompson@yahoo.com
Website: http://www.athletesforautismfoundation.org

Athletes for Autism seeks to enhance the quality of life for families affected by autism by supplementing traditional treatment therapies with health, wellness, fitness, and nutrition.

Autism Network through Guidance, Education & Life (ANGEL)
c/o Jennifer Larson
E4549 Sherwood Dr.
Spring Green, WI 53588
Email: jenny_larson@excite.com
Website: http://www.angelautismnetwork.org

Offers financial and emotional support to individuals with ASD.

Autism Society of South Central Wisconsin
Madison, WI 53711
Tel: (608) 213 8519
Email: autismsouthcentral@gmail.com
Website: http://www.autismsouthcentral.org

Autism Society of Southeastern Wisconsin, Inc.
3720 N 124th St. Suite O
Wauwatosa, WI53222

Tel: (414) 988 1260
Website: http://www.assew.org

Center on Disability Health and Adapted Physical Activity
108 Mitchell Hall
1725 State Street
La Crosse, WI 54601
Tel: (608) 785 8690
Email: cjambois@uslax.edu

Programs include: physical activity, motor development, adult therapeutic physical fitness, and a physical activity mentoring program.

Dial-A-Ride Transportation
1900 Kentucky St.
Racine, WI 53405
(262) 619 2438
Website: http://racinetransit.com/paratransit.html

Einstein Productions
161 W Winsconsin Ave #18
Milwaukee, WI53203
(414) 270 1081
Email: einsteinproductions2012@gmail.com
Website: http://www.einsteinproductions.org/index. html

Einstein Productions provides the opportunity for persons with high functioning autism to determine the activities they wish to pursue and then use those skills in a practice field environment before engaging in work which may impact their benefit levels.

Family Respite Care Services Inc of Rock County
205 N Main St Suite 106
Janesville, WI 53511
Tel: (608)-758-0956
Contact Name: Whitney Walraven
Email: family.respite@sbcglobal.net
Website: http://www.rockcountyrespite.org

Good Friend, Inc.
808 Cavalier Dr.
Waukesha, WI 53186
Tel: (414) 510 0385
Contact Name: Chelsea Budde
Email: chelsea@goodfriendinc.com
Website: http://www.goodfriendinc.com

Provides autism sensitivity training for first responders in a 2-hour workshop.

Have a Heart Inc.
W10356 State Rd 29
River Falls, WI 54022

Tel: (715)-425-7754
Contact Name: Kyle Johnson
Email: info@haveaheartinc.org
Website: http://www.haveaheartinc.org

Services include weekend respite care, supportive home care, adult family home placement, and adult day programming.

High Point Church
7702 Old Sauk Rd
Madison, WI 53717
Tel: (608) 836 3236
Website: http://www.highpointchurch.org

Metta Homes
W3490 Forest Trail
Montello, WI 53949
Tel: (608)-697-7698
Contact Name: Erin Bentley
Email: bentley.e@hotmail.com
Website: http://www.mettahomes.com

Native American Autism Resource Center
P.O. Box 251
Appleton, WI 549110251
Tel: (920) 840 5619
Email: nativeamericanautism@gmail.com

Addresses needs of tribal families with ASD regarding access to services, education, and treatment.

Opportunities, Inc.
200 E. Cramer St.
Fort Atkinson, WI 53538
Tel: (800) 314 4567
Website: http://www.oppinc.com

Paratransit Handivan Service
530 Doty St.
Fond du Lac, WI 54935
Tel: (920)-322-3650
Contact Name: Lynn Gilles
Email: lgilles@fdl.wi.gov
Website: http://www.fdl.wi.gov/departments.iml?DeptID=30&DeptPage=47

Shepherds Ministries
1805 15th Avenue
Union Drive, WI 53182
Tel: (262) 878 5620
Website: http://www.shepherdsministries.org

Students That Are Really Special (STARS)
Harry and Rose Samson Family JCC
6255 N Santa Monica Blvd.

Milwaukee, WI 53217
Tel: (414) 967 8206
Contact Name: Jody Margolis, Special Needs Coordinator
Email: jmargolis@jccmilwaukee.org

STARS, a program of the Jewish Community Center (JCC) provides several programs for children diagnosed with ASD.

Threshold, Inc.
600 Rolfs Avenue
West Bend, WI 53090
Tel: (262) 338 1188
Email: info@thresholdinc.org
Website: http://www.thresholdinc.org

Transit Plus
1942 N. 17th St.
Milwaukee, WI 53205
(414) 343 1700
Website: http://www.ridemcts.com/Programs/Transit-Plus/

VIP Services, Inc.
811 East Geneva Street
Elkhorn, WI 53121
Tel: (262) 723 4043
Contact Name: Angie Brunhart
Email: Angiebrunhart@vipservices-inc.org
Website: http://www.vipservices-inc.org

WI FACETS
600 W Virginia St. Suite 501
Milwaukee, WI 53204
Tel: (414) 374 4645
Tel: (414) 374 4635 TTD
Email: wifacets@execpc.com
Website: http://www.wifacets.org

Wisconsin Miss Amazing Pageant
De Pere, WI 54115
9208831810
Contact Name: Jade Strick
Email: jadestrick@missamazingpageant.com
Website: http://www.missamazingpageant.com/
Website: http://www.facebook.com/pages/Wisconsin-Miss-Amazing/264175403655527?ref=hl

Created for girls and young women with disabilities to build confidence and self-esteem in a supportive environment.

WYOMING

Therapy Services

Assistive Technology Solutions
19110 SE 47th Place
Issaquah, WY 98027
Tel: (425) 373 1315
Contact Name: Mark Russel
Email: mark@atsolutions.biz
Website: http://www.atsolutions.biz

Specialize in augmentative and alternative communication with individuals with severe communication impairments.

Emilee Tack
Casper, WY 82601
Tel: (989) 640 9432
Contact Name: Emilee Tack
Email: Emilee_Tack@yahoo.com

PLAY Project home consultant providing parent training and family support in relationship-based, play-based early intervention for families with children with ASD.

Jackson Hill Therapeutic Riding Association
PO Box 415
Teton Village, WY 83205
Tel: (307) 733 1374
Email: jhtra@bresnan.net
Website: http://www.jhtra.org

Equine assisted therapeutic and educational activities.

Jackson Hole Behavioral Services, LLC.
Jackson, WY 83002
Tel: (715)-829-5195
Email: jhbehavior@gmail.com
Website: http://www.jhbehavior.com

Provides ABA services to individuals with autism and related disabilities.

Jennifer Brown, MS, CCC-SLP
2201 Foothill Boulevard Suite B
Rock Springs, WY 82901
Tel: (307) 871 5732
Contact Name: Jennifer Brown
Email: jenannbrown@hotmail.com

Lincoln UINTA Child Development Association
(with 5 Child Development Centers across WY)
LUCDA Regional Office PO Box 570 Mountain View,
WY 82939 (307) 782 6602
Email: lucda@lucda.org

Steven D. Newman, PsyD, ABPP
2321 Dunn Ave Suite 6
Cheyenne, WY 82001
Tel: (307) 220 9099
Contact Name: Steven D. Newman, PsyD, ABPP
Email: drsnewman@yahoo.com
Website: http://drstevenewman.org/
DisabilityandCommunityInclusionServices.aspx

Trumpet Behavioral Health
1017 E. Lincolnway Ave.
Cheyenne, WY 82001
Tel: (970) 377 9401
Contact Name: Catherine Bladow, MS, CCC-SLP, BCBA
Email: cbladow@tbh.com
Website: http://www.tbh.com

Provides ABA-based therapies.

Schools and Educational Services

Big Horn Basin Children's Center
250 E. Arapahoe P.O Box 112
Thermopolis, WY 82443
Tel: (307) 864 2171 or Tel: (800) 928 2171
Contact Name: Carolyn Conner
Email: carolync@rtconnect.net
Website: http://www.nwboces.com

A cooperative educational / residential center providing services for school districts and the Department of Family Services across Wyoming.

Powell Sensory Learning Center
118 West 1st Street
Powell, WY 82435
Tel: (307) 754 3349
Contact Name: Barb Pearson
Email: drkim@bresnan.net
Website: http://www.sensorylearning.com

An innovative approach to developmental learning that unites three modalities (visual, auditory and vestibular) into one intervention.

Wyoming Department of Education
2300 Capitol Avenue
Hathaway Building, 2nd Floor
Cheyenne, WY 82002-2060
Tel: (307) 777 7690
Email: wdewebsite@wyo.gov
Website: http://edu.wyoming.gov/

Wyoming Institute for Disabilities
Department 4298 1000 E. University Ave
Laramie, WY 82071
Tel: (888) 989 9463 or Tel: (307) 766 2761
Email: wind.uw@uwyo.edu
Website: http://www.uwyo.edu/wind

WIND works to assist individuals with developmental disabilities, their families, professionals, and University of Wyoming students through education, training, community services, and early intervention.

Legal, Government & Financial Services

Developmental Disabilities Waiver
Wyoming Department of Health
401 Hathaway Building
Cheyenne, WY 82002
(307) 777 7656
Toll Free: (866)-571-0944

Equality Care
6101 Yellowstone Rd Suite 210
Cheyenne, WY 82002
(307)777-7531
Website: http://dfsweb.wyo.gov/economic-assistance/equality-care-medicaid

Helps pay for healthcare services for children, pregnant women, families with children and individuals who are aged, blind or disabled who qualify based on citizenship, residency, family income and sometimes assets and health care needs.

Pride, Inc.
261 Reed Ave
Cheyenne, WY 82007
Tel: (307) 286 3846 or Tel: (808) 208 1556
Contact Name: Ginny Barrett
Email: ginnyannb1@yahoo.com
https://www.facebook.com/pages/PRIDE-INC-a-voice-for-Autism/

Providing Medicaid waiver services for the Developmental Disabilities ABI, and the Mental Health Waivers in south east Wyoming.

Richard Gage P. C.
1815 Pebrican Ave PO Box 1223
Cheyenne, WY 82003
Tel: (307) 433 8864
Email: VaccineLaw@RichardGage.net
Website: http://www.RichardGage.net

Wyoming Department of Education
2300 Capitol Avenue Hathaway Building, 2nd Floor
Cheyenne, WY 82002-2060
Tel: (307) 777 7690
Email: wdewebsite@wyo.gov
Website: http://edu.wyoming.gov/

Wyoming Department of Workforce Services
122 W. 25th Street Hershler Building
Cheyenne, WY 82002
(307) 777 7389
Email: jmcint@state.wy.us
Website: http://www.wyomingworkforce.org/Pages/default.aspx

Wyoming Protection & Advocacy System
320 West 25th Street 2nd Floor
Cheyenne, WY 82001
Tel: (307) 632 3496 or Tel: (800) 624 7648
Contact Name: Jeanne A. Thobro
Email: hn4927@handsnet.org
Website: http://www.wypanda.com/index.asp

Community and Recreation Services

Casper Autism Society
P.O. Box 40132
Casper, WY 82604
Tel: (307) 232 8813
Contact Name: Derek Medlin
Email: CasperAutismSoc@bresnan.net
Website: http://www.casperautismsociety.com

Casper Area Transportation Coalition
1715 East 4th Street
Casper, WY 82601
Email: catcbus@catcbus.com
Website: http://catcbus.com/

Magic City Enterprises
1780 Westland Road
Cheyenne, WY 82001
Tel: (307) 637 8869
Email: lmckinney@mcewyo.org
Website: http://www.mcewyo.org

NOWCAP Services
Various Locations, WY
Contact Name: Cathy Ross
cross@nowcapservices.org
Website: http://www.nowcapservices.org

Parent Information Center
500 W. Lott Street Suite A
Buffalo, WY 82834
Tel: (307) 684 2277
Contact Name: Terri Dawson, Executive Director
Email: tdawson@wpic.org
Website: http://www.wpic.org

Special Olympics Wyoming
239 West 1st Street
Casper, WY 82601
Tel: (307) 235 3062
Email: office@specialolympicswy.org
Website: http://www.specialolympicswy.org/

START Paratransit Bus
P.O. Box 1687
Jackson, Wyoming 83001
Contact Name: Janice Sowder - Transit Coordinator
Email: jsowder@startbus.com

Alternate Email: info@startbus.com
www.startbus.com

Rehabilitation Enterprises of North Eastern Wyoming (RENEW)
Various Locations, WY
Sheridan: Tel: (888) 309 2020
Gillette: Tel: (888) 253 4653
Newcastle: Tel: (888) 693 9245
Website: http://www.renew-wyo.com

Provides a wide range of services for people with disabilities of all ages, including employment services.

CANADA

Doctors, Clinics, Hospitals, and Other Health Services

ErinoakKids Center for Treatment and Development
Burloak—Burlington
1122 International Boulevard, 5th Floor
Burlington, Ontario, L7L 6Z8

Bristol Circle—Oakville
2381 Bristol Circle, Suite 100
Oakville, Ontario, L6H 5S9

North Sheridan 1—Mississauga
2695 North Sheridan Way, Suite 120
Mississauga, Ontario, L5K 2N6

Milton
410 Bronte Street South
Milton, Ontario, L9T 0H9

Torbram—Brampton
8177 Torbram Road
Brampton, Ontario L6T 5C5

Orangeville —Orangeville
60 Century Drive
Orangeville, Ontario L9W 3K4

South Millway—Mississauga
2277 South Millway
Mississauga, Ontario, L5L 2M5

Guelph
340 Woodlawn Road West
Guelph, Ontario, N1H 7A6

Oaklands—Oakville
53 Bond Street, Suite 233 and 234
Oakville, Ontario, L6K 1L8

Howden—Brampton
375 Howden Blvd, Units 1 & 8
Brampton, Ontario, L6S 4L6

Tel: (905) 855 2690
Toll Free: (877) 374 6625
Website: http://www.erinoakkids.ca/

Glenrose Rehabilitation Hospital
Autism Clinic
10230 111 Avenue NW
Edmonton, Alberta T5G 0B7
Tel: (780) 735 6115
Website: http://www.albertahealthservices.ca/services.asp?pid=service&rid=1007810

Glenrose Rehabilitation Hospital's Autism Clinic provides support to children and their families with ASD.

Grandview Kids Children's Centre
Oshawa—Main Site
600 Townline Rd. S.
Oshawa, ON L1H 7K6
Tel: (905) 728 1673

Port Perry—Lakeridge Health Port Perry Hospital
451 Paxton St.
Port Perry, ON L9L 1L9
Tel: (905) 985 7321

Whitby—Whitby Mall
1615 Dundas St. E. Suite #203
Whitby, ON L1N 2L1
Tel: (905) 440 4573

Ajax—Grandview West
570 Westney Rd. S.
Ajax, ON L1S 6V5
Tel: (905) 619 6551

Bowmanville—Knox Christian School
410 North Scugog Court
Bowmanville, ON
Tel: (905) 728 1673

Toll Free: (800) 304 6180
Website: http://grandviewkids.ca/

Offers a variety of programs and services including: occupational therapy; physiotherapy; speech-language pathology; ABA-based autism services; medical services; social work services; audiology; preschool outreach program; specializing clinics (including orthopedics, orthotics, and muscle tone; and therapeutic recreation.

John Gannage, MD
Markham Integrative Medicine

300 Main Street Markham NorthMarkham, ON
L3P1Y8
Tel: (905) 294 2335
Website: www.integrative-medicine.ca

Kinark
Central Intake: (888) 454 6275
500 Hood Road Suite 200
Markham, Ontario L3R 9Z3
Tel : (905) 474 9595
Toll Free: (800) 230 8533
Email: info@kinark.on.ca
Website: http://www.kinark.on.ca/

McMaster Children's Hospital
1200 Main St. W.
Hamilton, ON L8N 3Z5
Tel: (905) 521 2100

Marlene Chapelle, DAc Allergy & Wellness Clinic
Bancroft, ON K0L1C0
Tel: (613) 474 3030
Website: www.allergyandwellness.ca

Ottawa Children's Treatment Centre
OCTC Central Ottawa Location – Main Site #1
395 Smyth Road
Ottawa, ON K1H 8L2
Tel: (613) 737 0871
Toll Free: (800) 565 4839

OCTC Central Ottawa Location – Main Site #2
Max Keeping Tower at CHEO
401 Smyth Road, Second Floor
Ottawa, ON K1H 8L1
Tel: (613) 737 0871
Toll Free: (800) 565 4839
Reception: (613) 737 2286

OCTC Western Ottawa Location – Kanata
Located in the Western Ottawa Community Resource
Centre
2 MacNeil Court
Ottawa, ON K2L 4H7
Tel: (613) 831 5098
Toll Free: (866) 391 2914

OCTC Eastern Ottawa Location
2211 Thurston Drive
Ottawa, ON K1G 6C9
Tel: (613) 688 2126
Toll Free: (800) 841 8252

OCTC Renfrew County Location – Renfrew
Located at the back of the Renfrew Victoria Hospital
499 Raglan Street North

Renfrew, ON K7V 1P6
Tel: (613) 433 8239
Toll Free: (888) 790 9166

OCTC Eastern Counties Location – Cornwall
The Children's Rehab Centre
600 Campbell Street, Suite 100
Cornwall, ON K6H 6C9
Tel: (613) 932 2327
Toll Free: (866) 558 2327

Surrey Place Centre
2 Surrey Place
Toronto, ON M5S 2C2
Tel: (416) 925 5141

West Satellite Office
2150 Islington Avenue, Suite 102
Toronto, ON M9P 3V4
Tel:(416) 925 5141

East Satellite Office
10 Milner Business Ct., Suite 102
Markham, ON M1B 3C6
Tel: (416) 925 5141

Kindercampus
St. Charles School, 50 Claver Avenue
North York, ON M6B 2W1
Tel: (416) 787 5707
Website: www.surreyplace.on.ca

Thames Valley Children's Centre–Autism Services
779 Baseline Rd.E.
London, Ontario N6C 5Y6
Tel: (519) 685 8700
Toll Free: (866) 590 8822
Website: http://www.tvcc.on.ca/

Therapy Services

Accent Music Therapy
PO. Box 21071, MTCC
Mississauga, ON L5N 6A2
Tel: (905) 870- 6895
Email: bill@accentmusictherapy.com
Website: http://accentmusictherapy.com/

Autism Partnership
Calgary Office:
2451 Dieppe Avenue SW, Bldg B1 Suite 12
Calgary, Alberta T3E 7K1
Phone: (403) 205 2749
Email: admin@autismpartnership.ca
Website: http://www.autismpartnership.ca/

Toronto Office
100 York Blvd, Suite 115
Richmond Hill, Ontario L4B 1J8
Phone: (905) 762 9909
Email: carol@acircleofsupport.com
Website: http://www.autismpartnershiptoronto.ca/

The Autism Program of Eastern Ontario
Children's Hospital of Eastern Ontario
401 Smyth Road
Ottawa, Ontario K1H 8L1
Email: webmaster@cheo.on.ca
Website: http://www.cheo.on.ca/En/autism

A program of the Children's Hospital of Eastern Ontario offering Autism intervention program, school support program, and ABA services and support program.

Central East Autism Program (CEAP)
600 Alden Road, Suite 200
Markham, ON L3R 0E7
Tel: (905) 479 0158
Toll Free: (800) 283 3377
www.kinark.on.ca

The Central East Autism Program (CEAP) provides individualized intensive behavioral interventions at home or in a clinical setting as well as transition support.

Gold Learning Centre
Autism spectrum disorders
5331 Ferrier
Montreal, Québec H4P 1M1
Tel: (514) 345 8330
Email: info@goldlearningcentre.com
Website: http://goldlearningcentre.com/

Kerry's Place
Kerry's Place Head Office
34 Berczy Street
Aurora, Ontario L4G 1W9
Tel: (905) 841 6611
Email: info@kerrysplace.org
Website: http://www.kerrysplace.org/

Le Parapluie Bleu
3 Boulevard Samson, suite J
Laval, Québec, H7X 3S5
Tel: (450) 314 4904
Email: info@parapluiebleu.ca
Website: http://www.parapluiebleu.ca/index_en.html

Provides ABA therapy, speech therapy and occupational therapy stressing early intervention.

One Kids Place

North Bay
400 McKeown Avenue

North Bay Ontario
P1B 0B2
Tel: (705) 476-KIDS (5437)
Toll Free: (866) 626 9100

Muskoka
100 Frank Miller Drive Suite 2
Huntsville, ON P1H 1H7
Tel: (705) 789 9985
Tel: (866) 232 5559

Parry Sound
70 Joseph Street Unit 304
Parry Sound, ON P2A 2G5
Tel: (705) 746 6287

Kirkland Lake
30 Second Street, Box #5, Unit 213
Kirkland Lake, ON P2N 1R1
Tel: (705) 572 5437

New Liskeard
Heritage Place
213 Whitewood Avenue West
New Liskeard, ON P0J 1P0
Tel: (705) 680 5437

Website: http://www.onekidsplace.ca/

Provides community-based rehabilitation and related support services for children and youth (up to the age of 19).

Pathways
Pathways for Children and Youth
1201 Division Street, Suite 215
Kingston, Ontario K7K 6X4
Tel: (613) 546 1422
Email: nseale@pathwayschildrenyouth.org
Website: http://www.pathwayschildrenyouth.org/

Offers both ABA and IBI programs and provides teaching in social, play, thinking, language, and self-developmental levels. Parent/caregiver education and engagement is an integral part of the autism services program. Also provides a school support program.

The Portia Learning Center
Head Office
48 Steacie Dr
Kanata, ON K2K 2A9
Tel: (613) 591 9966
Email: info@portialearning.com

Ottawa Center
201 - 1770 Courtwood Cr
Ottawa, ON K2C 2B5
Tel: (613) 221 9777

Durham Centre - Whitby
309 Beech St. W
Whitby, ON
(905) 493 7707
Toronto / Whitby: (905) 493 7707

Provides services based on Verbal Behavior, PRT (Pivotal Response Training), Floortime/DIR, ESDM (Early Start Denver Model), and Lovaas.

Society for Treatment of Autism
404 94th Avenue S. E.
Calgary, Alberta T2J 0E8
Phone: (403) 253 2291
Toll Free: (888) 301 2872
Email: autismtreatment@sta-ab.com
Website: http://www.autism.ca/index.php

Offers support, consultation and educational services for families and communities in Alberta.

Spectrum Intervention Group
19 Grenfell Crescent, Suite 100,
Ottawa, Ontario
Tel: (613) 723 0606
Email: info@spectrumig.com
Website: http://www.spectrumig.com/

An ABA/IBI treatment provider offering services to those 2–24 in home and in clinic, both 1:1 and in small groups.

Schools and Educational Services

Arrowsmith Schools
Arrowsmith School Toronto
245 St. Clair Avenue West
Toronto, ON
M4V 1R3
Tel: (416) 963 4962
Fax: (416) 963 5017
Email: reception@arrowsmithschool.org

Arrowsmith School Peterborough
366 Parkhill Road East
Peterborough, Ontario
K9L 1C3
Tel: (705) 741 4800
Fax: (705) 741 1832
Email: peterborough@arrowsmithprogram.ca
www.arrowsmithschool.org

Premised on the concept of neuroplasticity, the program identifies weak cognitive capacities and provides specific cognitive exercises to intervene and strengthen those areas and improve learning. In addition to the Toronto and Peterborough schools, the website identifies programs worldwide incorporating the Arrowsmith Program.

Avenue Road Academy
1650 Avenue Road, 2nd floor
Toronto ON M5M 3Y1
Tel: (647) 352 6060
Email: learn@avenueroadacademy.ca
Website: http://avenueroadacademy.ca/

Bright Start Academy
2950 Keele Street
Suite 102 and 202
Toronto, ON M3M 2H2
Tel: (647) 347 6122
Email: info@brightstartacademy.info
Website: http://www.brightstartacademy.info/

Brighton School
240 The Donway West (Lawrence & Don Mills)
Toronto, Ontario M3B 2V8
Tel: (416) 932 8273
Email: contactus@brightonschool.ca
Website: http://www.brightonschool.ca/

Centennial Academy
3641, avenue Prud'homme
Montréal, Québec H4A 3H6
Tel: (514) 486 5533
Email: info@centennial.qc.ca
Website: http://centennial.qc.ca/

Collège Sphere College
1095 chemin Quigley Hill Road
Ottawa (Cumberland), Ontario K4C 1H2
Tel: (613) 842 9111
Email: collegespherecollege@rogers.com
Website: http://www.collegespherecollege.com/

Eaton Arrowsmith School
Vancouver
204-6190 Agronomy Road at UBC
Vancouver, BC V6T 1Z3
Tel: (844) 264 8327
Email: admissions@eatonarrowsmithschool.com
E-mail: info@eatonarrowsmithschool.com
Website: http://www.eatonarrowsmithschool.com/

Victoria
200 – 3200 Shelbourne Street
Victoria, BC V8P 5G8
Tel: (250) 370 0046
E-mail: victoria@eatonarrowsmithschool.com

White Rock
300 – 1538 Foster Street, 3rd Floor
White Rock, BC V4B 3X8
Tel: (604) 538 1710

Eaton Arrowsmith School follows the Arrowsmith Program, strengthening areas that are the source of students' learning challenges.

Giant Steps
Giant Steps Toronto/York Region
35 Flowervale Road
Thornhill, Ontario L3T 4J3
Tel: (905) 881 3104
Email: info@giantstepstoronto.ca
Website: www.giantstepstoronto.ca

Provides a coordinated, comprehensive approach of specialized academics, therapies and inclusion.

The Good Samaritan School for Exceptional Students
6341 Mississauga Road
Mississauga, Ontario, L5N 1A5
Tel: (905) 814 5181 Ext. 101

The Good Samaritan School is a Christian private school that provides a structured academic environment for children with special needs.

Heritage Academy of Learning Excellence
207 Bayswater Avenue
Ottawa, Ontario K1Y 2G5
Tel: (613) 722 0133
Email: info@heritage-academy.com
Website: http://www.heritage-academy.com/

Kenneth Gordon Maplewood School
420 Seymour River Place
North Vancouver, BC V7H 1S8
Tel: (604) 985 5224
Email: jchristopher@kgms.ca, Dr. James Christopher, Head of School
Website: http://kgms.ca/

Kohai Education Centre
41 Roehampton Avenue
Toronto, Ontario M4P 1P9
Tel: (416) 489 3636
Email: kohai@bellnet.ca
Website: http://kohai.ca/

Landmark East
708 Main Street
Wolfville, Nova Scotia B4P 1G4
Tel: (902) 542 2237
Toll Free: (800) 565 5887
Email: admissions@landmarkeast.org
Website: http://www.landmarkeast.org/

Landmark East is a co-ed international school for students diagnosed with learning disabilities in grades 3 through 12.

Magnificent Minds
47 Glenbrook Avenue, Lower Level
Toronto, ON, Canada
Tel: (647) 404 6349 or (647) 985 7001
Email: MagnificentMindsToronto@Gmail.com
Website: http://www.magnificentminds.ca/

Offers programs for grades PS to 6 under a holistic framework and offers services including ABA, occupational therapy, and social/emotional skill development.

Mediated Learning Academy
550 Thompson Ave.
Coquitlam, BC
Tel: (604) 937 3641
Website: http://www.mediatedlearningacademy.org/

School for children from kindergarten to grade twelve providing mediated learning experiences and "brain-based" teaching.

Montessori House of Children
85 Charlotte Street
Brantford, Ontario N3T 2X2
Tel: (519) 759 7290 or 753-5770
Email: mails@montessorihouseofchildren.com
Website: http://www.montessorihouseofchildren.com/

Oakwood Academy
155 Queen St E., Mississauga
Ontario, L5G 2N1
Tel: (905) 486 1035
Email: info@oakwoodacademy.ca
Website: http://www.oakwoodacademy.ca/

Uses the DIR model methodology to provide individualized curriculum and developmental-based, multi-sensory experiences.

PALS Autism School
2409 East Pender Street
Vancouver, BC V5K 2B2
Tel: (604) 251 7257
E-mail: info@palsautismschool.ca
Website: http://palsautismschool.ca/site/school-program/

Uses ABA to provide core education, life skills, and social skills as a foundation for independence. Provides elementary, secondary, and adult (19–28) programs.

Renaissance Academy
8058 8th Line
Utopia, Ontario, Canada, L0M 1T0
Tel: (705) 423 9688
Email: rniedzwiecki@renaissanceacademy.ca
Website: http://www.renaissanceacademy.ca/

Offers residential and day programs, ranging from gifted to life skills with a variety of options; and supports are available including educational assistants, behavior consultants, music therapists, psychologists, and psychiatrists.

Robert Land Academy
6727 South Chippawa Road,
Wellandport, Ontario L0R 2J0
Tel: (905) 386 6203
Website: http://www.robertlandacademy.com/

A structured private boarding school program for boys with ADD/ADHD/ODD/NLD/NVLD and other learning disabilities.

Shoore Centre for Learning
801 Eglinton Avenue West, Suite 201 (Eglinton & Bathurst)
Toronto, Ontario M5N 1E3
Tel:(416) 781 4754
Email: info@shoorecentre.com
Website: http://www.shoorecentre.com/

Shoore Centre for Learning is a special needs, alternative, day school in Toronto, Ontario for grades 7 to 12.

Team School
275 Rudar Road
Mississauga, ON L5A 1S2
Tel: (905) 279 7200
Website: http://www.teamschool.com/

An academic program for elementary and secondary students with individualized academic programs.

Vanguard School
5935 chemin de la Côte-de-Liesse
Saint-Laurent, Quebec H4T 1C3
Tel: (514) 747 5500
Email: pjolibois@vanguardquebec.qc.ca
Website: http://www.vanguardquebec.qc.ca/

Vanguard School is a specialized school for elementary and secondary French and English speaking students with learning disabilities.

Whytecliff Agile Learning Centre
Whytecliff Learning Centre
20561 Logan Avenue
Langley, British Columbia V3A 7R3
Tel: (604) 687 8401
Email: focus@focusbc.org
Website: http://focusbc.org/learning-centres

Burnaby Centre
3450 Boundary Road
Burnaby, British Columbia V5M 4A4

Youth Futures Programmes, Located in Burnaby and Langley are therapeutic community programs for individuals ages 13–19, taking a holistic approach, blending education with therapeutics.

Wildwood Academy
250 Sheridan Garden Dr
Oakville, ON L6J 7T1
Tel: (905) 829 4226
Website: http://wildwoodadmin.wix.com/

The YMCA Academy
15 Breadalbane St., 3rd floor
Toronto, ON M4Y 1C2
Tel: (416) 928 0124 ext. 31400
Email: reception@ymcaacademy.org
Website: http://www.ymcaacademy.org/

Legal, Government & Financial Services

Canadian Autism Spectrum Disorders Alliance
Email: info@asdalliance.org
Website: http://www.asdalliance.org/

Developmental Services Ontario
DSO Toronto—Surrey Place Centre
2 Surrey Place
Toronto, ON M5S 2C2
Tel: (416) 925 4930
Toll Free: (855) 372 3858
Email: DSOTR@surreyplace.on.ca
Website: http://www.dsotoronto.ca/

Services in English and French to assist adults with developmental disabilities and their families to apply for services and supports.

Ministry of Children and Youth Services
Ministry of Children and Youth Services
ServiceOntario INFOline
M-1B114, Macdonald Block
900 Bay Street
Toronto ON M7A 1N3
Toll Free: (866) 821 7770
Email: mcsinfo@mcys.gov.on.ca
Website: http://www.children.gov.on.ca/

Ontario Association of Children's Rehabilitation Services
150 Kilgour Rd.
Toronto, Ontario M4G 1R8
Tel: (416) 424 3864
Website: http://www.oacrs.com/

Service Coordination des Services
200-150 Montreal Rd
Ottawa, ON K1L 8H2

Tel: (613) 748 1788
Email: admin@scsottawa.on.ca
Website: https://www.scsottawa.on.ca/

Developmental Services Ontario Eastern Region
200-150 Montreal Rd
Ottawa, ON K1L 8H2
Tel: (855) 376 3737
Email: admin@dsoer.ca

Service Coordination (SCS) is the initial contact for individuals who have a developmental disability or autism in the Ottawa region assisting people in accessing supports and services.

Community and Recreation Services

Ability Online
250 Wincott Dr.
RPO PO Box 18515,
Etobicoke ON Canada M9R 4C8
Executive Director: Michelle McClure
Tel: (416) 650 6207
Toll Free: (866) 650 6207
Email: information@abilityonline.org
Website: http://www.abilityonline.org/

Ability Online is a monitored and supportive online community for young people with challenges and their families to connect.

Alpha Camp and Retreat
A Helping Hand Always Inc.
3048 Barrie Hill Rd,
Springwater ON L4M 4S4
Tel: 1(705) 792 4133
Tel: 1(705) 770 5700
email: info@alphacampandretreat.com
Website: http://www.alphacampandretreat.com/index.html

Autism Canada Foundation
P.O. Box 366
Bothwell, ON, N0P 1C0
Tel: (519) 695 5858
Email: info@autismcanada.org
Website: http://m.autismcanada.ca/

Autism Ontario
1179 King Street West, Suite 004
Toronto, ON
M6K 3C5
Tel: (416) 246 9592
Toll Free: (800) 472 7789
Website: http://www.autismontario.com/

Autism Resources Miramichi Inc.
139 Duke Street, Miramichi, NB E1N 1H6
Tel: (506) 622 8137
Fax: (506) 622 3240
Email: arm@nb.aibn.com
Website: http://www.autismmiramichi.com/home

Autism Society Of Newfoundland and Labrador
Provincial Headquarters: Elaine Dobbin Centre for Autism, St. John's
PO Box 14078
St. John's, NL A1B 4G8
Tel: (709) 722 2803
Email: info@autism.nf.net

Eastern Regional Office: Clarenville
P.O. Box 9194
Clarenville, NL A5A 2C2
Tel: (709) 466 7177
Email: eastern@autism.nf.net

South & Central Regional Office: Grand Falls – Windsor
PO Box 133 Grand Falls – Windsor, NL A2A 2J4
Phone: (709) 489 4190 Email: southcentral@autism.nf.net

Western Regional Office: Corner Brook
Mailing Address:
40 Main Street
Corner Brook, NL A2H 1C3
Phone: (709) 637 7450
Email: western@autism.nf.net

Website: http://www.autism.nf.net/

The ASNL offers programing options for individuals with ASD and their family members at their regional office locations, including supportive employment, social thinking, structured teaching, therapeutic recreation, and more.

Autism Speaks Canada
Website: http://www.autismspeaks.ca/

Camp Kennebec
Special Needs Camp
1422 Cox Road
Arden, Ontario K0H 1B0
Tel: (613) 335 2114
Email: info@campkennebec.com
Camp Directors: Donna Segal & Rob Deman

Camp Kirk
Toronto Office—Open September to May
639A Mount Pleasant Road
Toronto, Ontario M4S 2M9
Toll Free: (866) 982 3310

Tel: (416) 782 3310

Kirkfield Camp Location—Open June to August
1083 Portage Road
Kirkfield, Ontario K0M 2B0
Tel: (705) 438 1353
Email: campkirk@campkirk.com

Camp Kodiak
Winter Office:
4069 Pheasant Run,
Mississauga, Ontario L5L 2C2
Tel: (905) 569 7595
Toll Free: (877)569-7595

Summer Address:
General Delivery
McKellar, Ontario, P0G 1C0
Tel: (705)389-1910
Fax: (705) 389 1911
Website: www.campkodiak.com
Serves campers ages 6-18.

Camp PEAK
90 Burnhamthorpe Rd. West
Suite 210A
Mississauga, ON L5B 3C3
Tel:(905) 949-0049 ext. 2388
Toll Free: (800) 668 1179
Email: info@camppeak.ca
Website: http://www.camppeak.ca/

Summer address:
5400 Eagle Lake Road
South River, ON P0A 1X0

Easter Seals Canada
40 Holly St, Suite 401 Toronto, Ontario M4S 3C3
Tel: (416) 932 8382 or (877) 376 6362
Email: info@easterseals.ca
Website: http://easterseals.ca/english/

Hands
The Family Help Network

North Bay
222 Main Street East
North Bay ON P1B 1B1
Tel: (705) 476 2293

East Nipissing—Mattawa
150 Water Street
Mattawa ON P0H 1V0
Tel: (705) 476 2293

West Nipissing—Sturgeon Falls
65 Queen Street

Sturgeon Falls ON P2B 2C7
Tel: (705) 476 2293

Powassan—Powassan Medical Centre
8 King Street
Powassan ON P0H 1Z0
Tel: (705) 384 5225

West Parry Sound—Parry Sound
2 May Street
Parry Sound, ON P2A 1S2
Tel: (705) 746 4293

East Parry Sound—Sundridge
37 Main Street, P.O. Box 596
Sundridge ON P0A 1Z0
Tel: (705) 384 5225

Muskoka—Bracebridge
23 Ball's Drive
Bracebridge ON P1L 1T1
Tel: (705) 645 3155

Timmins
60 Wilson Avenue, Suite 103
Timmins, ON P4N 2S7
Tel: (705) 476 2293

Toll Free: *(800) 668 8555*
Website: http://www.thefamilyhelpnetwork.ca/

Kinark Outdoor Center
Box 730
Minden, Ontario K0M 2K0
Tel: (705) 286 3555
Toll Free: (800) 805 8252
Email: info@koc.on.ca
Offers a variety of adapted traditional camp experiences and enhanced respite opportunities for children, teens, and young adults with ASD.

Reach for the Rainbow
20 Torlake Crescent
Toronto, Ontario M8Z 1B3
Tele: (416) 503 0088
Email: info@reachfortherainbow.ca
Website: http://www.reachfortherainbow.ca/
Programs provide environments of inclusion while offering respite for parents.

Respiteservices.com
112 Merton St
Toronto, ON M4S 2Z8
Tel: (416) 322 6317
Email: info@respiteservices.com
Website: http://www.respiteservices.com/

ACKNOWLEDGEMENTS

I would like to thank Tony Lyons and Skyhorse Publishing for their ongoing and unprecedented commitment to the autism community. I also would like to thank my editor, Maxim Brown, for his work on this book and all those at Skyhorse who spent many hours compiling the directory included with this book—it would not have happened without them. A special thanks to Louis Conte for giving me a call.

My son Henry is the reason I am an autism and vaccine safety advocate. As hard as I work on his behalf, he works harder every day. He is an incredible young man and I love him beyond measure. I am fortunate to have met amazing people who have become friends and colleagues on this journey. They inspire me and their knowledge and willingness to share information is invaluable. Looking for solutions to help my son led me to much of the information in this book and I hope that other families find these resources helpful for their own children.